GATEKEEPING IN THE INTENSIVE CARE UNIT

GATEKEEPING IN THE INTENSIVE CARE UNIT

Martin A. Strosberg
& Daniel Teres

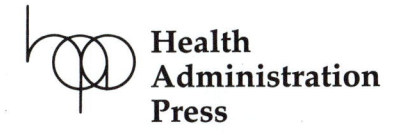

Health Administration Press

Chicago, Illinois

Copyright © 1997 by the Foundation of the American College of Healthcare Executives. Printed in the United States of America. All rights reserved. This book or parts thereof may not be reproduced in any form without written permission of the publisher. Opinions and views expressed in this book are those of the authors and do not necessarily reflect those of the Foundation of the American College of Healthcare Executives.
01   00   99   98   97   5   4   3   2   1

Library of Congress Cataloging-in-Publication Data

Strosberg, Martin A.
Gatekeeping in the intensive care unit / by Martin A. Strosberg
  and Daniel Teres.
    p.   cm.
  Includes bibliographical references and index.
  ISBN 1-56793-055-7 (pbk.)
  1. Intensive care units—Admission and discharge.   I. Teres, Daniel.
II. Title.
  [DNLM: 1. Intensive Care Units—organization & administration—
United States. WX 218 S888g 1997]
RA975.5.I56S76 1997
362.1'74—dc21
DNLM/DLC
for Library of Congress   97-7169
                                                                                  CIP

The paper used in this publication meets the minimum requirements of American National Standards for Information Sciences—Permanente of Paper for Printed Library Materials, ANSI Z39.48–1984. (TM) ∞

Health Administration Press
A division of the Foundation of the
  American College of Healthcare Executives
One North Franklin Street
Chicago, IL 60606
312/424–2800

*To Sharon and our children,
Nathaniel and Joshua Strosberg*

*To Evelyne and our children,
Rishona, Jeremy, Ilana, and Lorin Teres*

CONTENTS

Foreword ix

Acknowledgments xiii

Chapter 1 Introduction 1

Chapter 2 Background: Intensive Care Units, Critical
           Care Medicine, and Organizational Setting ... 23

Chapter 3 Gatekeeping: Decision Makers and
           Decision Making 61

Chapter 4 Six Patients: Gatekeeping at Anywhere
           Hospital ICU 89

Chapter 5 Management 147

Chapter 6 Public Policy for Critical Care
           Gatekeeping 173

Appendix A Guidelines on ICU Admission, Discharge,
           Triage, and Futility 205

Appendix B Examples of ICU Admission, Discharge, and Triage Policies.......................245

Appendix C Admission and Discharge Criteria Assessment Scale.......................254

Appendix D Components of Rapid Ethics Evaluation Process for ICU Patients with High Probability of Mortality...................256

Appendix E Role Playing the Simulation and Suggestions for New Rounds..............260

About the Author..263

FOREWORD

Much will be written about the amazing healthcare transformation currently happening in America. Managed care has been making steady gains in marketshare, and market forces have acted to create a major restructuring of American healthcare already underway prior to the ill-fated Clinton healthcare reform initiative. The influence of managed care and those who purchase medical services has controlled previously runaway costs, has highlighted opportunities for efficiency, and has probed and found weaknesses in many of our prominent hospitals, both academic and nonacademic. At the same time, the revolution has created enormous profits for stockholders, medical entrepreneurs, and officers of for-profit systems.

Anecdotes of poor care when nurse staffing is reduced or diluted, and stories of patients who are denied services or are told to go to a selected hospital to have a discounted operation or drive-through delivery are evidence of a consumer backlash aimed at a new system that has attempted to revolutionize the way medical care is delivered with mixed results.

Inexplicably, although healthcare in general has come under fire, there has been little discussion regarding intensive care delivered to our most fragile patients. Patients are moved out faster than ever before, to step-down or intermediate care units within the hospital, or rehabilitation units, or chronic ventilator hospitals outside of the acute care setting. The effects of such change are yet to be determined, but it is happening.

Gatekeeping in the Intensive Care Unit provides a contemporary description of life in the busy intensive care unit, with a focus on organizational patterns and policies that affect admission and discharge of patients and on allocation of resources. There is also a detailed analysis of current legal cases that bear on futility, and analysis of the role of the triage officer. While the nursing director or manager is well identified in the hospital hierarchy, the ICU medical director has not been well defined or identified within the complex medical politics that surround traditional medical boundaries such as departments of medicine, surgery, and anesthesia.

The key term used by the authors, *qualified critical care physician* (QCCP), was first described by the Society for Critical Care Medicine via the "Coalition for Critical Care Excellence." The QCCP not only coordinates care for the individual bedside patient (remember that prevention and early treatment are better than late treatment) but also shepherds the flock of critically ill patients and takes responsibility for the administration and efficient operation of the ICU. The QCCP functioning with the unit-based ICU team is a model that has great appeal for cost-efficient management of critically ill patients and the units they depend on for their survival.

The most exciting aspect of the book comes as one follows the medical discussion and decisions during what is typically called Triage Rounds. This is a daily function in a busy hospital and certainly reflects my experience as an ICU director in a tertiary center. I found myself reading ahead to find out: Who gets the bed? Who gets moved out? How are ethical issues regarding withdrawal of care playing out? These are common medical and ethical decisions faced on a regular basis but not open to public scrutiny. There have been excellent TV documentaries on the do not resuscitate (DNR) patient, and certainly famous legal cases such as Karen Quinlan, Brophy, and Helga Wanglie, but the comparative entitlement scenarios involved in allocating finite ICU beds have not been so clearly defined before, and they make compelling reading.

While the patients are getting sicker, the resources available to care for the critically ill are being constrained by the new forces at work to limit cost in the hospital. There is intense discussion about the patients, their changing medical status, prognoses, and family situations. Should the emergency room hold the next patient, how will we handle any overflow, do we transfer patients out of the system? How are decisions made when there are three emergency patients in the operating room who might require ICU beds, two patients in the emergency room with emphysema and respiratory failure, a gun-shot victim, and three patients on the medical floors who are doing poorly?

The decisions on Triage Rounds are difficult enough based on medical, ethical, and family issues and the too often existent medical staff politics. What about managed care influence? What is the physician's incentive to fight to keep a patient in the ICU, when the capitated plan may affect the year-end salary bonus? What about the continued pressure to limit ICU stay secondary to cost of care and capitation concerns? What about the increasing number of patients who are underinsured or have no insurance?

Strosberg and Teres present a unique approach, one that tries to preserve the doctor-patient relationship while attempting to evaluate the quality of the communication/interaction. This is the "rapid ethics evaluation process," which is distinct from the formal ethics committee. The evaluation is interesting and uses a small team of clinically experienced nurses, physicians, and social workers as well as a community representative who is not connected to an insurance payor to help guide decision making regarding the allocation of scarce ICU resources. But will the team be accepted by the family, the attending physician, the medical staff, or society at large and not be perceived as a hindrance?

Gatekeeping in the Intensive Care Unit is a welcome analysis of issues central to management of the ICU but very applicable in the wider context of medicine in general. Ethical and organizational analyses are woven together, and the resulting tapestry is rich in reality and the need to confront difficult issues while trying to do the right thing for "the guy in the bed."

Thomas Rainey, President
CriticalMed Inc.
Past President,
Society of Critical Care Medicine

ACKNOWLEDGMENTS

WE WISH to thank Dr. Paul Sorum of Albany Medical College and Professor Robert Baker of Union College for reading our manuscript and making many helpful suggestions; Union College Graduate Management Institute staff members Carolyn Micklas for helping with the graphics and Rhonda Sheehan for preparing the many versions of the manuscript; and Union College graduate assistants Melissa Zambri, Yun Ji, and Mitra Abbesi for their technical support. We would also like to thank Dr. James Strosberg for providing a timely, relevant, and endless supply of journal articles. Finally, thanks are owed to the dedicated and skilled critical care nurses and physicians of the ICUs at Albany Medical Center, Albany, New York; Baystate Medical Center, Springfield, Massachusetts; Ellis Hospital, Schenectady, New York; and Jewish General Hospital, Montreal, Canada for allowing coauthor Martin Strosberg to visit their facilities, interview the staff, and observe daily activities.

CHAPTER 1

INTRODUCTION

Gatekeeping at Anywhere Hospital: The Case of the Transfer Patient

The time is 8:30 A.M. It has been a stressful night for the administrative officer of the day at Anywhere Hospital—a large, tertiary, community teaching hospital. Today, for the first time in many months, an ambulance had to be diverted to another hospital because of a lack of critical care beds.

The administrative officer has called an emergency meeting of hospital staff so they can decide how to deal with the crisis. Assembled around a small conference table are nurses, administrators, and physicians, including nursing supervisors from the 12-bed combined medical-surgical (med-surg) intensive care unit (ICU), coronary care unit (CCU), and medical and surgical floors. One nursing supervisor is unable to attend because she is involved in resuscitating a patient. Also present are various administrators from the departments of medicine and surgery, the critical care division, the emergency room, and the admissions department, along with a community-based cardiologist designated by the ICU medical director to act as the "triage officer" of the CCU and ICU. Although the CEO is not present at the meeting, everyone is aware of the priorities of the hospital administration. Sensitive to financial pressures and relations with community surgeons, top management does not want to cancel elective surgery or turn away ambulances and risk losing its reputation as a regional trauma and referral center for the surrounding area. The question before the group is how to get through the day and develop a plan for the night.

2 Gatekeeping in the Intensive Care Unit

Reports of conditions on the floors and other units flow in by phone. Each participant offers an estimate on how many beds will be available for the day, which patients are scheduled for the operating room, how many patients could be safely moved to other parts of the hospital, and how many will likely die. The do-not-resuscitate (DNR) status is reviewed for each patient in critical care. Also of particular interest is the ongoing code (cardiopulmonary resuscitation), which is keeping the nursing supervisor busy on the floor. The physicians and nurses share their opinions.

The nursing supervisors report on the availability of staff nurses—how many called in sick and the likelihood of getting replacements for them. They speculate on how available critical care nursing can be stretched, for example, grouping a patient with high nursing needs with one with low nursing needs to help the nurse cope with a 1:2 nurse-to-patient ratio.

The staff trade "what-if" questions: What if a patient arrests on the floor and requires intubation (insertion of a breathing tube)? Will there be a code bed available in the unit? Together they consider feasibility of options for bedding the critically ill patients—the ICU, CCU, recovery room or post anesthesia care unit (PACU), the emergency room (ER), other hospitals. One participant reports that the house staff vehemently protests covering critically ill patients in the ER and they have recently gained the support of the Chair of Medicine. Also, it is well known that the PACU nurses object to going over their patient limit and that ICU nurses resist the idea of "mandatory overtime."

Collectively, they piece together scenarios for the day. The scenario considered most likely shows the availability of two critical care beds.

Along with the information sharing and scenario building is a discussion of a request to admit a patient from a hospital 20 miles away who requires a cardiac catheterization, a diagnostic procedure that involves the insertion of a catheter or tube into a coronary artery. The hospital requesting the transfer is part of a long-established system of referral arrangements with Anywhere Hospital. No other hospital in the region except Anywhere Hospital does cardiac catheterization.

The 48-year-old patient, in the other hospital's CCU awaiting transfer, has had two cardiac operations (one at Anywhere Hospital) and is apparently in serious condition. A physician at the meeting points out that a patient described over the phone often bears no resemblance to the patient directly observed. The cardiologist/triage officer says it would not be possible to personally evaluate the patient at the referring hospital. But he phones Anywhere Hospital's cardiac catheterization lab to get more information. At first he is put on hold. When he is finally able to talk to the physician in charge of the catheterization lab—the same physician who would actually do the catheterization—the cardiologist/triage officer recommends to the group that the patient be transferred by ambulance to the hospital and readied for cardiac catheterization. Evidently, the patient is stable enough for the procedure.

The administrators and the nurses point out that there is probably very little that can be done for the patient, given that he has already had two major cardiac operations and there is only a slim chance that cardiac catheterization would provide any useful information for prolonging his life. One participant says that a third heart operation would be medically futile. A physician expresses concern that the patient will destabilize and require a long-term-ICU stay—thus taking one of the two remaining beds projected to be available.

Although denying the transfer would free up a critical care bed at Anywhere Hospital and would perhaps reduce the risk of diverting ambulances or canceling elective surgery later in the day, the cardiologist/triage officer argues that as long as there is an open bed and the slightest chance of helping a dying patient, the patient must be admitted. Additionally, he would like more information on the condition of the patient's vessels. He states that if and when beds become completely filled later in the day, they will at that time make the tough decisions. Should the patient be admitted to Anywhere Hospital for cardiac catheterization and a potentially long stay in the ICU? Let's look at what the staff decided to do.

■　　■　　■　　■　　■

Decision: Admit the Transfer Patient to the Hospital

The argument of the triage officer prevailed: As long as there is a bed available and the slightest chance of helping a dying patient, the patient must be admitted.

The Outcome

The transfer patient was admitted to Anywhere Hospital for cardiac catheterization, destabilized, and was subsequently admitted to the ICU, taking up one of the two remaining beds. The patient died soon after.

The patient that was undergoing cardiopulmonary resuscitation died on the floor.

An Overview of Gatekeeping in the Triage and Non-Triage Mode

Decisions to admit and discharge patients to and from the ICU are made hundreds of times per year by hospital staff. Most, but not all, of the decision making is routine and free of conflict. Physicians request admission for their patients; phone calls are made; forms are filled out; orders are written and carried out; patients are admitted, transferred, or discharged; appropriate consults are given. The various steps have been programmed through standard operating procedures or through informal arrangements that have been negotiated over time.

The term "gatekeeping" is used to describe decision making with regard to ICU admission and discharge. Gatekeepers control who passes through the ICU doors and who gets an ICU bed. It should be noted that the term is being used differently than the usual notion of gatekeeper (i.e., a primary care physician who controls referrals to specialists).

Gatekeeping includes both "triage mode" and "non-triage mode" decision making. When beds are available in the ICU, non-triage mode decision making can be used. When there is full occupancy or high census, which is usually an intermittent phenomenon, the only way to admit a patient is to discharge another patient. "Triage" is the term used by ICU staff to connote the process of prioritizing access to beds during high census. Obviously, decisions to admit patients through the gates when there are available beds influences the likelihood of triage at a later point.

In the triage mode, ICUs should respond to scarcity of beds by carefully reviewing each possible admission and accelerating discharge both of the patient who can be safely transferred to another unit or floor as well as the patient who has not responded to intensive therapy (Teres 1989). In either of these two cases, the patients should be "triaged" out of the unit. No theoretical priority should be assumed for patients who are already in the unit. However, physicians performing triage sometimes find it difficult to discharge patients who have not responded to intensive therapy to make room for those who could benefit more. Even those who have achieved an adequate recovery can be difficult to discharge: Frequently, there are no suitable beds available in the intermediate care unit or on the regular floors. Attending physicians may also resist discharging a patient to a floor that they deem unsafe because of the low nurse-to-patient ratios. Or, families refusing to give up hope may resist the transfer of hopelessly ill patients. It may take a long time to make a decision about limiting care to these patients.

Frequently, a lack of consensus about prognosis among physicians and nurses exists. In addition, physicians cannot ignore the threat of a legal risk to premature discharge. One triage decision maker sums up the conflict by describing his job as "getting a patient to a safe floor without endangering another patient's life waiting to come in. It's constantly a game of shuffle—save this end, don't harm that end." The risks to patients in the triage mode include denying or delaying admission, diminishing the perceived quality of care through premature discharge, and/or diluting the quality of care to the remaining patients.

A Preview of the Book

To some degree, each gatekeeping decision raises issues of cost, access, and quality of care. Inevitably some decisions will be non-routine and controversial. This book is designed to provide understanding of:

- the medical, managerial, and ethical dimensions of ICU admission and discharge decision making;
- the organizational roles of various participants in the decision making;
- the organizational setting of the ICU and the constraints faced by decision makers; and
- managerial and public policy approaches to improving admission-discharge decision making.

Chapter 4 comprises sequential decision "rounds" embedded in case studies that simulate admission-discharge decision making, including triage and determination of medical futility. The case studies are the major vehicle for engaging many of the foregoing topics. Adult ICUs, as opposed to neonatal and pediatric ICUs, are the book's main focus.

In Chapter 2 we will provide an overview of intensive care units and critical care medicine in the United States. Chapter 3 raises some important management and organizational issues with regard to admission and discharge decision making. The simulation resumes in Chapter 4 with sequential decision rounds. Chapter 5 discusses approaches to improving the management of the ICU—in particular, approaches associated with managed care. Chapter 6 examines trends in public policymaking that respond to unresolved managerial and ethical issues, especially those generated by the shift to managed care. Now let's return to the case of the transfer patient (Round 1) and its implications for gatekeeping.

The Rationale for the Transfer Patient Decision

Triage Mode versus Non-Triage Mode Decision Making

It is an understatement to say that the participants in this case do not all feel comfortable with the decision; however, each participant has a different threshold for discomfort. Each understands the prognoses of the patients and the degree of potential risk involved in premature discharge, or delayed or denied admission slightly differently and each has different tolerance levels for those risks—including the risk of denying care to the unknown patient yet to show up at the hospital door or to a patient already in the hospital who might deteriorate on the floors.

All participants in the decision thought that the potential for hospital and ICU benefit was low for the cardiac transfer patient. The triage officer emphasized that it was greater than zero (i.e., there was still a slight chance that the patient's condition would improve). Others emphasized that virtually no benefit was to be gained or that probably a trauma or elective surgery patient would be arriving later in the day who could better use the bed. One might speculate that the triage officer's criteria for determining "slightest chance" of benefit might vary if no beds were available at the time of the decision. The availability of beds was an important factor in the decision. The triage officer's argument prevailed.

The events of this introductory case study illustrate the difference between operating in a triage mode and a non-triage mode of decision making. In triage mode, the question of comparative entitlement is raised: Who among two or more patients is more entitled to the bed? Which patient, relatively speaking, will derive the greatest benefit from being in that bed? If, for example, no beds were available at the beginning of the case, this clearly would have been a triage situation. If one bed was available with both the code patient and the transfer patient seeking admission, this also would have been a triage situation. As it turned out in the case, two beds were available. The nurse manager and the administrator, believing that the imminent arrival of other, more "deserving" patients was highly likely, raised the comparative entitlement questions, albeit in relation to unknown, "statistical" patients. The triage officer, in contrast, did not view the decision in terms of comparative entitlement—this was still a non-triage situation and he was not operating in a triage mode. If there were plenty of open beds and no bed pressure, it would be unlikely that the nurse manager and the administrator would be operating in a triage mode either. This attitude is common when there are open beds. In a 1988 survey of attitudes of critical care medicine specialists, under assumptions of empty ICU beds, 54 percent answered that they would admit a patient who had no hope of surviving more than a few weeks (Society of Critical Care Medicine Ethics Committee 1994a).

Once a patient is in a bed, ICU staff frequently perceive legal obligation to the patient and exhibit an emotional attachment. Length of stay and the amount of resources allocated to that patient ultimately influence the capacity of the unit and thus future admissions. For example, the amount of nursing time devoted to the patient (i.e, whether the nurse-to-patient staffing ratio is 1:2 or 1:3) influences the overall demand for nursing care. Frequently, when the supply of critical care nurses is limited, the number of patients who can be safely handled is constrained by the total hours of nursing time available in addition to the number of beds.

As will be explained, a higher level of prognostic certainty is frequently required to deny a patient admission in the non-triage mode as opposed to the triage mode. In the introductory case study there was not enough prognostic evidence to convince the triage officer that the patient did not have a chance to benefit, and therefore admission was approved.

Physician Socialization, Scarce Resources, and Medical Futility

Training and socialization incline all physicians, to a certain extent, to make an effort to save a life even if there is only a slight chance of recovery. Consider the triage officer, or any physician for that matter, who is deciding whether to admit or to continue treating a very sick patient. He or she may think back to prior experiences with twenty-five patients who were in a similarly serious condition and remember the one patient who actually recovered as a result of the treatment. Based on these odds, the triage officer or physician is inclined to admit the patient. Taken over the long run, for every patient who survives, twenty-four do not make it out of the hospital. They may linger in the ICU, perhaps suffering, but certainly consuming resources. Aside from this concern, what about the patient who is waiting for a bed that is occupied by someone with a one-in-twenty-five chance of recovery?

One participant in the transfer patient case study thought that a third heart operation would have been medically futile and so too the cardiac catheterization. In its narrowest sense, a medically futile intervention is one that is inefficacious (e.g., when it is absolutely certain that CPR will not restore cardiopulmonary function). Normally, physicians are under no professional obligation to provide patients with useless interventions. But what if the probability is more than zero but nevertheless extremely low? Where is the threshold? Or what if CPR has a good chance of restoring cardiopulmonary function but merely prolongs the dying process or extends poor quality of life? The concept of medical futility is highly problematic for bioethicists and clinicians (Baker 1995). One point for which there is general agreement is that the determination of medical futility should not be influenced by the number of beds that happen to be available at the time. However, beyond this point there is not much agreement over the definition of medical futility and whether it is necessary to include the patient or surrogate in the determination.

Ethical Dilemmas

Analysts of the healthcare system frequently refer to a set of four ethical principles to guide discussion of decision making in healthcare:

1. beneficence, the principle of helping people in need;
2. nonmaleficence, the principle of doing no harm;
3. autonomy, the principle of respecting patients' rights to make choices regarding their healthcare; and
4. justice, the principle of treating everyone in a fair manner (Beauchamp and Childress 1994).

Ethical dilemmas occur when providers make a decision based on a principle that conflicts with one or more of these four principles. For example, the principles of beneficence and nonmaleficence suggest that the patient (Patient X) with a one-in-twenty-five chance of recovery has a right to continued ICU treatment. But this conflicts with the principle of justice, since other patients are waiting to be admitted to the ICU. The principle of nonmaleficence is relevant in two ways. First, it could be argued that to the extent that Patient X is harmed because of withdrawal of treatment or discharge from the ICU, even to make way for another patient, this principle is violated. On the other hand, it could be argued that the *failure* to withdraw treatment is a violation if the professional believes that the treatment is harmful to the patient. From the perspective of Patient X, however, to withdraw care against his or her wishes is a violation of the principle of autonomy.

Defining Appropriateness

Guidelines for Non-Triage Mode Gatekeeping

An appropriate admission is one where the patient is neither too sick nor too well to benefit from treatment. In principle, these admission and discharge decisions should be based on criteria that are independent of the ICU occupancy rate at any particular point in time.

The Society of Critical Care Medicine (SCCM) Ethics Committee's (1994b) "Consensus Statement on the Triage of Critically Ill Patients" gives the following examples of patients who should be excluded from the ICU, whether beds are available or not:

- patients who completely decline intensive care or request that invasive therapy be withheld;
- patients declared brain dead who are not organ donors;
- patients in a persistent vegetative or permanently unconscious state.

Examples of terminally ill patients who "may" be excluded include:
- AIDS complicated by significant, irreversible neurological involvement;
- irreversible multi-organ failure; or
- metastatic cancer unresponsive to chemotherapy and/or radiation therapy except if in specialized ICUs or on specific protocols (for experimental purposes).

Most professionals would agree, however, that the prognosis becomes much clearer and the uncertainties reduced after the patient has been admitted (i.e., after the patient has been given a trial and a chance to declare himself or herself). Based on observation, the decision then can be made on continued stay, discharge, and/or withdrawal of life support.

With regard to criteria that could be used to deny admission to the "too sick," Chassin (1982) notes the difficulty in identifying specific subgroups of patients with a survival rate low enough to justify systematic exclusion from intensive care:

> . . . each intensive care patient represents a virtually unique combination of primary and secondary disease processes, therapeutic regimens, and complications of therapy and disease. While in some sense this may be true for all patients, the significance of the differences among patients with similar diagnoses seems magnified in an intensive care population. The uniqueness, which is reflected in the diagnostic diversity . . . makes the task of setting criteria for ICU exclusion even more difficult (p. 177).

Nevertheless, there has been great progress in developing prognostic models that could become the basis for setting criteria. Individual physicians, of course, use implicit prognostic (prediction) estimates and criteria in making admission decisions.

Prognostic Models

Over the past 15 years concerted efforts have been made to formalize and improve prognostic models. Two such efforts include the Acute Physiology and Chronic Health Evaluation (APACHE) system models (Knaus, Zimmerman, and Wagner 1981) and the Mortality Probability Model (MPM) system models (Lemeshow et al. 1985). The APACHE system presents a computer display of a hospital's ICU beds and, for each patient, the risk of death in the ICU and the risk of death during the entire hospitalization. The estimate of risk is based on predictive regression equations. Besides the obvious uses as a classification system for research purposes, institutional comparisons, and quality assessment, it has been suggested that prediction models play a role in admission and discharge decision making for individuals. With regard to discharge, Zimmerman et al. (1994) have developed a method based on the APACHE score and other variables to estimate the probability that a patient already in the unit will require ICU life support within the next twenty-four hours. Patients in the unit include "active treatment patients" on life support and "monitor patients" who are not receiving life support but are at risk of becoming critically ill and are under observation in case they need prompt intervention. The estimates can be used to help physicians decide whether the patient can be safely transferred.

Knaus (1989), a codeveloper of the APACHE models, advocates linking admission and discharge criteria with the probability of benefit from intensive care for the individual patient. Many critics doubt that prediction models will ever be accurate enough for the task (Civetta 1992). They also doubt whether agreement could be reached on what level of expected survival would be low enough to justify exclusion from the ICU: Five percent? One percent? (Chassin 1982). Furthermore, how would the views of patients and families, demanding treatment no matter what, be taken into consideration?

Guidelines for Triage Mode Gatekeeping

Perhaps those who would be hesitant in using formal or informal prediction models when there are available beds might be more willing to use them in making comparative entitlement decisions—in deciding which patient to discharge in order to make room for a new patient and which patient to admit in the first place. The SCCM Ethics Committee (1994b) states:

> The foremost consideration in triage decisions is the expected outcome of the patient in terms of survival and function, which turns on the medical status of the patient. In general, patients with good prognosis for recovery have priority over patients with poor prognosis. While uncertainty of prognosis is a crucial problem in critical care, providers should utilize predictive instruments with a full understanding of their strengths and limitations. Decisions to be made between patients with equivalent prognoses should be made on a first come, first served basis (p. 1201).

ICU decision makers would of course have to concede that they are actually making comparative entitlement decisions. Once (if) they did, what principles would guide their action? Englehardt and Rie (1986) argue, "Depending on what benefits are afforded a patient already in a bed, the time of discharge can be advanced hour by hour in order to make a bed available to a newcomer who may be in slightly greater need or have a slightly greater likelihood of benefiting by admission." As we will see, this advice is not universally accepted or followed.

Gatekeeping and Rationing

Participants in the National Institutes of Health Consensus Development Conference of 1983 concluded that, "It is not medically appropriate to devote limited ICU resources to patients without reasonable prospect of significant recovery when patients who need those services, and who have significant prospect of recovery from acute life-threatening disease or injury, are being turned away due to a lack of capacity" (NIH 1983). Leaving aside for now the definition of benefit and "reasonable prospect of significant recovery," it can be assumed that the first patient mentioned in the NIH example would be deprived of very little or no benefit if the resources of the ICU were devoted to the second patient. Conceptually, the tradeoff could be extended to include cases where there would be a diminishment in benefit for one patient in favor of another patient (i.e., triage or rationing implies a zero-sum game).

The technical term for a tradeoff that must be made in the face of scarcity is "rationing." Rationing is a term that frequently evokes emotionally charged debate. Rationing involves allocating resources so that everyone will receive a fair portion. Baker (1995) notes that European and American concepts of healthcare rationing differ. According to the tradition of European economists and philosophers, healthcare rationing is defined as any allocation of a medical resource that leaves some medical need unmet. Some American economists have redefined rationing in terms of the workings of a free market to mean withholding of healthcare from persons who would be willing and able to purchase it. In the European sense, rationing is the failure to meet the *needs* of patients as determined by some combination of patients, professionals, or society at large; whereas, according to the American redefinition, rationing is the failure to meet the *demands* of patients as registered in the marketplace (i.e., non-price rationing).

Common to both conceptions is the idea of scarcity. Scarcity can be considered at various levels of aggregation. "Commodity scarcity" is an absolute shortage of a certain item (e.g., an organ for transplantation). Benefit will be received by one person but may be denied or delayed to another. The tradeoff may be as stark as who shall live and who shall die. Another example is the case of kidney dialysis. When first made available on a nonexperimental basis in the early 1970s, it was in acute shortage. In Seattle, rather than let the market decide, access to dialysis was afforded according to a utilitarian criterion (Schupak and Merril 1965; Fox and Swazey 1978). The social worth of the candidate was considered (e.g., a working, middle class father received priority over a prostitute). Although in time universal financing alleviated the short-term shortage of dialysis machines, organs are still scarce and are allocated according to the United Network for Organ Sharing (UNOS) rationing criteria (1993).

In a larger sense, other resources—Medicaid budgets, payments by third party payors to hospitals, the amount that employers can afford to dedicate to health benefits—are scarce. How can scarce resources be used to bring greatest overall improvement in health status? As we will explain, this question is usually not one that is asked in the ICU at the bedside.

Is triage equivalent to rationing (i.e., failure to meet needs)? In busy ICUs, staff will admit to triaging—prioritizing access to beds to make way for new arrivals. Triage is an official function of the ICU medical director and designated triage officer, although it is sometimes delegated to others. But staff will be reluctant to admit to rationing—denying or delaying beneficial care or diminishing (diluting) its quality. The reasons for this reluctance—legal or psychological—will be explored in subsequent chapters.

Scarcity in the Triage and Non-Triage Mode

The hospital, perhaps more than any other institution in society, enjoys legitimacy and social support. This support comes from the widely shared belief that the hospital will strive toward maximizing the quality of patient care. Maximizing the quality of care for an individual patient is not the same thing as utilizing scarce resources to improve aggregate health status of the patients in a particular community or population. Exhibit 1.1 contrasts the perspectives of physicians, nurses, and administrators with regard to patient focus, time frame of action, and view of resources and scarcity. Whereas the administrator's focus is the institution and is constrained by resource limitations, the physician's focus is the individual patient and is relatively unconstrained by resource limitations (i.e., any expenditure is justified to preserve life or enhance quality of care). The nurse's focus is also the patient but is much more constrained by resource limitations. It is the physician's value system and perspective, supported by the patient and the community, that dominates the institution.

Given this dominant perspective, it is very difficult to embrace or sustain the notion of maximizing marginal utility when there are empty beds in the ICU. For the physician and patient there is no scarcity. It is hard for them to see who would directly derive the benefit from the savings accrued by denying a patient access to an ICU bed. However, the system—the hospital, the managed care organization and its members, the plan, investors, taxpayers, future ICU patients—might in fact benefit. Administrators, as representatives of these aggregations, should appreciate these system-wide benefits, but the incentives are not in place to encourage either the physician or patient to accept the logic of the tradeoff. In contrast, consider the hospital physicians in the British National Health Service (before the Thatcher reforms). Physicians, as employees of hospitals operating under fixed budgets, recognize that savings that accrue from denying beneficial services to one patient can be directly applied to another patient who could derive greater benefit from those services (Daniels 1986). Also consider the example of the Oregon Medicaid Demonstration Project. On a societal level, the State of Oregon, in a unique experiment, has prioritized various medical interventions on the basis of cost-effectiveness and other criteria to determine the content of the standard Medicaid benefits package. Funds saved by not covering intensive care for end-stage AIDS and cancer could go toward funding more cost-effective treatments.

In the United States, typically, when a patient is denied access to an available bed, it is on the basis of medical appropriateness or medical benefit criteria. Because it can be argued that there is at least some likelihood that the benefit of ICU intervention will be greater than zero,

Exhibit 1.1 Differences in Perspectives Among Participants (Triage Officers Not Included)

Attribute	Health Services Administrators	Nurses	Physicians
Patient focus	All patients in the organization and the larger community	Groups of patients in the nursing unit	Individual patients
Time frame of action	Medium- to long-range; gather information, analyze data; engage in long-run strategic planning	Medium- to short-range patient-care monitoring function	Generally short-range; cause-and-effect relations, although varies by specialty
View of resources	Limited; main challenge is one of allocating scarce resources	Recognize some limitations but more narrowly than administrators	Resources essentially unlimited; resources should be available to maximize quality of patient care

Source: Adapted from Shortell, S. M. *Health Care Management Review* 7 (4): 12. Copyright © 1982 by Aspen Publishers, Inc.

the use of an appropriateness argument to deny admission when there are empty beds must indeed be very compelling.

Managed Care: The New Perspective

Denial of admissions and the presence of empty beds may be markedly influenced by the advent of managed care. As the population of the nation shifts to managed care arrangements, the perspectives presented in Exhibit 1.1 will undoubtedly change. Some would even predict a paradigm shift brought on by the "managed care revolution." Although managed care is a very broad term encompassing a myriad of arrangements by which physicians and patients are restrained in providing or obtaining healthcare services, we will associate the term with health maintenance organizations and capitation. Under this scenario, physicians have the potential to undergo the most dramatic change in perspective. Patient focus will change from the individual to the population of covered lives to be cared for by resources constrained by a fixed budget. Some physicians, particularly primary care physicians, will be at financial risk for at least a portion of this budget. Will physicians be less likely to admit and manage ICU patients? Will they face ethical dilemmas in making tradeoffs between cost and quality? Managed care, according to the Council on Ethical and Judicial Affairs of the American Medical Association (1995), magnifies two ethical concerns involving conflicting loyalties. First, physicians practicing within the financial constraints of a managed care plan are expected to balance the interests of their patients with the interests of other patients covered by the plan. Second, the financial interests of physicians as manifested by bonuses, fee withholds, and other incentives may conflict with the needs of patients.

With regard to health services administrators, the attributes listed in Exhibit 1.1 will take on new significance under managed care, especially as healthcare systems become more integrated. However, the point of reference will change from the individual hospital and its ICU to the system level encompassing primary, secondary, and tertiary care delivery organizations accountable for providing care to identifiable populations of covered lives.

What will be the impact of managed care on ICU gatekeeping? One aspect of the managed care movement is the more efficient use of staff and resources, the streamlining of patients' flow through the hospital, and greater selectivity in ICU admission. One result could be a decrease in the demand for critical care and in the number of ICU patient days. On the other hand, industry consolidation, which frequently accompanies a shift to managed care, will bring a downsizing of hospitals, which will heighten the importance of admission and discharge decision making and raise concerns about the quality of care. Nurses at the bedside may be the first to feel the strain. Hospitals that serve the uninsured will be particularly vulnerable to downsizing and even closure.

The Triage Task: Uncertainty and the Need for Information

The decision whether to admit and discharge patients or to triage patients when beds are full is often complicated, stressful, value laden, and conflict ridden. Important factors to be considered, many of which are characterized by uncertainty, include:

1. the prognoses of the patients already in the unit, including estimate of hospital mortality as well as functional status, pain, and suffering;
2. the origins and prognoses of the candidates for admission;
3. the availability, capacity, and competency of the staff (e.g., nurses);
4. the capacity of the next best alternative unit (e.g., other ICUs, special care units, or intermediate care units, if available) either within the hospital or at another hospital;
5. demand from other hospitals generated by physicians known or unknown to the ICU staff or by physicians on the medical staff;
6. demand from emergency and elective surgery;
7. legal ramifications;
8. patient and family understanding of prognosis and their treatment choices;
9. preferences of private attending physicians;
10. physical plant or licensed bed capacity; and
11. hospital policies regarding the allowance of ventilator-dependent patients, including those with do-not-resuscitate orders, to be cared for on general floors.

The fact that there are many variables to be considered is an indication of the complexity of the decision-making environment. The extent to which these variables change unpredictably is an indication of its dynamic nature (Duncan 1972).

The complexity of the triage task also increases in proportion to the number of participants in the decision process (patients, families, attending physicians, hospital-based ICU physicians, risk managers, operating room directors, patient care advocates, and other administrators) and the severity of the constraints, particularly the number of beds and number of nurses. When beds are few and demand is great, in-depth knowledge about all these variables, including those found within the ICU itself and outside the boundaries—other units in the hospital and other hospitals—is required.

Not only are the number of variables important when making decisions, but also the dynamic and unpredictable ways in which the variables move. For example, an ambulance bearing a multiple trauma patient may arrive at the emergency room, nurses may call in sick, an infection may close a multi-bed room, and a new and inexperienced house staff may arrive on their rotation. By its very nature, the ICU patient population is an unstable one, and the knowledge base used for treatment is constantly changing. In such a dynamic environment, it is often difficult to plan in advance how illnesses will be managed and resources allocated.

The amount of information needed about these aforementioned eleven factors in part depends on the occupancy of the ICU. If the ICU is at 50 percent occupancy, these factors do not matter a great deal. The cost of making the wrong decision (e.g., admitting a patient who could be treated in another setting) is not as great as if the ICU were at full occupancy. When the ICU reaches full occupancy, the amount of information that is needed about each of these factors increases dramatically. Calculating the interaction among these factors becomes even more difficult and critical. As Galbraith (1977) suggests, "the greater uncertainty of the task, the greater the amount of information that has to be processed among decision makers during the execution of the task to achieve a given level of performance." Information that can reduce uncertainty about any of these factors is crucial to the task of admission-discharge decision making.

Obviously one solution to the problem of uncertainty surrounding the factors that must be considered in triage is to increase the resources—that is, increase the number of staffed beds in order to decrease the occupancy pressure. If this could be done, the factors or variables would recede in importance. Unfortunately, the pressure for beds coupled with budgetary restrictions are decreasing slack resources of ICUs.

Hospital Decision-Making Style and Performance Expectations

The case of the transfer patient presented earlier illustrates the importance of information collection and processing to decision making. A great many factors or variables were considered: What is the prognosis of the patient? Will cardiac catheterization provide useful information? What is the availability of staff nurses? Who can be safely transferred to another unit or floor? Who will likely die? Who is waiting to come in and what is his or her prognosis? Processing the information was an interdisciplinary task force assembled in a "NASA-like" command center (Strosberg 1991). This decision-making style was highly unusual for this hospital. Typically there are many fewer participants collecting and processing much less information. The task-force format was necessitated by a crisis situation. The crisis was defined as the failure to meet important performance expectations that the hospital had set for itself, namely that ambulances should not be diverted nor elective surgery be postponed or canceled.

What is infrequent in this particular hospital may be quite frequent at large, inner-city hospitals. There, elective surgery is routinely postponed, and critically ill patients are held in the emergency room. Shoemaker et al. (1992) present an extreme but dramatic case of an inner-city medical center in Los Angeles:

> King-Drew Medical Center may, on any occasion, have more than twenty patients who, though "admitted" to the hospital, are still occupying a bed in the emergency department observation area because a hospital bed is not yet available. In these instances, every hospital bed, critical-care-unit bed, and postanesthesia recovery bed are filled, which compels patients to recover in the operating room.
>
> During the past six months at King-Drew, there have been as many as eleven emergency department patients at one time on mechanical ventilation, and patient deaths have resulted from those acute inadequacies. At some point, the hospital shuts down for new admissions, but this often does not prevent paramedics from bringing in additional patients. Moreover, 40% of the patients arrive via their own transportation, and it is impossible to prevent their entry, although the hospital may be "officially" closed to ambulances. Moreover, when the other county facilities are also "closed," the center is of necessity "open," despite the inability to provide proper care.
>
> The snowball effect of delays not only increases shock and mortality but also increases the incidence of shock-related multiple organ failures, which can lead to multiple costs before the preventable death. Conjointly, delays tie up scarce and expensive resources and preclude their use for more salvageable patients (p. 16).

On the other hand, some small community hospitals, with low case-mix severity, seldom face the problem of having a shortage of critical care resources. It is doubtful that either the inner-city hospitals or the small community hospitals have adopted a task force arrangement to make decisions. If Anywhere Hospital had lower performance expectations or more open beds, it would not require such a decision-making style because it would not need so much information. It is quite possible that as the beds become more scarce or tolerance levels change, different decision-making styles and structures will evolve. This case of the transfer patient portrays a slice of organizational life at one point in time only.

Conclusions: Hard Choices Ahead at the Street Level and Public Policy Level

In the case of King-Drew Medical Center, gatekeepers share many of the characteristics of what Lipsky (1980) calls "street-level bureaucrats." Not unlike harassed inner-city teachers, policemen, social workers, and lower court judges, they have limited time and resources, an involuntary clientele with high needs, and contradictory performance expectations, yet they possess enormous discretion over the rationing and delivery of essential services, even life and death services. We usually think of a bureaucracy as a pyramid-shaped distribution of formalized roles with power and discretion diminishing in relation to altitude. At the bottom of the organization, the incumbents are harnessed in their positions by rules, regulations, and guidelines with little flexibility or discretion. But in a street-level bureaucracy, the pyramid is inverted with the bottom-level bureaucrats—the ones who directly serve the clients—having the greatest discretion and flexibility. According to Lipsky, street-level bureaucrats work in situations that are too complicated to be programmed by elaborate rules or that involve tasks that call for "sensitive observations and judgment, which are not reducible to programmed formats" (p. 15).

What is the difference between the street-level bureaucrat and a professional? They both require discretion to carry out their complex tasks. And most street-level bureaucrats rightly consider themselves to be professional. However, steadfast advocacy for the client, inherent in the fiduciary relationship, is considered the hallmark of the consulting professional epitomized by the physician.

Is street-level bureaucracy a construct that can be usefully applied to the ICU? It certainly can for describing the King-Drew Medical Center operating in the triage mode. For the uninsured patients entering involuntarily to the "hospital of last resort" through the emergency room, frequently in mentally incapacitated condition, a primary care physician or private attending physician advocate may be nowhere to be found. Family members may be confused, frightened, divided, or nonexistent. In situations of shortage, ICU staff, composed of hospital-based physicians including house staff and the nursing staff, fill the dual role of patient advocate/caregiver and implicit rationer of services. In principle, they could use well-accepted and unambiguous triage criteria based on guidelines promulgated by various professional associations and societies. But in practice, as will be shown in subsequent chapters, these criteria are often ambiguous, contradictory, open to legal challenge, or not particularly useful. ICU staff may very well consider themselves harassed street-level bureaucrats with stressful triage responsibilities. They must make difficult choices.

Most hospitals are not inner-city hospitals of last resort caring for the poor and the uninsured. But even in community hospitals such as Anywhere Hospital, facing a decrease in capacity and stricter control of access for routine hospital care under managed care, we can expect more pressure on ICU beds and increased necessity to triage. Ironically, ICU staff in the triage mode, negotiating with private attendings and family members or surrogates (frequently absent at inner-city hospitals), may also find themselves in a harassed and stressful position, facing contradictory performance expectations. They too must make hard choices. Managed care complicates matters. As plans strive to serve a defined population of covered lives within fixed budgets, different or even the same physicians operate under different sets of financial incentives depending on each patient's managed care plan.

Are the gatekeepers of the ICU destined to become street-level bureaucrats? As was pointed out, gatekeepers face complex and dynamic decision-making environments influenced by clinical and organizational uncertainty. There will always be intermittent periods of high census necessitating triage of beds. Those responsible for triage must exercise sensitive observation and judgment. Rules cannot completely eliminate the need for discretion and the nonroutine and controversial decisions that sometimes result.

This book explores the conditions that give rise to a complex and dynamic environment in hospital ICUs. Through the use of case studies we will show possible consequences for patients. We will also show how redesign of organizational structure and improvement in management practices could reduce nonroutine decision making and the necessity to make difficult choices. However, improving management and organizational structure can go just so far. We argue that, ultimately, society must decide how it will sort out competing claims to ICU resources and express its intentions through public policy. To be sure, changing societal norms with regard to end-of-life care will influence physicians, patients, and families in how hard they press on the gates of the ICU. However, the resolution of competing claims on ICU resources and the promulgation of public policies and instruments such as admission and discharge policies, guidelines, rules, and, as will be explained, insurance contracts, will require hard choices at the public policy level involving action in the legislative and judicial arenas. The marketplace alone cannot make these choices. If the difficult public policy decisions could be made, the subsequent availability of well-accepted and clear-cut policies, guidelines, and rules for non-triage mode decisions could reduce, but of course not eliminate, the necessity for triage-mode decision making.

In answer to the question posed earlier, the extent to which gatekeepers, at least those operating in the triage mode, will share characteristics with street-level bureaucrats will depend on whether society is willing to make the hard public policy choices.

References

American Medical Association Council on Ethical and Judicial Affairs. 1995. "Ethical Issues in Managed Care." *Journal of the American Medical Association* 273 (4): 330–35.

Baker, R. 1995. "Rationing, Rhetoric, and Rationality: A Review of the Health Care Rationing Debate in America and Europe." In *Allocating Health Care Resources,* edited by J. M. Humber and R. F. Almeder, 57–84. Totowa, NJ: Humana Press.

Beauchamp, T. L., and J. F. Childress. 1994. *Principles of Biomedical Ethics.* Oxford: Oxford University Press.

Chassin, M. R. 1982. "Costs and Outcomes of Medical Intensive Care." *Medical Care* 36 (1): 95–109.

Civetta, J. M. 1992. "Critical Care: How Should We Evaluate Our Progress?" *Critical Care Medicine* 20 (12): 1714–20.

Daniels, N. 1986. "Why Saying No to Patients in the United States Is So Hard." *New England Journal of Medicine* 314 (21): 1380–83.

Duncan, R. B. 1972. "Characteristics of Perceived Environments and Perceived Environmental Uncertainty." *Administrative Science Quarterly* 17 (3): 313–27.

Engelhardt, H. T., and M. A. Rie. 1986. "Intensive Care Units, Scarce Resources and Conflicting Principles of Justice." *Journal of the American Medical Association* 255 (9): 1159–64.

Fox, R. C., and J. P. Swazey. 1978. *The Courage to Fail,* 2nd ed. Chicago: University of Chicago Press.

Galbraith, J. R. 1977. *Organization Design.* Reading, MA: Addison-Wesley.

Knaus, W. A. 1989. "Criteria for Admissions to Intensive Care Units." In *Rationing of Medical Care for the Critically Ill,* edited by M. A. Strosberg, I. A. Fein, and J. D. Carroll, 44–51. Washington, D.C.: The Brookings Institution.

Knaus, W. A., J. E. Zimmerman, and D. P. Wagner. 1981. "APACHE—Acute Physiology and Chronic Health Evaluation: A Physiologically Based Classification System." *Critical Care Medicine* 9 (8): 591–97.

Lemeshow, S., D. Teres, H. Pastides, J. S. Aurunin, and J. S. Steingrub. 1985. "A Method for Predicting Survival and Mortality of ICU Patients Using Objectively Derived Weights." *Critical Care Medicine* 13 (7): 519–25.

Lipsky, M. 1980. *Street-Level Bureaucracy: Dilemmas of the Individual in Public Services.* New York: Russell Sage Foundation.

National Institutes of Health. 1983. *Consensus Development Conference on Critical Care Medicine: Summary.* Bethesda, MD: U.S. Public Health Service, National Institutes of Health.

Schupak, E., and J. P. Merril. 1965. "Experience with Long-Term Intermittent Hemodialysis." *Annals of Internal Medicine* 62 (3): 509–18.

Shoemaker, W., C. B. James, A. W. Fleming, E. Hardin, G. J. Ordog, R. Sterling-Scott, and J. Wasserberger. 1992. "DeFacto Rationing of Emergency Medical Services." In *Rationing America's Medical Care: The Oregon Plan and Beyond*, edited by M. A. Strosberg, J. M. Weiner, R. Baker, and I. A. Fein, 151–56. Washington, D.C.: The Brookings Institution.

Society of Critical Care Medicine Ethics Committee. 1994a. "Attitudes of Critical Care Medicine Professionals Concerning Distribution of Intensive Care Resources." *Critical Care Medicine* 22 (2): 358–62.

———. 1994b. "Consensus Statement on the Triage of Critically Ill Patients." *Journal of the American Medical Association* 271 (15): 1200–03.

Strosberg, M. A. 1991. "Intensive Care Units in the Triage Mode: An Organizational Perspective." *Hospital & Health Services Administration* 36 (1): 95–109.

Teres, D. 1989. "Triage: An Everyday Occurrence in the Intensive Care Unit." In *Rationing Critical Care for the Critically Ill*, edited by M. A. Strosberg and I. A. Fein, 70–75. Washington, D.C.: The Brookings Institution.

United Network for Organ Sharing. *Bylaws and Policies.* March 4, 1993. Policy 3.3.5.

Zimmerman, J. E., D. P. Wagner, E. A. Draper, and W. A. Knaus. 1994. "Improving Intensive Care Unit Discharge Decisions: Supplementing Physician Judgment with Predictions of Next Day Risk for Life Support." *Critical Care Medicine* 22 (9): 1373–84.

CHAPTER 2

BACKGROUND: INTENSIVE CARE UNITS, CRITICAL CARE MEDICINE, AND ORGANIZATIONAL SETTING

ICU Defined

The United States Office of Technology Assessment defines critical care medicine as:

> a multi-disciplinary and multi-professional medical/nursing field concerned with patients who have sustained or are at risk of sustaining acutely life-threatening single or multiple organ system failure due to disease or injury. These conditions necessitate prolonged minute-to-minute therapy or observation in an intensive care unit (ICU) which is capable of providing a high intensive therapy in terms of quality and immediacy (Berenson 1984, p. 13).

The care of critically ill patients is part of a continuum that "includes management at the scene of onset of critical illness or injury, during transportation, in the emergency department, during surgical intervention in the operating room, and finally in the ICU" (Safar 1984). The term "ICU" is often used interchangeably with the term "critical care unit." By convention, the abbreviation "CCU" has been reserved for coronary care unit.

The intensity of care refers to the amount of nursing, allied health professional, and physician care, and of special procedures, tests, and equipment that is devoted to the patient. In the hospital, there is a continuum of intensity that ranges from routine care on the regular floor to the highest level of intensity in the ICU. For example, on a regular floor, the average nurse-to-patient ratio might range from 1:8 to

1:12. In the ICU, the ratio is typically 1:2 or 1:3, although as hospitals are forced to cut costs under managed care this will likely change as technicians are substituted for registered nurses (RNs). Many hospitals have intermediate units with an intensity in between the ICU and the floors. These units are called intermediate care units, step-down units, or progressive care units. Nurse staffing is typically 1:3 or 1:4. The definition and functions are not uniform. However, a progressive care unit is often part of or adjacent to the ICU while an intermediate care unit is in a physically distinct location with separate unit management. Intermediate care units may be single function (neuro-observation, telemetry, postoperative) or multipurpose.

Typically, patients in the ICU are critically ill with life-threatening conditions associated with the failure of one or more organ systems. Examples include heart attack, major trauma (e.g., car accident, gun-shot wound), complications from major surgery, and overwhelming infection. The severity of these patients is high because they are at risk of death or major morbidity.

Also included in the ICU are patients at risk of becoming critically ill. These are the monitor patients. According to the National Institute of Health (NIH) Consensus Development Conference (1983):

> The purpose of intensive care in these instances is to prevent a serious complication that may occur. It is presumed that the prompt response to a potentially fatal complication made possible by continuous monitoring plus the concentration of specialized personnel in the ICU increases the probability of a favorable outcome (p. 3).

In a study by Zimmerman et al. (1995) of 17,440 ICU admissions in 40 U.S. hospitals with more than 200 beds, 46 percent were admitted for monitoring rather than active treatment. Of the monitored patients, 7.6 percent went on to active treatment.

Other reasons physicians seek admission to the ICU for their patients include providing preoperative and postoperative care for elective and emergency surgical cases, providing a setting for performing invasive procedures, and providing better nursing coverage than would be available on the floors.

Where does routine care end and intensive care begin? This question is raised for a variety of reasons. Historically, under cost-based retrospective reimbursement, ICU care has received a higher reimbursement rate than routine care, one cause for the rapid diffusion of ICUs. The designation of an ICU bed grouping, therefore, had special meaning for third party payors and for state regulators granting certificates of need. Along with this designation came special requirements for formalized admission-discharge criteria, staffing and equipment levels, administrative structure, physical space, quality assurance, and protocols for care (Myers et al. 1984).

Historical Roots and Evolution

The ICU, although it contains many technological wonders, is itself an organizational innovation. As Russell (1979) notes, the ICU is based on "the simple idea that critically ill patients need close observation, and constant nursing, and quick action in a crisis, and that the most efficient way to provide this kind of care is not to disperse these patients throughout the wards, but to bring them together in one place with the most sophisticated equipment and highly trained people in the hospital."

The SCCM, the professional association composed of critical care physicians and nurses, summarizes the major events in the history of critical care (1992):

> Florence Nightingale wrote about the advantages of a separate area of the hospital for patients recovering from surgery.
>
> During World War II, shock wards were established to resuscitate and care for soldiers injured in battle and undergoing surgery.
>
> The nursing shortage, which followed World War II, forced the grouping of postoperative patients in recovery rooms to ensure attentive care. The obvious benefits in improved patient care resulted in the spread of recovery rooms to nearly every hospital by 1960.
>
> In 1947–1948, the polio epidemic that raged through Europe and the United States resulted in a breakthrough in the treatment of patients dying from respiratory paralysis. In Denmark, manual ventilation was accomplished through a tube placed in the trachea of polio patients. Patients with respiratory paralysis and/or suffering from acute circulatory failure require intensive nursing care.
>
> In the 1950s, when the mechanical ventilator was developed, respiratory intensive care units (ICUs) were organized in many European and American hospitals. The care and monitoring of mechanically ventilated patients is more efficiently accomplished when they are grouped in a single location. General ICUs for very sick patients, including postoperative patients, were developed for the same reasons.
>
> In 1958, approximately 25 percent of community hospitals with more than 300 beds reported that they had an ICU. By the late 1960s, most United States hospitals had a least one ICU . . . (p. 2).

ICUs have evolved along a variety of paths. Age is certainly an important dimension. There are adult, pediatric, and neonatal ICUs. ICUs also have evolved along the two great medical branches, medicine (medical ICUs) and surgery (surgical ICUs). Within these branches there is also division according to subspecialty and organ system (e.g., cardiothoracic ICU, neurological ICU, and other specialized units such as the burn unit, trauma unit, and transplant unit).

ICUs are considered "special care units," which, according to the JCAHO, include ICUs, PACUs, and CCUs. A major function of the CCU is to employ special technology to monitor heart rhythms of patients at risk for heart attacks. In separating CCUs from the general category of ICU, the U.S. Office of Technology Assessment finds (Berenson 1984):

> ... CCUs treat patients with a relatively narrow range of diagnosis, primarily patients with suspected or actual heart attacks and related problems. CCU patients are not as ill, have fewer physiologic systems involved, require fewer therapeutic services, have better outcomes, have a greater need for a quiet, stress-free environment and pose different evaluation and policy issues than do patients in ICUs. In short, CCUs serve a different primary function from ICUs and most hospitals with more than 100 beds have separate CCUs and ICUs (p. 13).

Description of U.S. ICUs

Critical care is one of the most expensive components of hospitalization, accounting for 6 to 10 percent of hospital beds and consuming 20 to 34 percent of the hospital's budget (Chalfin, Cohen, and Lambrinos 1995). Cohen, Fitzpatrick, and Booth (1996) estimate that approximately 25 percent of hospitalized patients pass through the ICU at some point in their stay. Despite their importance, very little data have been collected on the distribution, operations, patient mix, and management of ICUs. To remedy the situation, the SCCM, in 1991, conducted a one-day census of U.S. ICUs. This SCCM survey included the CCU under the general category of ICU. The survey findings, which captured information on 39 percent of an estimated total of 7,434 ICUs (from 40 percent of the hospitals containing ICUs) are published in *Critical Care Medicine* (Groeger et al. 1992 and Groeger et al. 1993). The SCCM survey found wide variation in characteristics such as patient mix, referral patterns, number of beds, occupancy rates, and management. Much of the variation is correlated with the size of the hospital measured in terms of the number of beds. However, as will be explained later, some important managerial characteristics are not correlated with hospital bed size.

Hospital Size and Organizational Characteristics

In the organization theory literature, the size of the organization is an important contextual variable associated with variation in organization structure. For example, Robey (1982) describes the relationship between size, specialization, and differentiation:

> Specialization refers to the division of labor or number of distinct skills required at the task level. Differentiation refers to the grouping of specialists into departments, sections, or subunits at higher levels. As size increases, organizations develop more specialized rolls and more distinct groupings of specialists. In short, the organization becomes more complex and harder to control (p. 197).

Exhibit 2.1 shows that the number of ICUs per hospital increases with bed size. The range is from an average of one ICU per hospital with bed sizes of 100 or less to 3.4 ICUs per hospital with bed sizes of 500 or more beds.

The pattern of differentiation is clearly shown in Exhibit 2.2. In the smallest hospitals, the grouping of 1–100 beds, 76 percent of the ICUs consist of combined medical-surgical-coronary care units, by far the most common type of unit. As hospital size increases, this type of

Exhibit 2.1 Hospital Intensive Care Units

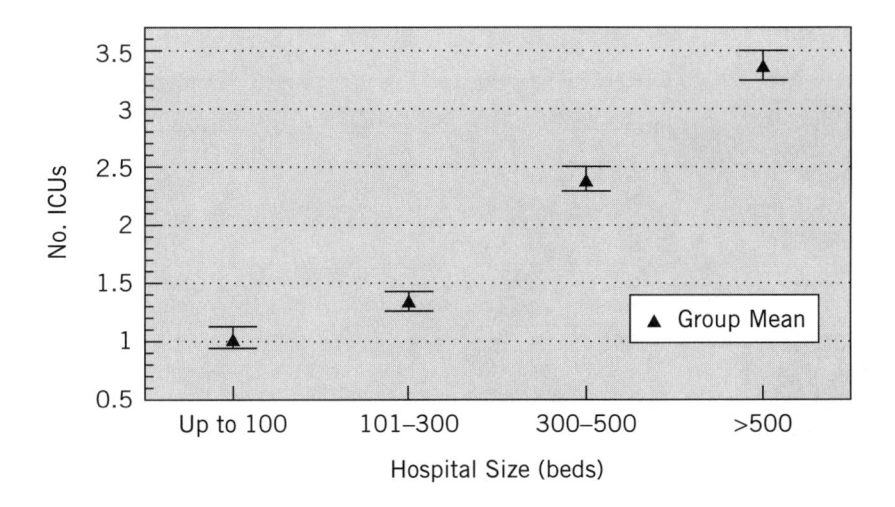

Source: Adapted from Groeger et al. 1992. "Descriptive Analysis of Critical Care Units in the United States." *Critical Care Medicine* 20 (6): 851.

Error bars overlap if the difference between group means is not significant at the 5 percent level. Significant differences are determined using Bonferroni simultaneous confidence intervals for all comparisons. Error bars represent nonsimultaneous 95 percent confidence intervals for each group based on the mean and SD for that group.

unit diminishes to 54 percent in the 101–300 bed grouping, 13 percent in the 301–500 bed grouping, and 5.6 percent in the above 500 grouping. As the undifferentiated medical-surgical-coronary care unit declines with increasing hospital size, other types of units emerge in predictable ways. For example, the medical-surgical ICU, separating from the coronary care unit, increases from 11.5 percent in the 1–100 bed grouping to 14.9 percent in the 101–300 bed grouping and 17.6 percent in the 301–500 bed grouping and then declines to 7.8 percent in the 500 or more bed grouping where separate medical ICUs and surgical ICUs dominate.

According to the SCCM survey, as hospital size increases, so does the number of ICU beds per unit and occupancy rate. With the exception of the smallest hospitals, the average size is approximately 10–14 beds. With regard to occupancy, on the particular day of the census, the overall average occupancy rate for all ICUs regardless of hospital size was 82 percent, ranging from an average of 66 percent in the 1–100 bed grouping to an average of 92 percent in the 500 or more bed grouping (Exhibit 2.3). What this means is that, especially in the larger hospitals, many ICUs will likely experience full occupancy on many days per year.

It should be pointed out that the traditional calculation of occupancy rate (ratio of patients to beds) may be somewhat misleading as an indicator of bed pressure. The SCCM survey asked about the number of patients awaiting a bed in the unit, the number of patients

Exhibit 2.2 Intensive Care Units* Distributed by Hospital Size**

Unit Group	1–100 Beds	101–300 Beds	301–500 Beds	500+ Beds	Total Units N	%
Medical	2.7%	4.9%	11.9%	17.8%	284	9.9%
Med/Surg	11.5%	14.9%	17.6%	7.8%	376	13.1%
Pediatric	0.6%	5.1%	6.9%	8.9%	172	6.0%
Neonatal	0.9%	5.6%	11.3%	11.4%	229	8.0%
CCU	2.5%	7.8%	16.1%	11.7%	294	10.2%
Med/Sur/CCU	75.6%	53.9%	13.1%	5.6%	971	33.8%
Neurological		0.6%	2.7%	6.0%	73	2.5%
Surgical		4.9%	17.6%	28.4%	391	13.6%
Other	5.7%	2%	2.1%	2%	86	3.0%
	N = 432	N = 935	N = 729	N = 780	2876	100%

* Some specialty units have been combined into broader categories.
** Adapted from Groeger et al. 1992. "Descriptive Analysis of Critical Care Units in the United States." *Critical Care Medicine* 20 (6): 851.

Exhibit 2.3 Occupancy of Individual Intensive Care Units Analyzed by Hospital Size

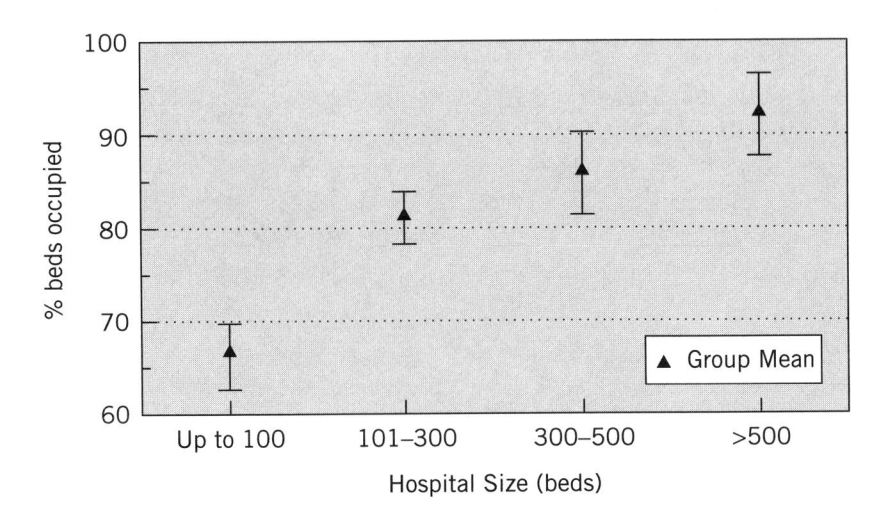

[Chart: % beds occupied vs Hospital Size (beds); Group Mean markers with error bars at Up to 100 (~67%), 101–300 (~82%), 300–500 (~87%), >500 (~93%)]

Source: Adapted from Groeger et al. 1992. "Descriptive Analysis of Critical Care Units in the United States." *Critical Care Medicine* 20 (6): 282.
See Exhibit 2.1 legend for additional information.

awaiting transfer out of the unit, the number of beds that were closed for various reasons, and the number of expansion beds (beds that could be staffed within 24 hours in a pinch). The average "effective occupancy rate" (Mallick et al. 1995) for all ICUs was 71 percent, rather than 82 percent, defined as [(patients in ICU) + (patients awaiting beds) − (patients awaiting transfer out)] ÷ [(beds in ICU) − (closed beds) + (expansion beds)].

Respondents to the SCCM survey were also asked about the number of ICU patients needing a different level of care: (1) patients who required a higher level of technology than available in their ICU; (2) patients who should be cared for in lower technology settings but who cannot be transferred due to lack of hospital beds; and (3) patients who need to be transferred but could not be for other reasons. Twenty-seven percent of ICUs contained at least one patient (6 percent of all patients) who should have been being treated at a lower level of care but could not be transferred out because of the lack of a suitable bed on the floor. Fifteen percent of all ICUs contained at least one patient (3 percent of all patients) who should have been transferred but could not be for other reasons including lack of facilities for chronic, long-term

Exhibit 2.4 ICU Points of Origin and Destination

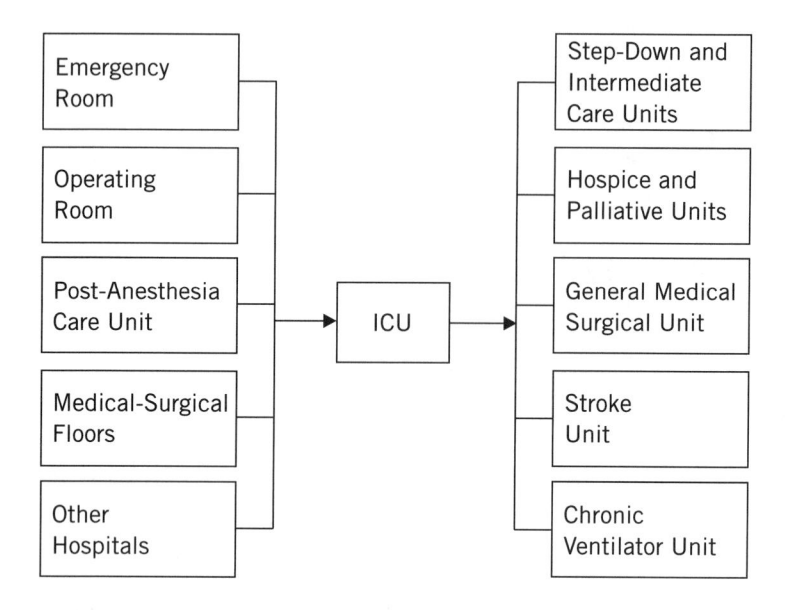

```
Emergency Room ─┐                    ┌─ Step-Down and Intermediate Care Units
Operating Room ─┤                    ├─ Hospice and Palliative Units
Post-Anesthesia Care Unit ─┼─► ICU ─┼─ General Medical Surgical Unit
Medical-Surgical Floors ─┤           ├─ Stroke Unit
Other Hospitals ─┘                    └─ Chronic Ventilator Unit
```

mechanically ventilated patients; unwillingness of family or physicians to authorize the transfer; or medicolegal considerations. These units may be characterized as inefficient to the degree that they allocate costly critical care resources to patients who could be adequately cared for at lower levels of intensity. Approximately 1 percent of all patients in 2 percent of ICUs require a higher level of technology, presumably in a major teaching hospital.

Admission Source

Exhibit 2.4 shows the multiple points of origin and destination for adult ICU patients. The source of admissions varies by the type of unit (Exhibit 2.5). For example, half of the admissions to the medical ICU came from the emergency room while only 2 percent came from the operating room/recovery room. On the other hand, 60 percent of the admissions to the surgical intensive care unit came from the operating room/recovery room for postoperative management. Nineteen percent came from the emergency room.

The surgical ICU contains both scheduled elective surgery patients (e.g., coronary artery bypass) and unscheduled emergency surgery patients. In some instances surgical patients are admitted preoperatively for

Exhibit 2.5 Admission Sources

Unit Type	Emergency Room	Operating Room Recovery Room	Hospital Floor	Other ICU	Other Hospital	Home	Delivery Room/Other	Total Patients
Medical	50.2%	2.5%	28.4%	5.9%	8.7%	1.8%	2.4%	2286
Med/Surg	35.4%	32.8%	21.1%	3.7%	3.4%	1.6%	2.1%	3329
Pediatric	25.5%	24.4%	17.7%	2.2%	23.9%	3.3%	3.0%	1290
Neonatal	0.4%	0.0%	3.6%	1.7%	34.4%	0.2%	59.6%	2796
CCU	57.3%	3.5%	14.5%	3.2%	12.2%	3.3%	6.0%	2243
Med/Surg/CCU	53.4%	20.0%	16.8%	0.9%	3.1%	2.7%	3.1%	7061
Neurologic	50.7%	25.6%	11.7%	3.6%	4.5%	2.4%	1.4%	418
Surgical	18.7%	59.7%	9.3%	2.2%	5.9%	2.5%	1.9%	3092
All Units	37.8%	21.8%	15.7%	2.5%	10.1%	2.2%	10.0%	22515

Source: Groeger et al. 1993. "Descriptive Analysis of Critical Care Units in the United States: Patient Characteristics and Intensive Care Unit Utilization." *Critical Care Medicine* 21 (2): 283.

Exhibit 2.6 Patients with Specific Interventions Performed in ICUs as a Function of Hospital Size (%)

	All Units	<101	101 to 301	301 to 501	>500
	24,927*	1,017	7,840	7,073	8,995
Continuous arteriovenous hemofiltration	0.5	1.2	0.5	0.5	0.6
Chest tube in place	11.0	3.4	8.2	11.0	14.4
Hemodialysis	3.5	0.8	2.9	4.1	3.9
Intravenous antiarrhythmic	12.3	19.2	12.3	12.9	11.0
Invasive arterial monitoring	30.3	10.9	22.7	29.8	39.4
Ventilator	33.9	15.8	29.5	33.6	40.0
Temporary transvenous pacemaker	3.9	1.7	3.4	4.0	4.6
Pulmonary artery catheter	16.1	6.3	11.6	17.4	19.9
Transfusion	13.7	7.9	10.9	12.7	17.6
Intravenous vasoactive or inotropic agent	20.0	15.9	17.7	20.1	22.5

*Total number of patients
Source: Groeger et al. 1993. "Descriptive Analysis of Critical Care Units in the United States: Patient Characteristics and Intensive Care Unit Utilization." *Critical Care Medicine* 21 (2): 286.

special preparation for operating room procedures. Combined medical-surgical units or medical-surgical-coronary care units face greater variability in admission source than separate medical ICUs or surgical ICUs.

Resource Utilization and Mechanical Ventilation

ICU patients have a wide array of diagnoses. The major categories for adult ICUs include arrhythmia, heart failure, ischemic heart disease, neurologic dysfunction, postoperative management, blunt trauma, and respiratory failure. Are ICUs in the larger hospitals treating sicker patients? Single diagnoses are not particularly good indicators of severity of illness or resource use, for the patients may have additional diagnoses, especially those patients with multiple organ system failure. Diagnosis Related Groups (DRGs) also do not capture the severity of illness of

ICU patients even though reimbursement is similar among patients. Using specific interventions as a rough proxy for severity, Exhibit 2.6 shows that interventions increase with hospital bed size. We emphasize the roughness of the proxy because it can be argued that large hospitals, with more equipment and personnel, are inclined to undertake more interventions, independent of patient severity level.

Nevertheless we note, in Exhibit 2.6, the large overall proportion (34 percent) of patients on mechanical ventilators. Mechanical ventilators present a special problem for ICUs. Developed in the 1950s and 1960s, mechanical ventilation expanded rapidly in later decades and facilitated many new high-risk surgical procedures such as cardiac surgery, which is now routinely performed. However, an increasing number of patients, especially those with multi-organ failure, require prolonged ventilatory support (Cohen and Booth 1994). While still a small proportion of total ICU population, these patients use up an extraordinary amount of resources. Wagner (1989) found that patients who required mechanical ventilation for one week or more used up 50 percent of all ICU resources, even though they constituted less than 10 percent of the population. Davis et al. (1980) estimate that an ICU patient on a mechanical ventilator costs twice as much as a non-ventilated patient in the ICU and eight times as much as a patient on a regular floor. The Health Care Financing Administration (HCFA) has established a heavily weighted DRG (number 483) for ventilated patients with tracheotomies.

What should be done with ICU patients who are placed on ventilators but cannot be easily weaned (gradually removed from ventilatory support) off them? Must they remain in the ICU taking up a bed for weeks and even months? Some hospitals reluctantly allow ventilator patients to be transferred to the floors. However, the nurse-to-patient ratios on these floors may not be adequate to provide the careful attention required by these patients. An increasing number of hospitals have established special respiratory care units. Other options include nursing homes, chronic care facilities, and even home care. However, in approximately 65 percent of hospitals, ventilator patients can only be cared for in the ICU. In these hospitals, the decision to intubate means automatic stay in the ICU.

The average length of stay in the ICU ranges from three to four days with around 20 percent of patients discharged within 24 hours. However, according to the SCCM survey, 17 percent of all critical care patients stayed 14 days or longer. Forty-nine percent of the units said that they had one or more patients remaining in the unit for 14 days or longer. The great majority of these long-stay patients are on mechanical ventilators.

Costs, Resource Use, and Outcome

Total ICU costs are composed of the direct costs of operating the unit and the indirect costs of services allocated to the unit. Direct costs are composed of the fixed costs of construction and maintenance and the variable costs associated with personnel, equipment, and supplies, which in turn depends on the number of patients and their severity of illness. Costs are difficult to assess, although it is generally agreed that the estimated ratio of ICU-day cost to hospital-day cost is 3:1 (Russell 1979; Wagner, Wineland, and Knaus 1983). ICU charges, although usually available, often do not accurately reflect true costs because they may have been artificially inflated to subsidize other parts of the hospital's operation. Interhospital comparisons based on charge information are problematic.

With regard to information on outcomes of critical care, no large database exists similar to the SCCM nationwide survey. Single and multi-institutional studies provide most of the information. The measurement of outcomes is problematic. Data on post-hospital survival, including functional status and quality of life, is difficult to collect, although survival to hospital discharge is easily and unambiguously measured.

A disproportionate number of patient days and resources are accounted for by a small percentage of the patients, many of whom either die in the hospital or are discharged with a short duration and poor quality of life (Wagner 1989; Fein et al. 1991; Oye and Bellamy 1991; Borlase et al. 1990; Cohen, Lambrinas, and Fein 1993). Although it is reasonable to try to identify ahead of time those ICU patients who will become high-cost high utilizers and whose outcome will be death or an extremely poor quality of life, the relationship between predicted outcome, actual outcome, and resource use is not at all clear cut. Detsky et al. (1981) found that patients who have outcomes that are opposite the predicted outcomes tend to be the high-cost patients, a finding confirmed by Rapoport et al. (1990). The two groups with longest stay are patients with massive injuries and poor prognosis who survive and those with an initially good prognosis who develop complications and die.

Esserman, Belkora, and Lenert (1995) studied resource use and long-term outcome (mortality) of 402 consecutively admitted critically ill patients at Stanford University Hospital during the period June 1988 and January 1989. Thirteen percent (52) of the patients died in the hospital. Ten percent (40) died within 12 months of hospital discharge, and 78 percent (314) survived longer than 12 months.

Esserman, Belkora, and Lenert have developed what they consider a promising model to identify "potentially ineffective care," defined as care given to patients who, despite prolonged intensive support, die either in the hospital or shortly after hospital discharge. In specific, these are patients who die in the hospital or within three months and who use resources (measured by charges) in the upper 25th percentile of all critical care patients. Thirteen percent of the patients in the Stanford University Hospital study met this definition and used 32 percent of the resources.

Cost-effectiveness analysis provides an economic framework for assessing costs and outcomes and for facilitating decision making that ensures the best possible outcome is obtained for the resources expended (Lambrinos and Papadakos 1987; Chalfin, Cohen, and Lambrinos 1995). A cost-effectiveness ratio provides a summary measure of the resources needed to achieve a certain outcome or certain level of health status. Some common examples are cost per survivor and cost per year of life saved (or gained). Faced with alternative approaches (e.g., two different ICU interventions, ICUs from different hospitals, or an ICU setting versus a non-ICU setting), it is desirable to choose the approach with the lowest cost-effectiveness ratio. Of course, survival is not a homogeneous measure of ICU outcome. Survival of a routine elective surgery patient is much different than the survival of a patient with multiple organ system failure. The latter uses more resources and represents a greater medical achievement. Cost-effectiveness ratios must be adjusted by the severity of illness of the patients (Rapoport et al. 1994).

Survival to hospital discharge and even duration of survival are limited as measures of ICU outcome. Cost-utility analysis, a subset of cost-effectiveness analysis, attempts to expand the assessment of outcome by incorporating a person's preferences for different health outcomes (i.e., a "utility") into a single summary effectiveness measure. A common quality-of-life measurement is the quality-adjusted life-year (QALY), which is a summary statistic that incorporates the mortality and morbidity effects of a particular medical intervention (O'Brien and Rushby 1990). If, for example, an additional year of healthy life is valued at one year, an additional year of less-than-healthy life would be valued at less than one year (depending on the extent of morbidity, disability, and discomfort).

Critical Care Nursing

Nurses are required to implement complex monitoring and treatment interventions and to provide educational and emotional support to the patient and family. The American Association of Critical Care Nurses (AACN) certifies RNs who have at least two years of experience in critical care nursing practice and have successfully completed an examination. The 1991 SCCM survey found that approximately 20 percent of the filled nursing positions in ICUs were held by certified critical care nurses. The proportion of certified nurses increases slightly as the number of hospital beds increases, ranging from 16 percent (fewer than 100 beds) to 21 percent (greater than 501 beds) (Groeger et al. 1992). In 1994, 52,200 nurses were certified in critical care, up 62 percent from 1989 (SCCM 1995).

Hospitals typically have extensive orientation programs for critical care nurses that may last as long as six months. These programs cover physiology, pharmacology, and the checking and testing of monitoring equipment. Nurses gradually assume clinical responsibility, usually under the guidance of an experienced nurse who serves as preceptor. The care of critically ill patients takes place in a high-pressure and emotionally charged environment. For an unstable ICU patient, there is no substitute for an experienced nurse.

Critical Care Teams

The intensive care unit requires a particularly close collaboration between bedside nurses and physicians. The AACN and the SCCM call for a "collaborative practice" between nurses and physicians who jointly share in the responsibility for managing the patients in the unit (Miccolo and Spanier 1993). In addition to nurses and physicians, the collaboration includes respiratory therapists, dietitians, social workers, critical care pharmacists, and occupational and physical therapists. Because of cost-containment pressures, an effort has been made to expand the team to include mid-level practitioners such as physician assistants or nurse practitioners, who can serve in physician-extender roles in acute care hospitals and critical care settings (Snyder et al. 1994). Cost-containment pressures also have expanded the domain of nurses to include case management for individual patients and non-bedside managerial roles in the interests of efficiency, collaboration, coordination, and continuity of care (Walleck 1994). We will return to this theme in Chapter 5.

Critical Care Medicine: Specialization and the Qualified Critical Care Physician

Critical care medicine specialists, or intensivists, are trained to deal comprehensively with a complex patient suffering from the malfunction of one or more organ systems. In a sense, intensivists are generalists for the critically ill not only because they have to deal with all organ systems but also because many life-threatening physiological disturbances are quite similar in critically ill patients, regardless of the underlying disease.

Specialization implies a division of labor. Medical care has been divided along the lines of age groups (e.g., neonatal, pediatrics, adult medicine), organ systems (e.g., cardiology, pulmonology), technologies (e.g., radiology), or combinations of categories (e.g., pediatric cardiology). Generally speaking, the divisions are contained within the traditional departmental structure of medical schools and hospitals: departments and sections of medicine, surgery, pediatrics, anesthesiology, etc. Critical care medicine differs from the typical pattern because it cuts across organ systems and the various departments although generally it does respect the separation between pediatric and adult medicine.

Robert Chase (1976) summarizes the process of medical specialization:

1. As a result of advances in a field or development of new technology, a new group develops special expertise in this area.
2. An organization or society is formed for an exchange of ideas and to display advances to one another.
3. Membership in the organization becomes a mark of distinction in the field, and, in an effort to externalize that recognition, certification of excellence in the field becomes established.
4. Institutions with responsibility for quality of health care soon accept certification as evidence of competence and limit care within that field to those certified (p. 498).

Most specialty groups aspire to reach the board certification state—a status that brings the specialist economic advantage along with a certain degree of control over technology, working conditions, and unique reimbursement rates. Faced with competition from rival groups and cries of monopolization, many budding specialty groups fail to reach this stage. To say the least, the process of specialization, which is not well understood by the general public, is only partially driven by scientific and technical advancement. The organizations that influence specialization have a major impact on the organization of U.S. healthcare. In the name of self-regulation, specialty societies, through interlocking directorates with parent and umbrella organizations, dominate the credentialing system, which in turn influences accreditation of graduate medical education programs, establishment of new specialties and subspecialties, and the distribution and practice patterns of specialists. Also affected are the policies, procedures, and organizational structure of the hospital; specification of physician qualifications; staff privileges and responsibilities; technology requirements for quality of care; organizational differentiation into departments, divisions, and sections; referral patterns and the cost of services; and incomes of practitioners—in short many of the essential characteristics of the U.S. healthcare system.

The development of critical care medicine followed the process described by Chase. The Society of Critical Care Medicine was founded in 1973. A central challenge facing the fledgling organization was how to establish an independent, multispecialty discipline that was not merely an extension of the older, well-established primary specialties such as surgery and anesthesiology, or the single-organ subspecialties of internal medicine. All of these groups laid special claim to treating the critically ill. In his 1974 presidential address, Dr. William Shoemaker (1975) highlighted some of the difficulties in establishing the legitimacy of critical care medicine:

> ... the Society having survived birth, the neonatal period, and infancy, now faces its puberty period with all the self-conscious doubts of the classic identity crisis. We have a hard time convincing ourselves as to who we are, what we are supposed to do, and where ultimately will be our place in the sun. We see ourselves beset by the over-powering parent disciplines who tend to regard departures from traditional ways as intrusions by irresponsible revolutionaries on the well established order. Even worse, efforts to organize critical care along multidisciplinary lines are often regarded as usurpation of the prerogatives of the parent disciplines. These incursions on the territorial imperatives are met with all the emotional intensity that outraged maternal instincts can muster when basic assumptions are challenged. It is little wonder that difficulty is encountered in defining the role of critical care medicine within the framework of the established health care system. If critical care is to be a department, is it to be in competition with the conventional departments in hospitals and medical schools? Can we afford to set up our units in a maverick fashion so as to challenge the function of more traditional specialties? (p. 1)

In the late 1970s and early 1980s, to consolidate their claims as a multidisciplinary specialty, the leaders of critical care medicine attempted to establish a "conjoint board specialty" with a common certifying examination to be taken by candidates from the primary specialties of internal medicine, surgery, anesthesiology, and pediatrics. The effort failed, primarily for the reasons suggested by Shoemaker. However, some interpret this failure as evidence of the lack of legitimacy of critical care medicine's claims that it cuts across primary specialty lines (Kelley 1988).

By 1985, critical care medicine's orbit was finally fixed in the U.S. specialty system. Critical care, as a subspecialty of other primary specialties, had achieved satellite as opposed to planetary status. The model of a broad-based intensivist trained by a multidisciplinary faculty with a common certifying exam has not yet been achieved. One prominent spokesman for the profession bemoans this fate (Civetta 1992):

> I believe that one of the saddest developments of the past few years has been the fragmentation of this initial multi-disciplinary commitment. This

fragmentation has occurred not within the SCCM; rather, as the primary disciplines have tried to develop isolated critical care subsections, both the professional and personal advantages of the multidisciplinary iterations were lost that transcended all single disciplines of medicine and other allied health care professions. Our founding fathers were correct in recognizing that this multi-disciplinary characteristic was one of the strengths of the SCCM and we should foster that aim, especially in the face of the popularity of "separatism" today (p. 1714).

According to the SCCM (1992), a Qualified Critical Care Physician (QCCP) is "a physician who is board certified in a primary specialty and has successfully completed either an ACGME-approved training program in critical care and successfully passed the examination or is a board certified specialist who has special qualifications in critical care medicine" (p. vii).

To become certified in critical care, a physician must first become board-certified in one of four specialties: anesthesiology, internal medicine, pediatrics, or surgery. Next, the physician must complete a fellowship approved by the Accreditation Council for Graduate Medical Education (ACGME) in critical care medicine lasting from one to four years. Finally, the physician must pass one of four critical care certifying examinations offered by the American Board of Anesthesiology, American Board of Internal Medicine, and American Board of Pediatrics, or the American Board of Surgery. In 1994, the number of physicians certified in critical care was 7,290, up 53 percent from 1989 (SCCM 1995).

Critical care physicians may also receive training as part of the subspecialties of pulmonary and trauma surgery. For example, many medical ICUs will be oriented toward pulmonary subspecialists who have added qualification in critical care medicine. The American Thoracic Society, in an official policy statement (1995), recognizes the role of the "pulmonary and critical care medicine physician." The vast majority of pulmonary fellowship training programs have expanded from two to three years (after three years of internal medicine) to include the internal medicine aspects of critical care. In the surgical ICU arena, trauma surgeons may choose to take care of patients in the SICU because trauma admissions constitute some of the high-profile admissions and because critical care is a component of their training. However, many pulmonologists and trauma surgeons spend the majority of their time in the pulmonary office or in the trauma arena (prehospital, emergency room, operating room).

Other primary pathways by which a small number of physicians obtain formal training in critical care include a background in family practice, general surgery, emergency medicine, neurology, and nephrology followed by a fellowship in critical care medicine. In small community hospitals, the majority of patients with an acute illness are evaluated and managed by general internists, family practitioners, cardiologists, or general surgeons.

Providing Critical Care: Options for Hospitals

There are a variety of arrangements by which hospitals might engage physicians, many of whom are not QCCPs, to provide critical care. Examples include:

- rotating private practice surgeons who are on call in the trauma unit/ICU one to two months per year during which time they cut back on other responsibilities;
- hospital-based intensivist who has developed a call schedule with a private pulmonary medicine group;
- senior residents and fellows, particularly in academic medical center hospitals, who are assigned to the ICU rotation;
- moonlighting fellows;
- group of in-house intensivists who have a contract to run the ICU, much like physician groups who contract to run the emergency department;
- pulmonary medicine or multispecialty group on a rotational basis;
- in-house anesthesiologists who primarily cover the operating room but also provide backup for the ICU; and
- physician assistants or nurse practitioners, with telephone coordination by an intensivist or a senior physician.

Claims for Critical Care Medicine

Although the SCCM was blocked in its efforts to establish a conjoint board with a common examination, it has continued to press its claims for the scientific and medical validity of critical care medicine as a multidisciplinary specialty organized around the common physiological processes manifested by the critically ill patient (Weil, Shoemaker, and Rackow 1988).

In a 1993 policy statement, the SCCM defended the role of the qualified critical care physician (QCCP) or intensivist who:

> Assesses and responds to the complex, interactive features characteristic of critical illness or injury. Other specialists may care for patients with conditions that fall within a single organ system. The QCCP is prepared to care for seriously ill patients whose illness or conditions may disturb one or more organ systems resulting in physiologic instability (SCCM 1992, p. 5).

Interdependence, Uncertainty, and Conflict

The hallmark of a professional organization such as the hospital is professional autonomy, discretion, and certainty of action. Professionals apply their repertoire of skills and routines and oversee those of allied health personnel. The critical professional skill comes into play in deciding in what diagnostic categories to place the patient and then what set of therapeutic routines to apply to the patient. From a distance, the treatment process is composed of a stable set of diagnoses and interventions. But a closer look shows the set is in flux. There is a great deal of conflict over the shape and size of the diagnostic categories which Minzberg (1979) euphemistically calls "pigeonholes" and in whose jurisdictions they lie. Which critically ill patients are to be managed by which specialists? The contestants include the pulmonologist without critical care training, cardiologist, anesthesiologist, general surgeon, and internist. What is the role of the intensivist? The battle rages over numerous fronts including credentialing, reimbursement, and the organization of work into departments, sections, and units—all common flash points in ICU governance. The trend toward managed care will accentuate these conflicts, but, as will be explained, managed care will also bring resolution.

The fact is, given clinical uncertainty, the treatment of patients often requires interdependent action among a variety of clinicians. Strauss et al. (1985) conceptualize interdependency and uncertainty in terms of the "illness trajectory." The illness trajectory, as opposed to illness, refers "not only to the physiological unfolding of a patient's disease, but to the total organization of work done over that course, plus the impact of those involved with that work and its organization." Under this conception, it is more appropriate to think of managing the trajectory rather than managing the illness:

> ... under conditions of contemporary hospital practice, it's not always a simple matter to say who is in charge of managing the trajectory. In a routine case, the principal physician is primarily responsible for visualizing the trajectory: for ordering, evaluating, and acting on utilizing the ward's organizational machinery. When the course of illness becomes problematic, however, when things get out of hand, when other chronic illnesses impinge on the primary one—and even begin to take priority—then the trajectory management begins to get shared with other medical specialists. And ... these specialists may disagree or their orders may conflict, so that the problems of coordination can play havoc with house staff and, not incidentally, also with patient care. Lack of coordination amounts to a blurring of the division of labor, with untoward consequences then flowing from unclear or disagreed upon conceptions of responsibility ... An additional complication is that precedence in the trajectory management is directly affected by the existence of multiple illnesses.
>
> ... One feature of highly problematic trajectories, especially when there are several deeply interested parties or even trajectory managers, is what might be called *trajectory debates*, which involve not merely technical but also ideological

issues. As the trajectory (or trajectories) goes badly awry, many voices are heard, some soto voces, but some loud and clear, expressing different views on why the illness is out of hand, why the new symptoms or illness have appeared, and what lines of action ought to be taken, who ought to be brought into the act, and who pulled out, and so on (Strauss et al. 1985 p. 27–28).

The Doctor-Doctor and the Doctor-Patient Relationship

Intensivists can have three types of roles in patient care: primary, concurrent, and consultative (SCCM 1992b). The primary attending is the physician responsible for the period of hospitalization and may not be the patient's primary care physician. The intensivist could become the primary physician (or the attending of record) when the patient is admitted to the ICU and transferred to the critical care service composed of ICU-based intensivists. In this case, primary responsibility for patient care has been delegated to the ICU-based intensivist. When no such delegation has been made and when responsibilities are shared between the primary attending physician and the ICU-based intensivist, a concurrent relationship exists (e.g., the primary attending physician and the intensivist jointly develop a treatment plan which is coordinated by the intensivist). The relationship is considered consultative when the majority of care is provided by physicians other than those on the critical care service. The intensivist serves as a consultant. Of course, when no intensivist is involved, 100 percent of the care is provided by the primary attending physician, either alone or in consultation with non-ICU-based specialists.

Consultation traditionally implies that the consultant gives advice to the primary attending physician, who may or may not accept the advice. Traditionally, it is the primary attending who writes the orders. In practical application, however, complex decisions regarding major illnesses and operations are shared by, if not taken over by, subspecialists or surgeons who perform major procedures and/or critical care physicians. The consultant manages that one aspect of care (i.e., the pulmonologist writes orders for the ventilator, the infectious disease specialist writes orders for antibiotic therapy, the surgeon manages the drains and the wound, and the nephrologist writes orders for fluid balance and for dialysis). The main problem with the consultation approach, however, is that the primary physician may not recognize early enough that a complication is occurring, which can result in a delay before the consultant can respond and evaluate the situation.

Exhibit 2.7 is constructed from two questions on the SCCM survey: (1) All patients admitted to the critical care unit are transferred to the service of the ICU medical director or designee (yes or no?); and

(2) Medical orders for critical care patients may be written only by critical care unit staff (yes or no?). What is seen is that 74.3 percent of the respondents answered no to both questions; their unit policies are categorized as "open orders, remain on service of primary MD." These respondents are from ICUs in which the intensivists (if available) have consultative roles. The average number of attendings certified in critical care per unit is 2.2, ranging from 1.1 in units in hospitals with 100 beds or fewer to 2.9 in units in hospitals with 500 beds or more.

The number of hours per day that these physicians are available to provide coverage varies greatly among ICUs. In half of the ICUs, certified physicians are available six hours per day or less (Groeger et al. 1992). Two points should be made: (1) at the time of the survey, the certifying exams had been in existence for only six years; and (2) there are many physician intensivists who are not certified.

Respondents who answered yes to both questions represent the most restrictive type of unit, the closed unit where the intensivist becomes the primary physician. Only 11.3 percent of the units fall into this category. For patients that remain on the services of the non-ICU primary physician (the second and fourth columns in Ex-

Exhibit 2.7 Policy of Unit Operation

Unit Type	Closed Orders[1] Transferred to Unit Staff (%)	Open Orders[2] Remain on Service of Primary MD (%)	Open Orders Transferred to Unit Staff (%)	Closed Orders Remain on Service of Primary MD (%)
Medical	29.4	48.1	2.9	19.4
Medical/Surgical	2.8	85.8	1.4	9.9
Pediatric	12.1	71.9	6	9.7
Neonatal	47.6	32.2	10.2	9.3
CCU	7.4	77.5	1.5	13.3
Med/Surg/CCU	1.5	87.9	2.1	8.3
Neurology	5	78.3	6.6	10
Surgical	14.4	69.4	6	9.7
All units	11.3	74.3	10.6	3.6

*Closed vs. open units for order writing and whether patients remain on service of primary physician or are transferred to service of ICU medical director or designee.
[1] Closed orders—medical orders in ICU that can only be written by ICU staff
[2] Open orders—medical orders in ICU that can be written by any physician
Adapted from Groeger et al. 1992. "Descriptive Analysis of Critical Care in the United States." *Critical Care Medicine* 20 (6): 859.

hibit 2.7), the survey does not reveal whether the intensivist is occasionally involved as consultant or participates regularly in concurrent care.

As the data indicate, the transfer of primary responsibility to the intensivist is infrequent. However, in Europe, Australia, and New Zealand the closed unit is the norm. How has this been achieved? First, in these countries there is a traditional separation between hospital and office-based practice. General internists and family practitioners do not manage their hospital patients. Also, surgeons give intensivists primary responsibility. Second, in contrast to the United States, critical care medicine is recognized as an independent, primary specialty. Along with this recognition comes an independent power base that is reflected in the organization of the ICUs.

In the United States, the primary care physician (family physician or general internist) is expected to follow and manage or at least coordinate the care of his or her patient throughout the hospitalization. The general, vascular, and cardiothoracic surgeons are expected to follow and manage all aspects of care in the postoperative period. There are also several subspecialists who actively participate or consult in the ICU including cardiology, pulmonary, and nephrology. As was explained, critical care training is a substantial part of pulmonary fellowship training with particular emphasis on patients on mechanical ventilator support. Similarly, trauma surgeons undergo extensive critical care training during their fellowship years. Furthermore, a full-time intensivist is often competing with other attending physicians not only for the right to provide critical care but also for the reimbursements for the treatment of individual patients, especially the reimbursement for procedures. Finally, little third party reimbursement is available for their managerial duties not directly associated with patient care. It has been difficult politically and economically to maintain a full-time intensivist.

Constructing the Gates to the ICU

Every hospital has formal policies governing the ICU. Furthermore, the Joint Commission on Accreditation of Healthcare Organizations (JCAHO) in its *Accreditation Manual for Hospitals, 1994* (1993), mandates the presence of an ICU medical director:

> ... a physician member of the active medical staff who has received special training, acquired experience, and demonstrated competence in a specialty related to the care provided in the unit ... The director is responsible for making decisions, in consultation with the physician responsible for the patient, for the disposition of a patient when patient load exceeds optimal operational capacity (p. 206).

Also, the Society of Critical Care Medicine Task Force on Guidelines (1988) in its "Recommendations for ICU Admission and Discharge Criteria" assign managerial responsibilities concerning gatekeeping to the ICU director or designee.

> It is the responsibility of the patient's attending physician to request ICU admission and to promptly transfer patients who meet discharge criteria; it is the responsibility of the ICU director (or designee) to decide if the patient meets eligibility requirements for the ICU; in case of conflict regarding admission or discharge criteria, the ICU director (designee) will decide which patient should be given priority (p. 2).

Medical directors may be part time or full time, unpaid or paid as direct employees of the hospital, as members of a faculty practice plan, or under contract for providing management services to the ICU. The SCCM survey found that 51 percent of medical directors are unpaid for administrative duties, 61 percent are part time, and 56 percent do not bill for critical care services.

Describing the Gatekeeping Decision-Making Process: Centralization and Decentralization

Paterson (1969) provides a useful framework for understanding the five steps of the decision-making process involving ICU admission and discharge:

1. Information: What can be done.
2. Advice: What should be done.
3. Choice: What is intended to be done.
4. Authorization: What is authorized to be done.
5. Execution: What is in fact done.

To the extent that some of these steps are shared with or controlled by others, decision making is decentralized. It is most centralized when decision makers unilaterally control all the steps. They collect information on the potential admittee (e.g., go to the emergency room or recovery room to make on-the-scene judgments); analyze that information in relation to admission criteria or in comparison with information they have on the patients currently in the ICU or with other candidates for admission; make the choice to admit, not admit, or discharge; need no authorization; and execute the decisions themselves. Centralizing decision making shortens lines of communication and increases the ability to quickly process information and respond to a dynamic environment. These characteristics are exhibited in what Mintzberg calls the "simple structure" with a single, well-informed decision maker typical of the small, flexible, albeit autocratic, entrepreneurial firm (Mintzberg 1979).

Legitimately, however, in the complex task environment surrounding admission, discharge, and triage decisions, many participants are competitively enmeshed in all five stages of the decision process. These participants include hospital-based and private attending physicians who represent individual patients as well as different specialties and subspecialties; nursing, medical, and administrative managers of different rank and power; and, if in a teaching hospital, house staff of different rank and specialty. Frequently, the decision maker must depend on others for the collection of information. The interpretation of that information, which has perhaps been selectively filtered and reported, sets the premises—that is, what should be done for the actual choice (Mintzberg 1979). Rules are useful in structuring information collection, interpretation, and subsequent action.

Where there is only a part-time or weak medical presence, decision making is often delegated to the nurse who becomes the de facto medical director even if the physician is "only a phone call away." In this decentralized environment, the nurse, although an expert at formulating nursing diagnoses and determining how much nursing care and other resources would be required for an admitted patient, is a junior partner when formulating medical diagnoses and prognoses (although experienced ICU nurses may be quite competent at these tasks). The ICU medical director or triage officer is limited to authorizing (usually by phone) the decision of the nurse. While this situation may be stressful for the nurse, the maintenance of a decentralized decision-making process may be seen as advantageous to individual attending physicians seeking to maximize access for their patients.

To the extent that centralizing or closing the unit removes various participants from admissions decisions and empowers a single decision maker, dependence on information from outside the ICU's boundaries will be diminished, thus reducing the possibilities of information distortion and strategic misrepresentation. To the extent that closing the unit also involves controlling therapy, there will be greater flexibility in discharging as well as admitting patients. Of course, as a consequence of centralizing decision making, ICU staff and intensivists will face an increased workload and must become more involved at the bedside and in the emergency room, recovery room, and other units. This may be an option that smaller hospitals cannot afford.

An ever-present danger of the closed unit strategy is that it may lead to the balkanization of intensive care into one or more self-contained fiefdoms, impeding the sharing of resources and the flow of patients across the boundaries of different units. Subspecialty ICUs may be more prone to such a narrow focus as compared to general, broad-based ICUs.

At the ends of a continuum, the terms "open" and "closed" describe the increasing centralization of management functions as they relate to admission, treatment, and discharge decision making. Rie (1995) draws a stark contrast between the American open ICU, "where physicians are the marketing instruments for a hospital in bringing their patients to the hospital, caring for their patients, and then commandeering intensive care resources for the use by their patients without regard to the use by other patients," and the European closed unit, "where an intensive care team may function both as resource allocator and primary care giver and decision maker for the individual patient." However, in the United States a great deal of latitude exists between these two extremes.

Exhibit 2.8 describes three organizational arrangements: open unit, semi-closed unit, and closed unit. In the open unit, all qualified physicians, approved by the hospital credentials committee, may admit and care for their patients in the unit without the review or approval of the medical director. It should be pointed out that qualified physicians, although most likely board certified in some specialty, are not necessarily QCCPs. The director and/or associates consult on patients only when requested. Patients still must meet the criteria spelled out in the admissions policy. Generally, however, admission and discharge criteria are broadly defined, leaving a great deal of discretion to the attending physician. Thus, particularly in hospitals where private attending physicians have a great deal of influence, patients may be admitted with little difficulty as long as there is a bed available. Of course, under managed care, physicians may face pressures not to admit.

In an open unit, the types of illnesses, the degree of severity, and the reasons for admission tend to vary greatly. For example, consecutive admissions might include an elderly nursing home patient admitted through the ER in terminal multi-organ system failure with no advance directive or designated DNR status, followed by a patient from the regular floor whose physician is worried about lack of nursing coverage and believes that the ICU coverage will lessen his or her potential legal liability. Typically, in an open unit, physicians other than the intensivists are the primary providers of care for their patients. When beds are filled, the medical director or designee (i.e., triage officer) is responsible for triaging the beds.

In the closed unit, the director and/or associates are responsible for patient care. In general, full-time and paid medical directors are more likely to be found nearer to the closed side of the continuum (Groeger, Strosberg, Halpern et al. 1992). In the closed unit (see Exhibit 2.8),

Exhibit 2.8 Gatekeeping Arrangements for ICU Admission, Discharge, and Treatment

Unit Type	Admission	Treatment	Discharge
Open	All Qualified Attendings[1]	All Qualified Attendings[2]	All Qualified Attendings[1]
Semi-Closed	Medical Director and Associates Review and Approve	All Qualified Attendings[3]	Medical Director and Associates
Closed	Medical Director and Associates Review and Approve	Medical Director and Associates Assume Primary Responsibility for Patient Care	Medical Director and Associates

[1] Except in triage situations when medical director or triage officer makes decision
[2] Medical Director and/or associates consult upon request
[3] Medical Director and/or associates may consult on all patients, consult upon request, or work concurrently with primary physician

Based on I. A. Fein, M. A. Strosberg, S. L. Fein. 1993. "Organization of Critical Care Units." In *Principles and Practices of Medical Intensive Care*, edited by R. W. Carlson and M. A. Gehab. Philadelphia, PA: W. B. Saunders Co.

patients are transferred upon admission to the service of an intensivist for direct patient care. Instead of coming in from their offices or the operating room for relatively short periods of time, these intensivists are physically present in the ICU and therefore are better able to monitor and direct treatment. Typically, this type of closed unit arrangement requires the services of several full-time intensivists who may be employees of the hospital, members of a faculty plan, or part of a group that contracts its services to the hospital. This type of arrangement facilitates a greater degree of collaboration between doctors and nurses (Carson et al. 1996). Ideally, patient care is given by a team led by an ICU-based intensivist including the nurses and other ICU staff, and the attending physician of the patient. Exhibit 2.9 presents the advantages and disadvantages of the three kinds of arrangements.

Gatekeeping arrangements, even when formalized by written policies, must be viewed as part of the overall negotiated order of the hospital. According to Strauss et al. (1963), a negotiated order is a set of understandings, agreements, and informal contracts among various professionals and nonprofessionals. In contrast to written rules backed by formal sanction (the traditional notion of the hierarchy), unwritten

Exhibit 2.9 ICU Structure Advantages and Disadvantages

	Open Unit	Semi-Closed Unit	Closed Unit
Advantages	Invites active participation of medical staff; medical director may be full-time or volunteer. Better long-term continuity of care.	Improved control of patient flow and bed availability. Improved accountability for quality assessment, risk management, and cost containment. Staff participation facilities collaborative practice between physicians and nurses.	Absolute control and accountability for beds and patient flow, quality assessment, risk management, and cost containment. Easiest situation to create collaborative practice between physicians and nurses.
Disadvantages	Patient thru-put and bed availability may be difficult to maintain. Accountability for quality assessment, risk management, and cost containment may be difficult. May be difficult to implement collaborative practice.	Requires 24-hour availability of medical director or designee.	Requires 24-hour availability of medical director or designee. May alienate medical staff if not properly managed. May be harder to get patient admitted quickly. May diminish coordination with other levels of care and continuity of care.

Based on I. A. Fein, M. A. Strosberg, S. L. Fein, 1993. "Organization of Critical Care Units." In Principles and Practices of Medical Intensive Care, R. W. Carlson and M. A. Gehab (eds.) Philadelphia, PA: W. B. Saunders Co.

understandings, sometimes implicit and arrived at through negotiation and renegotiation, govern relationships in the hospital. As an example of the negotiated order, consider the variety of tactics that can be used in controlling not only admission of patients to the unit but also in countering the influence of other physicians. Start with written admission policies that might include the following proviso: The surgical intensive care unit will serve surgical patients who require preoperative insertion of invasive monitoring devices for preoperative monitoring. These admissions are subject to space availability and can be canceled if a critically ill patient must be admitted.

This policy does not give the ICU director or designee control over admissions or control over who can perform what procedures. But the ability to make beds available does engender bargaining as the following conversation illustrates:

> **Surgeon**: "Do you have any beds available?"
> **ICU physician**: "I don't know, I'll see. By the way, if I do, do you want me to manage the ventilator and the lines postoperatively?"

One issue is, of course, who will manage the monitoring catheters (lines) and the ventilator—the ICU-based intensivists, or other credentialed specialists, such as the cardiologists or pulmonologists? Subtle pressure is placed on the surgeon to tip the balance in favor of the ICU physicians. Of course, ICU physicians can legitimately argue that if they are being asked to provide the beds, they should be able to influence patient care.

The Medical Director as Manager: Working Versus Paper Medical Directors

Fein and Spanier (1991) outline various models of medical director involvement in unit management:

1. Open unit with no physician director ("paper director" only).
2. Open unit with a part-time physician director.
   A. Non-salaried volunteer staff physician as director.
   B. Paid part-time staff physician director.
3. Open unit with a full-time physician director and open medical staff.
4. Open unit with a full-time physician director and full-time medical staff.
5. Semi-closed unit with full-time physician director and full-time medical staff.
6. Closed unit with a full-time physician director and full-time medical staff. (p. 1974)

Full-time medical staff in models 4, 5, and 6 above may be: (a) direct employees of the hospital; (b) employees of a corporation that contracts with the hospital for management of the critical care unit(s); or (c) members of a faculty practice plan.

Formal policies and the designation of open and closed units present an incomplete picture of the structure of the ICU gates and the role of medical directors. The descriptors "working" and "paper" medical directors show that medical directors can exercise or fail to exercise leadership in a variety of structures along the continuum from open to closed units (Adler 1984). Working directors take an active part in ICU operations, including quality assurance, education, policy development and enforcement, triage, and bed allocation. Regardless of employment status, paper directors may delegate important management functions to the nurse director and/or house staff.

Hospital Bed Size and Medical Director Functioning

A 1988 survey of ICU nursing supervisors showed that a surprising 21 percent did not perceive there to be any medical director, even though the JCAHO clearly requires one (Strosberg et al. 1990). This same survey showed that over 30 percent of ICU nursing supervisors perceived a lack of availability of the medical director or attending level designee to make admission/discharge/transfer decisions and resolve conflict at night. These findings, which hold for both teaching and non-teaching hospitals, suggest that many ICUs lack physician leadership in ICU management and resource allocation even in units with supposedly full-time directors. When there is a leadership vacuum in the medical directorship, this responsibility by default falls to the nursing staff or the house staff.

Groeger et al. (1992), in their 1991 national SCCM study, confirmed the findings of the 1988 survey. Approximately 80 percent of the respondents from adult ICUs reported being supervised by a medical director and only 50 percent reported that a medical director or unit attending physician (not nursing or house staff) was available at night to resolve conflicts involving admissions, discharges, and transfers. These findings hold across all sizes of hospitals. If one uses "medical director supervision" and "availability at night to resolve conflict" as proxies for a working medical director, then a considerable number of ICUs are headed by paper medical directors.

Admittedly, in the smaller hospitals with lower occupancy rates and low case-mix severity there may be little need for a senior-level physician to be available at night to resolve conflict concerning admissions, treatment, and discharges. But in the larger hospitals, or in hospitals with high occupancy rates, this default position may have implications for access, fairness, and quality (Mallick et al. 1995). All hospitals must recognize the implications for efficiency.

Drawing on data from the study of nine ICUs (five teaching and four non-teaching hospitals), Zimmerman et al. (1993) noted that one of the greatest challenges facing ICUs was coordinating admission, discharges, and triage. They identified a number of practices that facilitated these processes:

> Admission and discharge policies were most useful when they conformed to published guidelines that emphasize both the need and priority for ICU care. Charge nurse or residents were effective for routine control, but a physician (usually the ICU medical director) was needed for enforcement and to resolve conflict. Patient triage was most effective in units with good physician-nurse collaboration and where throughput was also facilitated by early physician control, and by minimizing guesswork in admission planning (p. 1448).

The researchers also identified some of the problems in coordinating patient triage faced by some of the lower performing ICUs:

> These problems included the lack of clear criteria and priorities for admission and discharge, decision-making by physicians with no knowledge of unit status, and an over reliance on nurses to deal with triage pressures in the absence of clear policies or support. Charge nurses often had responsibilities that greatly exceeded their authority and were frequently diverted from patients by multiple phone calls about triage. A charge nurse in one unit felt that admission was ultimately determined by "who yelled the loudest" (p. 1448).

In Chapter 3 we will examine in detail the organizational dynamics shaping ICU gatekeeping, impeding the implementation of admission and discharge policies, and leading to a situation where those who yell loudest have a say in decision making. We conclude this chapter with a discussion of severity-of-illness models.

Prognosis and Severity: A Primer

Upon admission to the ICU, the acutely ill, unstable patient receives resuscitation, assessment, and treatment. Concurrently, physicians develop a working differential diagnosis and initiate diagnostic testing. Shortly after these efforts are started, they formulate the patient's prognosis. The patient and the patient's family want to know the diagnosis, the treatment options, and the chances of survival.

The field of prognostication has grown rapidly in the past 15 years with the use of computers and advanced statistical techniques. Although an experienced physician augmented by the assessment of consultants and a medical literature review can provide an accurate prognosis, ICU severity models bring a greater level of objectivity to the process because they are based on large patient databases.

The field of ICU prognostication started with a simple scoring system ranging from zero to four points, based on deviation from normal physiological states during the first 24 hours following ICU admission. As an example, if the serum potassium value was abnormally high, then a certain number of points would be added. The sum of the points at the end of 24 hours constituted the Acute Physiology Score, which was the basis of the original APACHE system as well as the pediatric score, Physiology Stability Index (PSI), and a French version called the Simplified Acute Physiology Score (SAPS). It was shown that the higher the score, the more unstable the patient and, therefore, the higher the likelihood of hospital mortality. This approach captured the imagination of clinical researchers and physicians in the ICU arena and created enthusiasm and energy for expanding the field. These physiology-based scores have been widely applied for clinical studies as well as for a general measure for severity of illness.

However, it soon became evident that not all variables contributed equally to a hospital mortality outcome. For example, it was shown that coma contributed much more toward severity and hospital mortality than did an elevation of the heart rate (Teres, Brown, and Lemeshow 1982). It was also clear that a score collected at a different time interval would have a different meaning than one based on the first 24 hours following ICU admission (e.g., for the same score, the probability of dying would be greater if taken later in the ICU stay). Also, the significance of a score varied among different categories of patients; a cardiac surgery patient would have a very high physiology score postoperatively but a low probability of mortality. This type of surgery causes a lot of physiological unstability, but the patient generally does well. Families and medical teams want to know the patient's probability of surviving or probability of dying, rather than just a physiology score.

A major shift then occurred toward developing techniques for providing a probability of hospital mortality. With the addition of the primary precipitating factor (i.e., the reason that brought the patient into the ICU), and a chronic health evaluation, it was then possible to convert the physiology score to a probability of hospital mortality. Likewise, it was possible to convert the pediatric physiology score to a probability of hospital mortality, called Pediatric Risk of Mortality (PRISM) Score. The same was true with the European version, now called SAPS II. In addition, an alternative approach called the Mortality Probability Model (MPM) was developed. Instead of using a numerical score derived from laboratory tests and vital sign measurements (temperature, heart rate, blood pressure, respiratory rate), this approach requires adding up the number of important risk factors present. In addition to a probability at 24 hours, the MPM approach also provides a probability available directly at ICU presentation as well as at 48 and 72 hours. MPM is the only system that can generate a probability of mortality at ICU presentation (Lemeshow et al. 1993).

The cardiac surgery models use the same type of approach as the MPM. Large databases that provide a risk assessment prior to the start of cardiac surgery are now available. Such models are being used for comparing the quality of performance of one cardiac surgery unit to another. For example, the comparative "report cards" on cardiac surgery mandated by the New York Department of Health have been published and critiqued in the medical literature and the media (Hannan et al. 1994). Other models include trauma scores, which incorporate physiology plus degree of anatomic injury caused by the precipitating trauma. Trauma scores are collected for trauma registries but have not been developed as an adjunct to clinical decision making.

Applications

The main application of the general ICU severity models has been for aggregate or group analysis. By knowing the average expected probability of a large consecutive group of ICU patients, it is possible to measure the observed outcome of these patients. The ratio of the observed-to-expected mortality forms the basis of a quality performance measurement and can be used to compare one ICU to another or one ICU to itself over time. It should be noted that the MPM II and SAPS II are available in the public domain and can be adapted for utilization review and clinical research studies.

The model-building field is advancing in three different directions. The first direction has to do with special models, such as the cardiac surgery example, based on a large number of patients undergoing a common procedure (Higgins et al. 1992). For clinical trials that involve ICU patients, particularly for those with severe infection, it is important to have a highly accurate model so that placebo control and treated patients can be compared. This is a more difficult process than one would imagine since many hospitals are involved in these multi-hospital trials and have varying admission criteria and different case mixes. For example, a great deal of interest has been expressed in biotechnology agents such as monoclonal antibodies for patients with severe sepsis. Accurate models are required. The general ICU severity models (APACHE III, MPM II, SAPS II) are not accurate enough to meet the high standards of the Food and Drug Administration for this subgroup of patients. Specialized sepsis models—the APACHE, MPM, and SAPS sepsis models—have developed as valid methods for testing new agents and are a major component of current clinical trials (American College of Chest Physicians et al. 1997).

The second direction has to do with the availability of probabilities over time. It is one thing to have an estimated probability for a large number of patients at or near admission to an ICU. It is another to say how the probability is changing over the first two or three days or even out to one week. The APACHE III can generate probabilities of hospital mortality for out to one week. MPM II goes out to 72 hours. Neither system has been independently validated for these later times. However, it is now possible to project a trajectory of an individual patient's trend over time. For example, a patient is admitted with a critical illness and a 40 percent chance of dying. The next day the probability of dying is 60 percent and four days later it is 80 percent. Could this approach mean that probability models can be used for individual patients? To begin with, remember that if an individual patient's prognosis is a 45 percent likelihood of dying, this means that out of 100 similar patients, 45 of these patients would die and 55 would live. The model cannot predict if this individual patient will be among those who live or those who die. Also, the probability only tells you the patient's prognosis at the moment, not necessarily what it will be in the future. However, with probability over time, much more information is available to project into the future and to serve as an adjunct to an experienced clinical decision maker, but the same limitation holds. In addition, the probabilities calculated well outside the 24-hour window still need rigorous testing and independent validation. The probability should also be presented with a confidence or probability interval to show the range of accuracy.

Finally, with the increasing availability of larger databases, it is now possible to look at additional end points rather than just hospital mortality. Although the patient's family wants to know about mortality, it is often not the end point that is most important to decision making. A patient may survive a massive stroke but be left severely disabled. Patients and families may not want to pursue an aggressive hospital course if the most likely outcome is a very poor functional state.

With individual patient application on the horizon, a possibility exists that ICU severity models could serve as adjuncts to clinical decision making for a wide variety of purposes, including the initial evaluation of whether a patient should be admitted to an ICU. Although models are based on patients who were admitted to the ICU (patients who were denied ICU admission were not included in these studies) potential exists to determine what groups of patients generally should or should not be admitted to an ICU. For the present time, the most obvious approach to the in-flow of patients would be the early discharge of a high-risk monitor patient who has done well from elective surgery or an emergency admission who has improved. If a patient has a low physiology score after 24 hours or 48 hours of admission, a low probability estimation of mortality, and a low therapeutic measure in terms of nursing resources (e.g., the score on the Therapeutic Intervention Scoring System [TISS]) (Cullen et al. 1974), he or she should be a candidate for early discharge.

Partly based on these types of analyses, it is now much more common in high-volume ICUs for high-risk elective patients to be monitored in a post-anesthesia care unit or a surgical step-down or intermediate bed/rather than in the ICU. Included in this group are patients having peripheral vascular surgery, carotid artery surgery, well-defined elective neurosurgery, and partial lung resection or lobectomy (assuming that the patients do not have severe underlying chronic heart or lung disease). A moderate proportion of all these patients now can be cared for safely outside of the ICU environment; if these patients are admitted, it should be for a short time period or based on significant underlying co-morbid conditions or for complications that occurred during surgery.

Regarding the outflow of patients from the ICU, there are several groups of patients for which ICU severity modeling may also provide an adjunct to clinical decision making and has stimulated the development of a new type of model to measure organ failure or organ dysfunction. If a patient has an acute critical illness with multi-organ involvement the patient may be projected to spend a long time in the ICU. If the patient starts showing steady organ system improvement and has a stable physiology except for the necessity of mechanical ventilation, it could be argued that a lower cost option should be found for this patient. The patient may be a candidate for a respiratory step-down or chronic ventilator unit. On the other hand, if a patient has multiple problems following an acute illness with the development of multi-organ dysfunction, the patient will have a steady rise in daily probability of mortality. If the multi-organ dysfunction progresses to multi-organ failure, the patient's chances of survival become much reduced. How much effort and resources should be expended toward an individual patient who has a very marginal chance for a meaningful recovery? Is it possible to utilize an ICU severity model as a clinical adjunct for determining end-of-life decisions? This usage is being discussed and even advocated as a cost-containment measure. We will return to this discussion in Chapters 5 and 6.

References

Adler, D. C. 1984. "Hospital Management of Critical Care." In *Major Issues in Critical Care Medicine*, edited by J. E. Parrillo and S. N. Ayres, 265–70. Baltimore: Williams and Wilkins.

American College of Chest Physicians, National Institute of Allergy and Infectious Disease, and National Heart, Lung, and Blood Institute Workshop. 1997. "From the Bench to the Bedside: The Future of Sepsis Research." *Chest* 111 (3): 744–53.

American Thoracic Society. 1995. "Role of the Pulmonary and Critical Care Medicine Physician in the American Health Care System." *American Journal of Respiratory and Critical Care Medicine* 152 (3): 2199–2201.

Berenson, R. A. 1984. *Health Technology Care Study 28: Intensive Care Units (ICUs): Clinical Outcomes, Costs and Decisionmaking*. Washington, D.C.: Office of Technology Assessment.

Borlase, B. C., J. T. Baxter, P. N. Benotti, et al. 1990. "Surgical Intensive Care Unit Resource Use in a Specialty Referral Hospital." *Surgery* 109 (6): 687–93.

Carson, S. S., C. Stocking, T. Podsadecki, and J. Christenson. 1996. "Effects of Organizational Change in the Medical Intensive Care Unit of a Teaching Hospital: A Comparison of Open and Closed Formats." *Journal of the American Medical Association* 276 (4): 322–28.

Chalfin, D. B., I. L. Cohen, and J. Lambrinos. 1995. "The Economics and Cost-Effectiveness of Critical Care Medicine." *Intensive Care Medicine* 21 (11): 952–61.

Chase, R. A. 1976. "Proliferation of Certification in Medical Specialties: Productive or Counterproductive." *New England Journal of Medicine* 294 (9): 498.

Civetta, J. M. 1992. "Critical Care: How Should We Evaluate Our Progress?" *Critical Care Medicine* 20 (12): 1714–20.

Cohen, I. L., and F. V. McL. Booth. 1994. "Cost Containment and Mechanical Ventilation in the United States." *New Horizons* 2 (3): 283–90.

Cohen, I. L., J. Lambrinos, and I. A. Fein. 1993. "Mechanical Ventilation for Elderly Patients in Intensive Care: Incremental Charges and Benefits." *Journal of the American Medical Association* 269 (8): 1025–29.

Cohen, I. L., M. Fitzpatrick, and F. V. McL. Booth. 1996. "Critical Care Medicine: Opportunity and Strategies for Improvement." *Journal of Quality Improvement* 22 (2): 85–103.

Cullen, D. J., J. M. Civetta, B. A. Briggs, and L. C. Ferrara. 1974. "Therapeutic Intervention Scoring System: A Method for Quantitative Comparisons of Patient Care." *Critical Care Medicine* 2 (2): 57–60.

Davis, H., S. S. Lefrak, D. Miller, and S. Malt. 1980. "Prolonged Mechanically Assisted Ventilation: An Analysis of Outcomes and Charges." *Journal of the American Medical Association* 243 (1): 43–45.

Detsky, A. S., S. C. Stricker, A. G. Mulley, and G. E. Thibault. 1981. "Prognosis, Survival and the Expenditure for Patients in an Intensive Care Unit." *New England Journal of Medicine* 305 (12): 667–72.

Esserman, L., J. Belkora, and L. Lenert. 1995. "Potentially Ineffective Care: A New Outcome to Assess the Limits of Critical Care." *Journal of the American Medical Association* 274 (19): 1544–51.

Fein, I. A., E. Cole, and S. Socaris. 1991. "Assessing Resource Utilization in a Surgical Critical Care Unit." *Chest* 100 (Abstract): 805.

Fein, I. A., A. H. Spanier, et al. 1991. "Organization and Management of Critical Care Units." In *Intensive Care Medicine*, edited by J. M. Rippe, R. S. Irwin, J. S. Alpert, and M. P. Fink, 1970–1977. Boston: Little, Brown, and Company.

Groeger, J .S., K. K. Guntupalli, M. A. Strosberg, N. Halpern, R. C. Raphael, F. Cerra, and W. Kaye. 1993. "Descriptive Analysis of Critical Care Units in the United States: Patient Characteristics and Intensive Care Unit Utilization." *Critical Care Medicine* 21 (2): 279–91.

Groeger, J. S., M. A. Strosberg, N. S. Halpern, R. C. Raphael, W. Kaye, K. K. Guntupalli, D. L. Bertman, D. Greenbaum, T. P. Clemmer, T. J. Gallagher, L. D. Nelson, A. E. Thompson, F. B. Cerra, and W. R. Davis. 1992. "Descriptive Analysis of Critical Care Units in the United States." *Critical Care Medicine* 20 (6): 846–63.

Hannon, E. L., H. Kilburn, M. Racz, E. Shields, and M. R. Chassin. 1994. "Improving the Outcomes of Coronary Artery Bypass Surgery in New York State." *Journal of the American Medical Association* 271 (10): 761–66.

Higgins, T. L., F. G. Estafanous, F. D. Loop, G. J. Beck, J. M. Blum, and L. Paranandi. 1992. "Stratification of Morbidity and Mortality Outcome by Preoperative Risk Factors in Coronary Artery Bypass Patients: A Clinical Severity Score." *Journal of the American Medical Association* 267 (17): 2344–48.

Joint Commission on Accreditation of Healthcare Organizations. 1993. *Accreditation Manual for Hospitals, 1994.* Oakbrook Terrace, IL: The Commission.

Kelley, M. 1988. "Critical Care Medicine—A New Specialty?" *New England Journal of Medicine* 318 (21): 1613.

Lambrinos, J., and P. J. Papadakos. 1987. "An Introduction to the Analysis of Risks, Costs, and Benefits in Critical Care." In *Managing the Critical Care Unit*, edited by I. A. Fein and M. A. Strosberg, 358–370. Rockville, MD: Aspen Publishers.

Lemeshow, D., D. Teres, J. Klar., and J. S. Avrunin. 1993. "Mortality Probability Models (MPM II): Based on an International Cohort of Intensive Care Unit Patients." *Journal of the American Medical Association* 270 (20): 2478–86.

Mallick, R., M. A. Strosberg, J. Lambrinos, and J. Groeger. 1995. "The ICU Medical Director as Manager: Impact on Performance." *Medical Care* 33 (6): 611–24.

Miccolo, M. A., and A. H. Spanier. 1993. "Critical Care Management in the 1990s: Making Collaborative Practice Work." *Critical Care Clinics* 9 (3): 443–53.

Mintzberg, H. 1979. *The Structuring of Organizations.* Englewood Cliffs, NJ: Prentice-Hall.

Myers, L. P., S. A. Schroeder, S. A. Chapman, and J. Leong. 1984. "What's So Special About Special Care?" *Inquiry* 21 (Summer): 113–27.

National Institutes of Health. 1983. *Consensus Development Conference on Critical Care Medicine: Summary.* Bethesda, MD: U.S. Public Health Service, National Institutes of Health.

O'Brien, D., and J. Rushby. 1990. "Outcome Assessment in Cardiovascular Cost-Benefit Studies." *American Heart Journal* 119 (3.2): 740–48.

Oye, R. K., and P. E. Bellamy. 1996. "Patterns of Resource Consumption in Medical Intensive Care." *Chest* 99 (3): 685–89.

Paterson, T. 1969. *Management Theory.* London: Business Publications Limited.

Rapoport, J., D. Teres, and S. Lemeshow. 1990. "Explaining Variability of Cost Using Severity of Illness Measure for ICU Patients." *Medical Care* 28 (4): 338–48.

Rapoport, J., D. Teres, S. Lemeshow, and S. Gehlbach. 1994. "A Method for Assessing the Clinical Performance and Cost Effectiveness of Intensive Care Units: A Multicenter Inception Cohort Study." *Critical Care Medicine* 22 (9): 1385–91.

Rie, M. A. 1995. "Ethical Issues in Intensive Care: Criteria for Treatment within the Creation of a Health Insurance Morality." In *Critical Choices and Critical Care*, edited by K. W. Wildes, 23–56. Dordrecht, The Netherlands: Kluwer Academic Publishers.

Robey, D. 1982. *Designing Organizations.* Homewood, IL: Richard D. Irwin.

Russell, L. 1979. *Technology in Hospitals: Medical Advances and Their Diffusion.* Washington, D.C.: The Brookings Institution.

Safar, P. 1984. "The Critical Care Medicine Continuum, from Scene to Outcome." In *Major Issues in Critical Care Medicine*, edited by J. E. Parrillo and S. N. Syres, 71–84. Baltimore, MD: Williams and Wilkins.

Shoemaker, W. C. 1975. "Interdisciplinary Medicine: Accommodation or Integration?" *Critical Care Medicine* 3 (1): 1–4.

Snyder, J. V., C. A. Sirio, D. C. Angus, M. T. Hravnak, S. N. Kobert, E. H. Sinz, and E. B. Rudy. 1994. "Trial of Nurse Practitioners in Intensive Care." *New Horizons* 2 (3): 296–304.

Society of Critical Care Medicine. 1992. *Critical Care in the United States: Coordinating Intensive Care Resources for Positive and Cost-Efficient Patient Outcomes.* Anaheim, CA: SCCM.

Society of Critical Care Medicine Coalition of Critical Care Excellence. 1995. *ICU Cost Reduction: Practical Suggestions and Future Considerations.* Anaheim, CA: SCCM.

Society of Critical Care Medicine Task Force on Guidelines. 1988. "Recommendations for Intensive Care Unit Admission and Discharge Criteria." *Critical Care Medicine* 16 (8): 807–08.

Strauss, A., L. Schatzman, and D. Ehrlich. 1963. "The Hospital and its Negotiated Order." In *The Hospital in Modern Society*, edited by E. Freidson, 147–169. New York: Free Press of Glencoe.

Strauss, A., S. Fagerhaugh, B. Suczek, and C. Weiner. 1985. *Social Organization of Medical Work.* Chicago: University of Chicago Press.

Strosberg, M. A., D. Teres, I. A. Fein, and R. Linsider. 1990. "Nursing Perception of the Availability of the Intensive Care Unit Medical Director for Triage and Conflict Resolution." *Heart and Lung* 19 (5): 452–55.

Teres, D., R. Brown, and S. Lemeshow. 1982. "Predicting Mortality of Intensive Care Unit Patients: The Importance of Coma." *Critical Care Medicine* 10 (2): 86–95.

Wagner, D. P. 1989. "Economics of Prolonged Mechanical Ventilation." *American Review of Respiratory Disease* 140 (2.2): 514–18.

Wagner, D. P., T. D. Wineland, and W. A. Knaus. 1983. "The Hidden Costs of Treating Severely Ill Patients: Charges and Resource Consumption in an Intensive Care Unit." *Health Care Financing Review* 5 (1): 81–86.

Walleck, C. A. 1994. "Nursing and Labor Cost Reduction." *New Horizons* 2 (3): 291–95.

Weil, M. H., W. C. Shoemaker, and E. C. Rackow. 1988. "Competent and Continuing Care of the Critically Ill." *Critical Care Medicine* 16 (3): 298.

Zimmerman, J. E., S. M. Shortell, D. M. Rousseau, J. Duffy, R. R. Gillies, W. A. Knaus, K. Devers, D. P. Wagner, and E. A. Draper. 1993. "Improving Intensive Care: Observations Based on Organizational Case Studies in Nine Intensive Care Units: A Prospective, Multicenter Study." *Critical Care Medicine* 21 (10): 1443–51.

Zimmerman, J. E., D. P. Wagner, W. A. Knaus, J. F. Williams, D. Kolakowski, and E. A. Draper. 1995. "The Use of Risk Predictions to Identify Candidates for Intermediate Care Units." *Chest* 108 (2): 490–99.

CHAPTER 3

GATEKEEPING: DECISION MAKERS AND DECISION MAKING

PARTICIPANTS IN ICU admission, discharge, and triage decision making bring different perspectives based on their backgrounds, professional socialization, and the positions they hold in the hospital. This chapter introduces four important organizational decision makers—the attending physician, the triage officer, the ICU nurse manager, and the hospital administrator—and describes the conditions they typically face.

In subsequent sections, we analyze managerial roles of ICU staff, the application of decision criteria to admission and discharge of ICU patients, and the organizational dynamics shaping the application.

Four Important Decision Makers

The Attending Physician

The attending (admitting) physician's primary focus is his or her individual patient. Typically, the attending physician's relationship with the patient is long-term as opposed to the ICU staff, who interact with the patient only during the duration of the ICU stay. The doctor-patient relationship, according to Hippocratic tradition, transcends other institutional concerns. The physician's role is to diagnose and make treatment decisions based on risk-benefit analysis. This ability is unique to the physician. Administrators and nurses, because of their lack of certified expertise, do not have a legitimate basis for making these decisions.

The usual method of physician reimbursement is fee-for-service. One advantage of fee-for-service is that the reward is closely linked to output of services. Economists have noted that one disadvantage of fee-for-service compensation is that it provides incentives for overservicing the patient.

Increasingly, physicians are participating in managed care arrangements, which may include capitated payment (i.e., physicians share some financial risk for the costs of services that exceed a fixed budget amount). One criticism of capitation is that it may produce incentives for underservicing the patient and place the physician in a conflict of interest.

The Triage Officer

The triage officer is typically the designee of the ICU medical director. The JCAHO mandates that there be an ICU medical director responsible for implementing policies on admissions and discharges. Furthermore, according to the SCCM (1988):

> It is the responsibility of the ICU director (or designee) to decide if the patient meets eligibility requirements for the ICU. In cases of conflict regarding admission or discharge criteria, the ICU director (designee) will decide which patient should be given priority (p. 2).

Physicians are asked to fill a number of roles: clinician, teacher, researcher. Most also serve on committees of the organized medical staff. However, the managerial role of triage officer, with the responsibility to decide which patient should be given priority, moves well beyond the traditional doctor-patient relationship, even though it is often filled concurrently with other roles. There are a variety of ways in which the physician may be engaged in the triage role ranging from a full-time salaried intensivist to a part-time attending physician serving voluntarily as triage officer on a rotating basis.

The ICU Nurse Manager

The ICU nurse manager, next to the administrator, has the broadest institutional perspective. The nurse manager makes resource allocation decisions in a complex and often dynamic environment. Chief among managerial responsibilities is the staffing function, making sure that appropriate nurse-patient ratios are maintained. The JCAHO manual (1990) states that "a sufficient number of permanently assigned qualified registered nurses shall be on duty within the unit at all times when patients are in the unit." (p. 253)

Working within the constraints of the personnel budget, the nurse manager must balance the necessity of "stretching" nursing coverage to meet the increasing demand for ICU services against the need to maintain minimum levels of quality. The nurse manager must be cognizant of the relationship between stretched nursing staff and the increased propensity for personnel turnover, which may lead to the closing of beds. Some common stressors include: excessive workload, high patient-nurse ratios, little time to deal with patients' or families' emotional needs, dealing with the futile prolongation of life, unpredictable schedules, and administrative conflicts (Gonzales and Stern 1991).

One common theme arising from the impact of managed care on hospitals is the replacement of highly trained nurses and respiratory therapists with less-skilled workers. As ICUs begin to change their ratio of nurses to patients from 1:2 to 1:3, other personnel are substituted such as cross-trained nursing assistants. Agency nurses are also more frequently used. Similarly, changes on the regular floors of the hospital have increased pressure to transfer patients to the ICU, thus increasing the necessity to triage.

The Hospital Administrator

The administrator has the broadest institutional perspective of all decision makers. He or she must be sensitive to the external forces buffeting the hospital. From a strategic perspective, the administration desires to maintain and enhance its competitive position by remaining responsive to physicians. (The administrator is also interested in appearing responsive to the community and protecting the public image of the institution.) But administration is also facing cost-containment pressures building up from managed care plans and payors. Budgets are becoming tighter, including the one for nursing services. The challenge to administration and governance is to utilize resources more efficiently while at the same time remaining attractive to physicians who will be demanding more critical care services for their patients. Many of these physicians, who are competitors among themselves, have the option of sending their patients to competing hospitals if not satisfied. The challenge cuts to the core of many issues involving the organization of a critical care service (e.g., granting privileges, credentialing, operating an open versus a closed unit, establishing dedicated special care units, employing full-time intensivists).

Typically, an administrator does not get involved in routine admission and discharge decisions. Only in extraordinary circumstances will an administrator directly participate. Nevertheless, other decision makers are usually aware of the interests of administration.

Exhibit 1.1 summarizes these perspectives for three of the four decision makers discussed above: hospital administrator, nurse, and attending physician. While administrators and nurses have clearly delineated roles within the organization and its hierarchy, the relation of the physician to the organization is more complex. Most physicians are not part of the formal hierarchy of the hospital. They are, according to Blair and Fottler (1990), "interface stakeholders" who function both internally and externally to the organization. They are powerful because they admit patients, control patient care processes and use of resources, and provide services. They value clinical quality, patient access, support services, physician autonomy, and medical training. It is management's job to manage this interface stakeholder in terms of these values, in other words, to offer sufficient inducements so that physicians continue to make appropriate contributions (e.g., admit patients) to the hospital (Blair and Fottler 1990). In a managed care environment, the added challenge is to expand the definition of appropriate to include the cost-effective use of resources.

The Triage Officer: In Context

What can be done to improve the capacity of the organization to collect, process, and share information? In pursuing the answer, we adopt Galbraith's (1977) "information processing" approach to organization design. Improving the organization's ability to cope with uncertainty is an important aspect of organizational design. Decision makers are needed who are able to quickly collect and evaluate complex physiological and organizational information. These decision makers must be authoritative about staffing, patient case load, and have working relationships with ER, PACU, and other units in the hospital. They must be an important part of the negotiated order of the ICU. Exhibit 3.1 lists the elements of the triage officer role as well as the requirements for communication.

Organizationally, the triage officer must be an integral part of a rich communications network designed to process difficult-to-interpret information from diverse sources. To cope with the uncertainty of the triage decision, the triage officer requires online information sharing and scenario building with nursing staff. It is the triage officer's responsibility to integrate that information.

In Exhibit 3.2, Dawson (1993) outlines the daily responsibilities of the triage officer. Below we describe the factors that impede the carrying out of these responsibilities.

The organized medical staff and its standing committees, a standard fixture in American hospitals, occupies a central place in the governance of the hospital. Symbolically, committee policies have legitimacy because representation, voting, appeals mechanisms, written rules, official

Exhibit 3.1   THE TRIAGE OFFICER: OFFICIAL ROLE
According to the *Consensus Statement on the Triage of Critically Ill Patients of the Society of Critical Care Medicine Ethics Committee*

1. On a daily basis, a single individual should have the authority to implement hospital triage policy.
2. When all critical care units are filled to capacity, the hospital triage officer, with the cooperation of the ICU directors, should have access to all critical care units and have responsibility and authority to admit patients to and discharge patients from these units. The triage officer has the ultimate responsibility and discretion to implement hospital policy by arranging transfer of patients in and out of ICUs.
3. If there is an irreconcilable disagreement between the triage officer and other interested parties, the ICU committee should have a mechanism for reviewing appeals.
4. The triage officer should be a senior, experienced, and respected physician. The officer may delegate routine decisions to other physicians and non-physicians as appropriate. The officer should make decisions in consultation with others who have appropriate expertise.
5. When a physician acts as both health care provider and triage officer, conflicts of interests are inevitable. Physicians serving in both roles must be aware of possible conflicts. Where adequate facilities exist to assign different personnel to each role, institutions should so. When dual assignments are unavoidable, triage officers should balance both responsibilities impartially and should seek the advice of others. The triage officer's decisions may have to be monitored by the ICU committee.
6. Agreements between physicians and their patients regarding availability of ICU care are subject to the oversight and possible modification of the triage officer.
7. Hospital triage officers should have general knowledge of the various conditions treated in the hospital's ICUs, treatments commonly employed, and their associated range of outcomes. They should also be familiar with the various prognostic models and their uses and limitations.
8. Regardless of the patient's circumstances, the process of triage has the following common elements:
    a. patient assessment;
    b. urgency determination;
    c. priority of care based on urgency;
    d. resource analysis;
    e. documentation;
    f. disposition.
    Triage involves a common logic which includes:
    a. probability estimates of outcomes;
    b. judgments of the benefit and burden to the patient and the system;
    c. judgments of the value of the outcome to the patient and to the system.

Methods Of Communication
1. The hospital should keep those who need to know informed about the status and availability of ICU beds. Physicians whose patients may require ICU services have a responsibility to know what is available and communicate their patients' needs to the appropriate individual.

Continued

> **Exhibit 3.1 Continued**
>
> 2. Hospital triage officers should communicate effectively with those care givers affected by triage decisions. The triage officer should engage in active and explicit negotiation and consultation with other care givers when making decisions which may include postponing elective procedures for patients who normally require assignment of ICU beds (p. 1202).

minutes, and other manifestations of due process have been painstakingly built into policymaking. Organization members are reassured of the process's accountability and legality (Delbecq and Gill 1985). The Critical Care Committee, appointed by the medical staff and composed of physicians and other representatives, adopts policies governing the ICU, including the admission, discharge, and triage policies. The ICU medical director oversees the carrying out of the policies.

> **Exhibit 3.2 Triage Officer's Daily Responsibilities**
>
> —Review present occupancy status with charge nurse
> —Perform rapid triage rounds on patients
>   Extubated? Off monitor? Orders Written? Other pertinent factors?
> —View admission list for unit (assumes prebooking)
>   Check daily admits for expected numbers
>   Scan weekly lists for potential high census based on current knowledge
> —Contact "front door" units for potential emergent admits
>   If operating room or post-anesthesia care unit discuss add-on cases, possible overload
>   Discuss potential triage pathway
> —Contact admitting or floor units to identify potential
>   Bed availability in stepdown or floor
>   "Back door" block due to high census on general floors or discharge delays
> —During clinical rounds, formalize
>   Do-not-resuscitate, discharge, withdrawal decisions with caregivers
>   Plans for presenting information to family
> —Develop triage list
>   Category 1: Will leave today, normal discharge
>   Category 2: May leave today—accelerate discharge
>   Category 3: Prefer to retain; triage if bed needed
>   Category 4: Remain in unit, not dischargeable
> —If triage situation develops
>   Contact "front door" units; discuss situation and plan
>   Inform administration (nursing and hospital)
>   Consider closure to electives, bypass emergency room
>   Contact "back door" units for bed availability
>   Accelerate discharge (Category 2)
>   Triage out Category 3 (p. 572)

Exhibit 3.3 presents a typical hospital organization chart with its dual administrative structure: the functional departments organized hierarchically and the medical staff organized horizontally along specialty lines. Whereas a very clear chain of command exists in the nursing hierarchy ranging from the Vice President for nursing down to the bedside nurse, the medical chain of command is often incomplete and truncated with blurred lines of accountability.

As was mentioned in Chapter 2, nurses frequently distinguish between working medical directors who actively participate in the management of the unit and paper directors who may sit on JCAHO-mandated committees but take little part in the day-by-day operations, unless they are taking care of their own patients (Adler 1984). One management function that is the responsibility of the medical director or designated senior level physician is the application of the admission-discharge policies on a case-by-case basis. This function is fulfilled by either the medical director or the designee acting as triage officer. How seriously do medical directors/triage officers carry out this responsibility? It varies from unit to unit. Recent studies, as mentioned in the previous chapter, have shown that in almost half of all ICUs, the medical director or designee is unavailable at night (when many of these decisions are made) to make admission, transfer, and discharge decisions and resolve conflict (Strosberg et al. 1990; Groeger et al. 1992). The nurse, in effect, becomes the de facto triage officer. In teaching hospitals, house staff may take over this role. Typically, physicians are not well paid for their managerial involvement because triage and other managerial activities do not involve direct patient care and are usually not reimbursable.

Managerial Roles and Role Conflict

Both the nurse manager and the medical director are vested with formal authority over the ICU, although for different types of tasks. They jointly share in the overall management. Ruelas and Leatt (1985), in their analysis of physician executives holding various managerial positions in the hospital heirarchy, explore the underlying sources of conflict and stress for managers with regard to their "role sets" (those individuals who are essential to the performance of manager's role, e.g., subordinates, supervisors, peers, and individuals external to the organization). For the ICU medical director or physician executive, the role set would include the chief of service or division chair, other physician managers and administrators, nursing managers at various levels in the hierarchy, nurses, risk managers, laboratory, infection control, physicians, families, and patients. The general approach to role analysis used by Ruelas and

Exhibit 3.3 Sample Organization Chart of a Hospital ICU

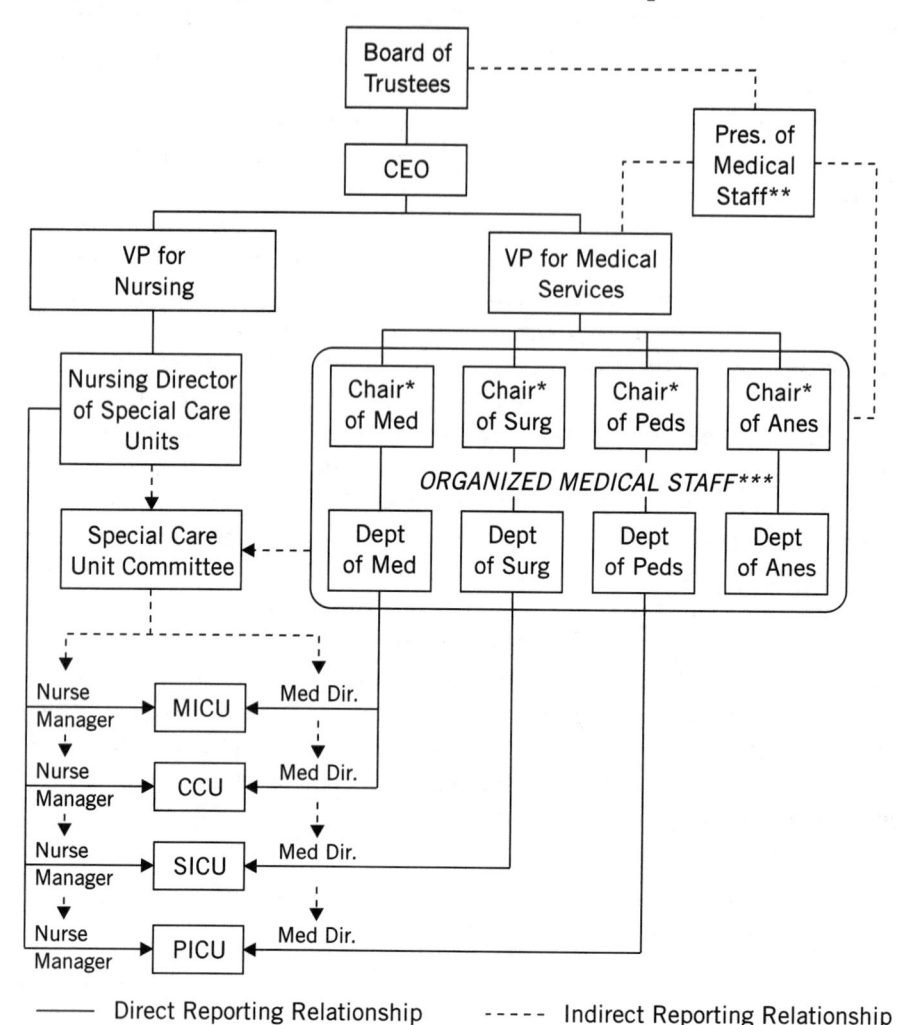

————— Direct Reporting Relationship   - - - - - Indirect Reporting Relationship

* Chiefs typically nominated by department and appointed by board of trustees
** Elected by attending staff
*** Includes attending staff who hold department membership

Leatt is equally applicable to nurse managers, who will of course have a different role set, including managers and staff of other nursing units, (e.g., operating room, emergency room, post anesthesia care unit, step down units, medical and surgical floors).

Following are examples of five different sources of stresses facing ICU medical directors as delineated by Ruelas and Leatt (1985, p. 158):

1. ***Ambiguity****. Information regarding the scope of responsibilities or the expectations from others is uncertain.* A clear delineation of responsibility for carrying out the triage task between the medical director and/or triage officer and the nurse manager may not exist.

2. ***Overload****. Inability to meet demands simultaneously or within prescribed time limits.* For physicians, the time committed to patient care which generates income, subtracts from the time needed to carry out managerial activities. Thus, the nurse manager may be forced to carry out the tasks for an absent "paper" medical director.

3. ***Intersender role conflict****. Demands from one individual are in conflict with those from other individuals.* Private attendings demand access to beds and autonomy in treatment while others in the role set emphasize cost-containment, maximization of opportunities to perform elective surgery, or maintenance of appropriate nurse-to-patient ratios. (See Exhibit 1.1 for other examples.)

4. ***Interrole conflict****. Demands from one role are in conflict with those for another role played by the same physician-executive.* Many physicians serving as medical directors or acting as triage officers have patient care responsibilities with heavy time commitments both inside and outside of the ICU. Collegial relationships must be maintained in the interests of ensuring continued referrals upon which their incomes may depend. The triage task, in addition to other managerial tasks, may interfere with these responsibilities and these relationships.

5. ***Person-role conflict****. Role requirements violate the needs, values, or capabilities of the physician-executive.* For both the medical and nursing manager, triage and gatekeeping functions may conflict with their notions of quality of patient care. Physicians and nurses may see themselves as caregivers first and managers second. On the other hand, demands by attending physicians or families may lead to what they consider the futile prolongation of life not in the best interests of the patient and conflicting with their personal values.

The task of admission-discharge and triage is a complex one. The person performing the task must weigh the competing claims of attendings, consultants, or nurses made on behalf of patients and make difficult judgments. He or she must be proficient at obtaining information quickly and reliably and must be courageous in the face of medical uncertainty, conflicting values, legal uncertainties, and demands from others in the role set. Obviously, good interpersonal skills are required. Most specialists in critical care medicine, coming out of fellowship training, are ill-equipped to undertake the management responsibilities inherent in the position of medical director. Most learn on the job and are surprised and frustrated by the complexity of the job.

A Role for Patients?

What is the role of the patient in decision making? In an era that emphasizes patient autonomy and self-determination, the patient should be considered the most important decision maker. Typically, however, patients lack decision-making capacity—the ability to understand the consequences, to communicate, and to reason with regard to a particular medical decision (AMA Council on Ethical and Judicial Affairs 1992). A surrogate, usually a family member, may be appointed to act on behalf of the patient who lacks capacity.

ICU staff frequently do not see patients in terms of their full-blown humanity but in terms of disease processes and numerical values for physiological states. For the clinician, "personhood" comes back into the picture in terms of abstract notions of informed consent concretized by DNR orders, surrogate decision making, and other advance directives (Zussman 1992). The preferences of families and surrogates can be highly influenced by the manner in which physicians present information on prognosis.

Chapter 4 presents a variety of ways in which patients and surrogates participate in clinical decision making.

Policies and Guidelines

All hospitals are required to have admission and discharge policies for their ICUs. A typical hospital policy is presented in Exhibit 3.4. The criteria of this policy are very general. An example of more elaborate and discriminating criteria are presented in Appendix B. See Appendix C for an assessment scale with which to evaluate criteria.

Various professional associations have also developed guidelines for admission, discharge, and resource allocation in triage situations. For example, the AMA Council on Ethical and Judicial Affairs (1995) outlines acceptable criteria for comparative entitlement decisions (see Appendix A):

> Five factors relating to medical need may appropriately be taken into account when organs or other scarce medical resources, such as spaces in the ICU, are allocated. These include (1) the likelihood of benefit to the patient, (2) the impact of treatment in improving the quality of the patient's life, (3) the duration of benefit, (4) the urgency of the patient's condition (i.e., how close the patient is to death), and in some cases (5) the amount of resources required for successful treatment. Each of these criteria serves to maximize the following three primary goals of medical treatment: number of lives saved, number of years of life saved, and improvement in quality of life (i.e., the criteria maximize quantity of life, quality of life, or both) (p. 29).

The AMA Council suggests ways in which these criteria might be specifically applied to the allocation of scarce ICU beds (see Appendix A). Very few hospital policies address the specific application of these criteria in a triage situation.

Decision Rationales for Gatekeeping

Underlying ICU admission, discharge, and triage decision making are three different rationales and concomitant sets of criteria:
1. non-triage mode (bed availability);
2. triage mode/comparative entitlement (no bed availability); and

---

Exhibit 3.4 Admission and Discharge Criteria

Admission Criteria

Intensive Care Unit
1. Patients requiring mechanical ventilation for respiratory or ventilatory failure.
2. Patients requiring intravascular and/or invasive hemodynamic monitoring.
3. Patients with cardiogenic, septic, hypovolemic, or other types of shock.
4. Patients who have undergone successful cardiopulmonary resuscitation.
5. Patients who must receive intravenous vasoactive medications.
6. Patients requiring massive transfusions.
7. High-risk surgical patients who require preoperative physiologic assessment and/or management.
8. Postoperative patients who require mechanical ventilation, hemodynamic monitoring, intensive nursing care, or surgical monitoring.
9. Patients with impending respiratory/ventilatory failure who need intensive medical management to prevent intubation.
10. Patients with drug intoxications who either satisfy the above criteria or need intensive medical care for detoxification and/or treatment.
11. Patients undergoing diagnostic and therapeutic procedures that, for the individual patient, can logistically only be safely performed in the ICU. These include endoscopy, bronchoscopy, dialysis, continuous arterio-venous ultrafiltration, pacemaker insertion, thrombolytic therapy, etc.
12. Patients with metabolic, endocrine, or electrolyte abnormalities requiring close physician and nursing surveillance and care, such as diabetic ketoacidosis, hyperosmolar states, severe dehydration, hypothermia, hyperthermia, etc.

Discharge Criteria

Patients will be discharged from the ICU when the criteria for admission are no longer present, in other words, the patient has improved, or the patient's condition has deteriorated to the extent that he/she has no medically reversible condition. In the latter event, the patient will be transferred to an appropriate floor where comfort care will be continued.

3. medical futility, a special subset of the admissions-discharge criteria, often ill-defined and controversial because it may imply the unilateral withholding or withdrawal of treatment.

The determination of medical futility can be made either in the triage or non-triage mode but should not be influenced by bed availability in the ICU.

As was mentioned in the beginning of Chapter 1, agreement on which mode (triage mode or non-triage mode) is operative is not always achieved. Obviously they are linked: loose admission and discharge criteria increase the likelihood that triage and comparative entitlement decisions will be made at a later time. Also, disagreement and confusion frequently occur over the concepts of futility and benefit because they have not been adequately defined in the criteria.

Included in the admission criteria presented in Exhibit 3.4 is a general statement requiring that a patient be discharged "when his/her condition has deteriorated to the extent that he/she has no medically reversible condition." Presumably a patient should also not be admitted with such a condition. The decision to withhold or withdraw ICU care is one that it is frequently made. Some recent studies have estimated that 40 percent to 65 percent of ICU deaths have been preceded by decisions to withhold or withdraw life support. (Smedira et al. 1990; Lee et al. 1994). The American Hospital Association (1989) estimates that approximately 70 percent of hospital deaths occur after a decision has been made to forgo treatment.

How should it be decided that the patient has reached the point of withholding or withdrawal? Who should decide? These are issues that are frequently considered in connection with medical futility. Medical futility is a confusing and controversial topic. Approaches to its definition can be arrayed along a continuum. The most restricted approach is sometimes called physiological futility—care that cannot be expected to have any physiological benefit to the patient. For example, CPR cannot possibly restart the heart when there is a cardiac rupture; it has a 0 percent chance of working. Schneiderman and Jecker (1993) provide a quantitative or probabilistic definition (e.g., less than one chance in 100):

> that when physicians conclude (either through personal experience, experience shared with colleagues, or consideration of published empirical data) that in the last 100 cases a medical treatment has been useless they should regard the treatment as futile (p. 437).

The definition of medical futility also has qualitative dimensions that take into consideration the quality of life of the patient. Even if the particular intervention is successful, will it produce any benefit for the patient beyond the mere prolongation of life? Schneiderman and

Jecker, for example, state that "if a treatment merely preserves permanent unconsciousness or cannot end dependence on intensive care medicine, the treatment should be considered futile." (p. 438)

Both the quantitative and qualitative approaches have been criticized. First, assuming that a probability can be reasonably estimated, why arbitrarily choose 1 percent? Some patients would consider a 1 percent chance worth taking, considering the alternative. Second, toward what end or objectives are interventions considered medically futile? Some patients or families, valuing the "sanctity of life," would regard the addition of any time (e.g., in an ICU and/or in a persistent vegetative state [PVS]) as worthwhile. Cut-off percentages and quality-of-life considerations are value judgments.

The quantitative and qualitative approaches are problematic only when there is disagreement between the patient or family and the physician or triage officer who is applying the admission and discharge criteria. In the vast majority of cases agreement is achieved; futility is obvious to all parties. But when can the primary attending physician and, in some instances, the triage officer unilaterally make a decision even if it conflicts with the values of the patient or surrogate? If we reserve the term medical futility for those cases where the decision maker can unilaterally apply a criteria, there will be only a tiny subset of decisions where there could not possibly be a disagreement over values (i.e., those interventions that offer no physiological benefit). Moving beyond this point, unilateral decision making is problematic as the cases in the next chapter will show. Possible solutions will be discussed in Chapter 6.

Models of Organization Decision Making

To the extent that they capture the "reality" of the process, models are useful in improving understanding of the constraints faced by decision makers. Two models of decision making, which are frequently juxtaposed at opposite ends of a continuum, are the "rational model" and the "political model."

In the rational model, goals are clear and agreed-upon and the alternatives for reaching those goals are well understood. Decisions are made in the name of maximizing some single value (e.g., benefit to patients) or set of values. The rational model assumes that criteria exist for judging the correctness of a decision. It is management's job to monitor outcomes, compare them to criteria and standards, and take corrective action if necessary.

Clearly, the rational model has great appeal as an approach to organizing the ICU decision-making process. Embedded in the official policy statements governing ICUs is the rhetoric of rationality—efficiency and appropriateness. Also, a widely shared belief exists that decision making should be based on ethical principles that guide the allocation of scarce resources with appeals to such concepts as justice, fairness, and equity.

The political model assumes that participants disagree about goals and have poor information about alternatives. They bring to decision making separate interests, goals, and values. Information is ambiguous and incomplete. Disagreement, conflict, and bargaining are normal, so power and influence are needed to reach a decision. As opposed to the rational model, decision making is disorderly and characterized by the push and pull of interests (Pfeffer 1981).

Using the characteristics of the models as benchmarks, it is instructive to ask where ICU decision making falls on the continuum between these two poles. How realistic is the rational model for the ICU? To what extent is there agreement on organizational and therapeutic goals (ends) and to what extent is there an understanding of the means (e.g., treatment effectiveness) of achieving those goals?

Means: Examples of Uncertainty

For many classifications of patients, uncertainties exist over the benefits of treatment and what is medically indicated. For example, the NIH Consensus Development Conference (1983) has identified a group of patients:

> ... with a low probability of survival without intensive care whose probability or survival with intensive care may be higher—but potential benefit is not as clear. Clinical examples include patients with septic or cardiogenic shock. The weight of clinical opinion is that ICUs reduce mortality for many of these patients, though this conviction is supported only by uncontrolled or poorly controlled studies. Often these studies do not allow one to distinguish between ICU effectiveness and/or differences in cointerventions that do not require the ICU (p. 2).

For these patients, it is not at all clear that ICU care, as a discrete technology, offers any definitive advantage over treatment in non-ICU settings, thereby calling into question the cost-effectiveness of treatment. Even if enough information exists to accurately estimate probabilities of benefit and establish confidence limits, it is possible for an individual patient to fall outside of the confidence interval. What constitutes certainty: 90 percent, 95 percent, 99 percent? Who decides?

Uncertainty also occurs with regard to diagnostic procedures. There is no more controversial example of the technical uncertainty of a diagnostic procedure than the pulmonary artery or Swan-Ganz catheterization often performed in the ICU. The Swan-Ganz catheter, a pulmonary artery catheter (PAC), is used for providing information on heart functioning. It was first introduced in 1970. Like many other innovations, it was widely diffused without a formal evaluation of its efficacy (use under ideal circumstances), and effectiveness (use under usual circumstances). And yet the national expenditure on Swan-Ganz catheterization amounts to billions of dollars. The catheter itself is relatively inexpensive. But there are physician charges for the insertion of the catheter, maintenance of the catheter, the changing of the catheter (every five or six days the catheter should be changed to reduce the risk of infection, clots, and other complications), the collection and interpretation of the information, and the removal of the catheter. Nursing assignment usually goes up for a patient with pulmonary artery monitoring. A measurable complication rate exists. Iberti et al. (1990) found wide variation in the ability of physicians to correctly and safely interpret and apply the information that is provided. Questions abound. If the PAC information is available, is it useful? Is treatment altered, and if treatment is altered is patient outcome improved? Connors et al. (1996), in a prospective cohort study, found that the PAC was associated with increased mortality and increased use of resources.

The inability to definitively answer these questions has led to calls for a moratorium on the use of the PAC (Robin 1987; Dalen and Bone 1996). Most intensivists propose a less radical approach by calling for an appropriately designed prospective randomized controlled study and the development of guidelines for the appropriate use of the PAC (Naylor et al. 1993; SCCM 1996).

Ends (Goals): Examples of Disagreement

There are a variety of sources of disagreement over the goals of ICU treatment.

1. Outcomes. Is the goal of ICU care the preservation of life and is survival to hospital discharge an appropriate indicator? Should quality of life be considered, and if so, how should it be defined and measured? Is the goal of ICU care preserving life at all costs regardless of the quality of that life?
2. Patient preferences. It is often unclear just how aggressively patients want their physicians to pursue intervention. In the ICU, it is often the case that patients lack decision-making capacity and cannot make their wishes known. Advance directives are generally not available or, if available, not heeded. Living wills are often incomplete. Physicians often overestimate the patient's desire for

intervention, while at the same time families or surrogates often underestimate the patient's desire for aggressive treatment (Danis et al. 1988). What happens if patients and/or surrogates disagree with physicians?
3. Family preferences. What happens when there is no family, a distant family, or a dysfunctional or stressed family? In these cases it is difficult to make decisions for critically ill patients in need of invasive procedures, tests, or surgery.
4. Legal uncertainty. Physicians, especially in situations of uncertainty over patient preference, may feel unsure about what the law requires them to do, especially as it relates to the withdrawal of treatment. Many physicians, fearing legal consequences, choose to treat aggressively because they feel that it is the least risky alternative.
5. Allocation rules for comparative entitlement decisions. Given the Hippocratic tradition and the fiduciary relationship with patients, an individual physician finds it difficult to accept the notion of comparative entitlement when he or she believes that the quality of care for his or her patient is being compromised. Furthermore, the institution also faces contradictory expectations. Should patients already in the unit take priority over those waiting to come in from other parts of the hospital or from outside the hospital? Many feel that there is a contract with patients already in the unit and to discharge them prematurely is tantamount to abandonment. Others, including Englehardt and Rie (1986), argue that hospitals have the responsibility to allocate a scarce bed according to the ability to benefit and an ICU patient should be discharged to make room for someone who could derive greater benefit. However, malpractice law generally requires that the community standard of care be available to all patients regardless of the economic hardships faced by the hospital. The quality of care cannot be diminished because of scarcity or the lack of beds.
6. Institutional priorities under managed care. Are hospitals with managed care contracts under any obligation to give admission priority to plan members?

Political Power, Medical Provincialism, and Income Maximization

Marshall et al. (1992), in a study of bed rationing in a surgical ICU undergoing temporary bed closure due to a nursing shortage, hypothesized that as bed availability decreased, the severity of illness of patient admittees would increase. This hypothesis was based on the research of Singer et al. (1983) and of Strauss et al. (1986), who showed that physicians responded to temporary ICU bed shortages by admitting the sicker patients and decreasing length of stay. Using the APACHE II scoring system to assess severity of illness, Marshall et al. found that severity actually decreased. In specific, they found that cardiothoracic surgical patients were being given admission priority over general surgical patients who had higher APACHE II scores. They concluded that "political power, medical provincialism, and income maximization" influenced bed allocation more than patient need. Apparently, the cardiothoracic surgeons used their influence to maintain their referral pattern and flow of patients through the ICU. Typically, elective open-heart surgery, which requires postoperative treatment in the ICU, generates large amounts of revenue for physicians and hospitals.

From the point of view of the cardiothoracic surgeons attempting to build a regional cardiothoracic program and the administrators and surgeons who would reap economic gains for the institution, the postponement of surgery or the diversion of patients to competing centers would in the long run be detrimental for the patients and the institution (Teres 1993). The strength of this position is exemplified by the fact that the cardiothoracic surgeons ultimately obtained a separate ICU totally dedicated to the postoperative care of cardiothoracic patients (Marshall et al. 1992). This solution, although satisfactory to the cardiothoracic surgeons, further fragments the hospital's organizational structure, generates a new set of coordination problems, and raises costs. In an era of cost constraint, small, distinct units are often very expensive and encourage overuse with lower severity patients or long-stay patients.

Inter-Unit Coordination and Sub-Optimization

From a managerial perspective, the boxes on the organizational chart indicating the grouping of beds, equipment, and personnel into organizational units are a fundamental means of achieving coordination. Grouping has four major effects (Mintzberg 1979):

1. establishes a system of common supervision among positions and organizational units;
2. requires positions and units to share common resources (e.g., budget and equipment);
3. creates common measures of performance; and
4. encourages mutual adjustment (e.g., face-to-face communication, feedback, and socialization).

Generally, as organizations become more and more differentiated into units, the units become separated by spatial, social, and psychological distance with different time perspectives, orientations, pay scales, and goals. Social solidarity within units can cause "we-them" phenomena among organizational units (Mintzberg 1979). However, it is frequently the case that in this interdependent critical care system, one unit's outputs become another unit's inputs, thus creating an environment for intergroup conflict.

Examine the flowchart in Exhibit 3.5, which updates an earlier version by Gosselin (1978). The components of the flowchart, which constitute part of the process of diagnosing and treating patients with heart disease, can all be traced to boxes or positions on the organizational chart. The flowchart shows that the process is fragmented among several boxes (unit groupings); different units have different and sometimes contradictory policies. For example, the policy of the recovery room might be to help maintain the operating room schedule. The policy of the ICU may be to smooth admissions from the operating room by requiring a certain period of advance notice. Thus, the possibility exists of two units, system-linked but physically separate, to hold contradictory policies. These contradictory policies are like two continental plates, unobtrusively pressing against each other beneath the surface until a threshold is reached and an earthquake (conflict) makes the contradictions immediately apparent.

At some level in the hierarchy, someone in the chain of command is ultimately responsible for making sure that the interaction among various units is coordinated. But frequently there is not enough power emanating from the hierarchical system of authority to command things to happen. Quite simply, the hierarchy is not strong enough to harness all the boxes to work for some overall common objective of the institution. The institution may not even be sure of its major objectives: Should it promote elective surgery, which is a big revenue producer but serves a limited set of patients and physicians? Should it promote the trauma service or burn units, which are typically big money losers, but nevertheless serve the general community? Even with the presence of overall objectives and with the best of intentions, managers of units may overemphasize their own particular goals to the detriment of the institution's goals (Strosberg 1987).

Cohen, Fitzpatrick, and Booth (1996) aptly describe the frustration often experienced by ICU managers:

> Critical care processes tend to be fragmented by conventional administrative structures. The result of the disjointed system is often familiar and predictable—before significant improvement or changes can be made, two or three centers of authority may have to be convinced if the change crosses organizational divisions. Typically, if a crisis occurs (this often means that some individual becomes upset), a letter, a memorandum, or an incident report is generated. The issues goes up and down several departmental channels. The event is "looked into," assurances are made, and little changes. Most critical care leaders are

Gatekeeping: Decision Makers and Decision Making 79

Exhibit 3.5 Flowchart of Patients with Acute Coronary Disease

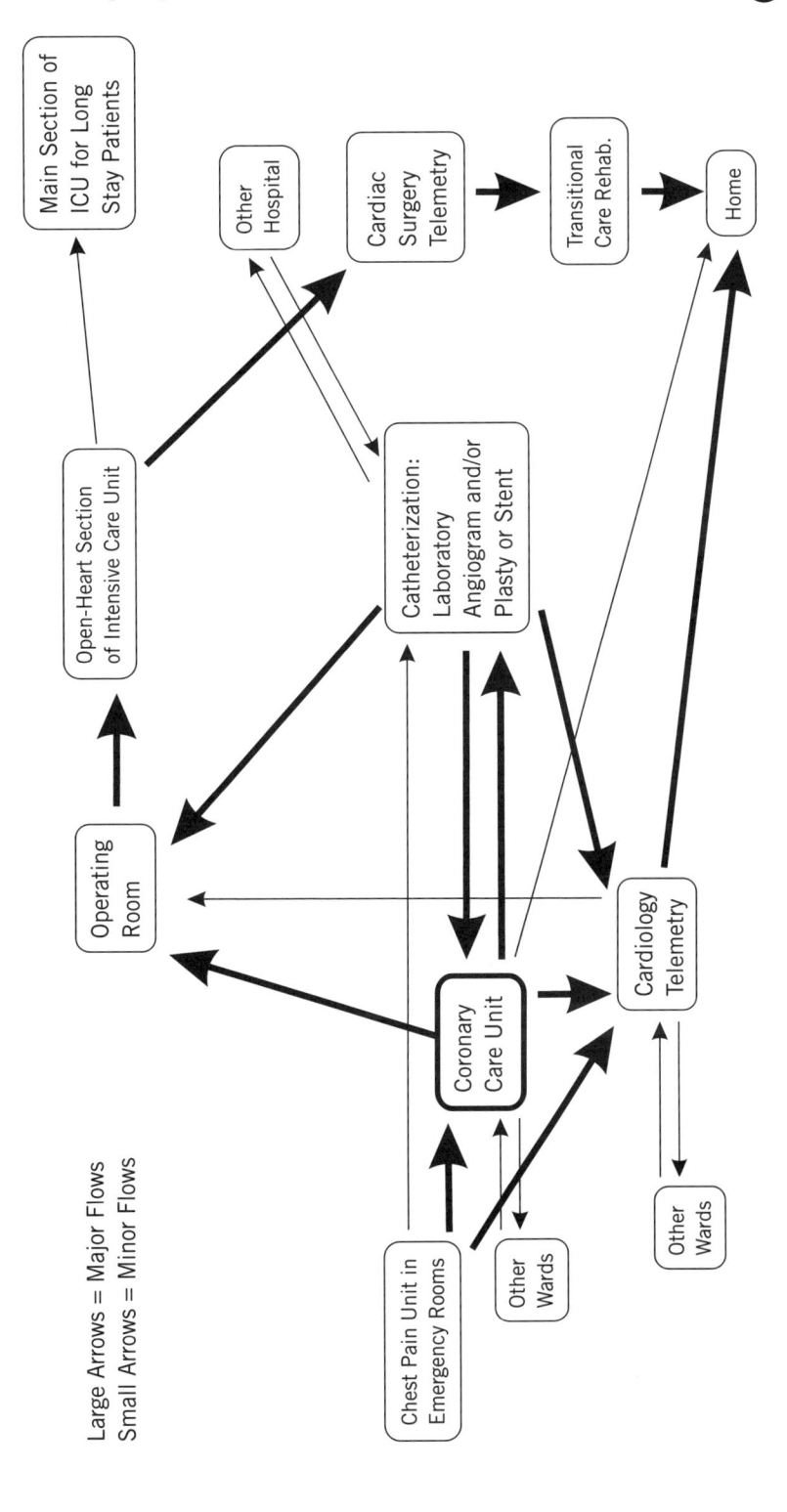

Large Arrows = Major Flows
Small Arrows = Minor Flows

familiar with the impasses that appear to block even the most rational process or structural change (p. 88).

Total quality management (TQM) or continuous quality improvement (CQI) offers an approach for breaking down some of the boundaries between units by emphasizing and analyzing the processes that transcend boundaries. The development of care maps, practice guidelines, and benchmarking will go a long way toward streamlining and standardizing critical care processes (Berwick 1994; Cohen, Fitzpatrick, and Booth 1996). Product line management is another way to cross divisions and departments. Furthermore, the JCAHO mandates a single Special Care Unit Committee because the problems tend to be so similar among units (Teres and Turner 1995). Nevertheless, it is often extremely difficult to overcome the centrifugal forces influencing the hospital organization.

Making an Admission/Discharge Decision

Lumb (1993) compares the role of the ICU gatekeeper to the air traffic controller who directs aircraft landing and takeoff. In the interests of overall safety and system efficiency, pilots readily accept air traffic controller direction. Aircraft schedules, flight plans, priorities for arrival and departure, and rules for handling contingencies (e.g., "Mayday" emergencies) have become routine for the entire nation, and much of the world, which is possible because most of the activity in the airline industry is predictable and schedulable. In support of the air traffic controller analogy, Cohen, Fitzpatrick, and Booth (1996) argue that much in critical care is predictable and therefore schedulable. In Buffalo General Hospital, for example, one-third of patients entering ICUs do so as a result of elective surgery. And at least some of the nonelective admissions could be anticipated through careful analysis of patient flow patterns from points of origin. Theoretically, with proper scheduling, managers at most hospitals could minimize delays, cancelation of elective surgery, and the necessity to triage. Unfortunately, however, in most ICUs the air traffic controller analogy is limited in how far it can be extended to critical care gatekeeping. Organizational fragmentation limits the ICU gatekeeper's view of incoming patients (flights). Whereas air traffic controllers know when an aircraft has entered the airport's airspace extending out hundreds of miles, the illness trajectories of patients are frequently obscured from ICU gatekeepers' radar. And politics, as Marshall et al. (1992) show, allow some primary physicians (i.e., pilots) to trump the gatekeepers.

How then will the decision makers decide? One prominent theorist suggests that instead of trying to maximize any particular value or objective, decision makers "satisfice" (Simon 1964). That is, they try to meet at least the minimal level of expectations for a variety of stakeholders (attending physicians, patients, families, third party payors, regulators, nursing staff, etc.) For example, we could conceive of a participant deciding in such a way so as to:

- meet the formal requirements of institutional policies;
- keep powerful physicians satisfied and contributing (e.g., admitting patients);
- keep the nurses from quitting or burning out;
- keep the hospital and physician out of legal and regulatory difficulty; and
- keep the quality assurance review process from being triggered.

In times of resource shortage (e.g., in a triage situation), decision makers search for that stakeholder for whom a lower level of performance would be least objectionable, or for that stakeholder who has the least power to object.

The satisfiable mode of decision making is well expressed by the "Triage Flowchart" (Exhibit 3.6) created by a physician who frequently functioned as a triage officer in a large, tertiary teaching hospital. In spite of the intended humor, the chart does capture the flavor of the search process and the interconnection between non-triage and triage mode decision making. The starting point of the flow sheet is the request for admission: "Do you have a bed? If yes, fill it—problem solved for now." Presumably, prior questions were asked such as, "Does this patient meet admission criteria, or would it be possible to exclude the patient on other grounds?" However, when beds are available, the path of least resistance frequently is to admit the patient.

Problems grow in complexity when no beds are available (i.e., during triage). (Of course, by automatically filling the beds, the triage officer assures the necessity of triage.) If there are no beds available, the question becomes, "Did you say you did?" If you didn't, then you can begin to calculate the political consequences of approving or denying admission (i.e., "Are you in hot water?"). If in fact you are not, you have the discretion to admit (and discharge another patient), refuse admission, or "turf" (send to some other unit in the hospital). On the other hand, if you are in "hot water," you cannot diminish satisfaction to this particular stakeholder and you have to hope that someone will either die or get better. Or you can "DNR your way out of it," perhaps implying an attempt to speed up a decision to determine medical futility or that an intervention would be inappropriate. The worst of all possible worlds is to say you had a bed when you really did not, a situation which might happen when a patient scheduled for extubation and transfer becomes unstable. The overwhelming expectation is that if a bed is available it will be filled.

Both the rational model and the political model require calculation. In the rational model, decision makers calculate which alternative best maximizes a certain, well-agreed upon goal. In the political model, decision makers calculate political consequences: "Whom do I make glad; how glad? Whom do I make mad; how mad?"

Accountability and Fairness

Although the decision of who gets admitted and discharged is obviously important and triage is the central preoccupation in many ICUs, it generally has not been conceptualized as an administrative task with defined performance standards. Criteria for triage decisions vary among hospitals, among units within the same hospital, and by personnel within each unit. Very little research has been conducted on what criteria triage

Exhibit 3.6 Triage Flowchart: The Dawson Model

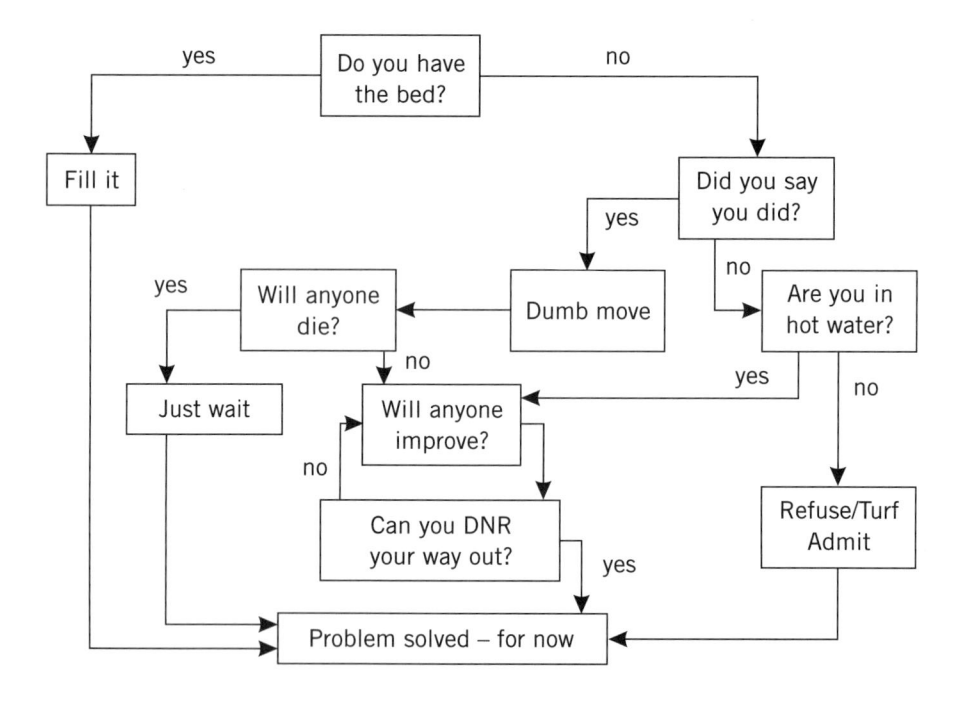

```
                    Do you have
         yes ───────  the bed?  ─────── no
          │                              │
          ▼                              ▼
      ┌──────┐                    ┌──────────────┐
      │Fill it│                    │ Did you say  │
      └──────┘          yes ──────│  you did?    │
                         │         └──────────────┘
                         │                │ no
                         ▼                ▼
          yes  ┌──────────┐  ┌──────────┐    ┌──────────────┐
          ┌───│Will anyone│◄─│Dumb move │    │ Are you in   │
          │   │   die?    │  └──────────┘    │  hot water?  │
          │   └──────────┘                   └──────────────┘
          │         │ no                       yes │    │ no
          ▼         ▼                              ▼    ▼
     ┌─────────┐  ┌──────────────┐              ┌──────────────┐
     │Just wait│  │ Will anyone  │◄─────────────│ Refuse/Turf  │
     └─────────┘  │  improve?    │              │   Admit      │
          │       └──────────────┘              └──────────────┘
          │         no │  ▲
          │            ▼  │
          │       ┌──────────────┐
          │       │ Can you DNR  │
          │       │ your way out?│ yes
          │       └──────────────┘
          │              │
          ▼              ▼
        ┌────────────────────────────┐
        │ Problem solved – for now   │◄──
        └────────────────────────────┘
```

Source: J. Dawson. 1993. "Admission, Discharge, and Triage in Critical Care," *Critical Care Clinics: Critical Care Unit Management* 9 (3): 570.

decision makers use in making their decisions, although one study suggests that triage decision makers, when independently evaluating the same patients, often arrive at different estimates of the potential for discharge, that is, suitability for triage (Shear et al. 1988). Triage decision makers may bring different values to their definition of appropriate outcome (e.g., return to productive activity versus short-term survival). Some may respond differently to pressures from the family, primary physicians, or specialists. Racial and social status differences and age discrimination may also play a role. In managed care settings, cost considerations may covertly enter the decision-making process.

With regard to the unplanned readmission of discharged patients, information is sometimes collected, but it is not clear how it is used to evaluate the appropriateness of ICU discharge policy. Similarly, little is known about denied or delayed admissions originating from within the hospital or from outside the hospital, and hospitals usually do not examine the implicit or explicit criteria used in decision making to see if consistent application occurs among patients with similar conditions. Especially in open, decentralized units, individual physicians, fortified by the Hippocratic tradition and their fiduciary relationship with their patients, are under no compulsion to consider micro tradeoffs (i.e., savings that accrue from denying beneficial care to one patient might bring even greater benefit to another patient). In short, comparative entitlement decisions are frequently not relevant.

Singer et al. (1983) report that attending physicians, faced with a substantial reduction in beds in a combined medical ICU-CCU, spontaneously adjusted their individual admission and discharge decisions to achieve a more efficient use of a smaller number of beds by limiting admission of the less severely ill. No central direction or explicit administrative rules were required. "Mutual adjustment" of an adhocratic nature was sufficient (Mintzberg 1979). However, Singer and his colleagues point out the dangers of cutting back on resources without providing explicit guidelines for their use. If beneficial services are indeed being denied, diminished, or delayed, issues of accountability and fairness draw sharply into focus.

The ICU that Singer et al. describe is an open unit. At the other end of the spectrum is the closed unit with centralized decision making. When necessary, decision makers in such a unit, who are also the attending physicians of record, are able to achieve micro-level tradeoffs through considerations of comparative entitlement. End-of-life decision making can also be made with more appropriate involvement of families. The reduction in the influence of private attendings eliminates a layer of complexity facing decision makers.

A centralized, closed-unit approach is certainly one way of empowering decision makers to make difficult judgment weighing the competing claims of patients to ICU resources. Decision makers have political independence. Does this approach, however, necessarily lead to more accountable decision making? As other voices are eliminated from the decision-making process, there is a danger that the remaining empowered decision makers will not exercise their gatekeeping responsibilities in such a way that advances the overall objectives of the patient or the unit.

Roles and Rules

The open unit and the closed unit require different coordinating mechanisms. With many participants and many interests, the decentralized structure requires mutual adjustment as described by Singer et al. In the centralized unit, with fewer stakeholders to worry about and less complexity, a single person or just a few people can make the decision. Coordination and communication are more easily achieved (Mintzberg 1979). In both instances, we could describe these organizational structures as non-bureaucratic. Bureaucracy, although it is a term with an unfortunate negative connotation, is an organizational structure designed to make decision premises explicit, ensure that like cases are treated alike, and filter out arbitrary and capricious behavior. To the extent the aforementioned is not happening in admission, discharge, and triage decision making, we may wish to consider the establishment of rules that guide resource allocation and support well-recognized performance expectations about access to ICU beds. Political pressures from those who "yell loudest" should be minimized. Roles will also need to be structured to support decision makers in applying rules or, where necessary, in exercising discretion in an appropriate manner. This will be a difficult challenge given disagreement on goals and means for achieving them, competition for resources, and unstable illness trajectories. We will examine the structuring of roles and the improvement of management in Chapter 5. In Chapter 6 we will discuss approaches to public policymaking that can help resolve disagreement over goals and generate a consistent and explicit set of rules. But now we return to the unfolding events at Anywhere Hospital.

References

Adler, D. C. 1984. "Hospital Management of Critical Care." In *Major Issues in Critical Care Medicine,* edited by J. E. Parrillo and S. N. Ayres, 265–70. Baltimore, MD: Williams & Wilkins.

American Hospital Association. 1989. *Brief of the American Hospital Association as Amicus Curiae in Support of Petitioners Nancy Beth Cruzan, L. Lester, and Joyce Cruzan.* Chicago: American Hospital Association.

American Medical Association Council on Ethical and Judicial Affairs. 1995. "Ethical Considerations in the Allocation of Organs and Other Scarce Medical Resources Among Patients." *Archives of Internal Medicine* 155 (Jan 9): 29–40.

American Medical Association Council on Ethical and Judicial Affairs. 1992. "Decisions Near the End of Life." *Journal of the American Medical Association* 267 (16): 2229–33.

Berwick, D. M. 1994. "Eleven Worthy Aims for Clinical Leadership of Health Care System Reform." *Journal of the American Medical Association* 272 (10): 797–802.

Blair, J. D., and M. D. Fottler. 1990. *Challenges in Health Care Management: Strategic Perspectives for Managing Key Stakeholders.* San Francisco: Jossey-Bass.

Cohen, I. L., M. Fitzpatrick, and F. V. McL. Booth. 1996. "Critical Care Medicine: Opportunity and Strategies for Improvement." *Journal of Quality Improvement* 22 (2): 85–103.

Connors, A. F., T. Speroff, N. V. Dawson, and C. Thomas. 1996. "The Effectiveness of Right Heart Catheterization in the Initial Care of Critically Ill Patients." *Journal of the American Medical Association* 276 (11): 889–97.

Dalen, J. E., and R. C. Bone. 1996. "Is it Time to Pull the Pulmonary Artery Catheter?" *Journal of the American Medical Association* 276 (11): 916–18.

Danis, M., M. S. Gerrity, L. I. Southerland, and D. L. Patrick. 1988. "A Comparison of Patient, Family, and Physician Assessments of the Value of Medical Intensive Care." *Critical Care Medicine* 16 (6): 594–600.

Dawson, J. A. 1993. "Admission, Discharge, and Triage in Critical Care." *Critical Care Clinics* 9 (3): 555–74.

Delbecq, A. L., and S. L. Gill. 1985. "Justice as a Prelude to Teamwork in Medical Centers." *Health Care Management Review* 10 (1): 45–51.

Engelhardt, H. T., and M. A. Rie. 1986. "Intensive Care Units, Scarce Resources and Conflicting Principles of Justice." *Journal of the American Medical Association* 255 (9): 1159–64.

Galbraith, J. R. 1977. *Organization Design.* Reading, MA: Addison-Wesley.

Gonzales, J. J., and T. A. Stern. 1991. "Recognition and Management of Staff Stress in the ICU." In *Intensive Care Medicine,* edited by J. M. Rippe, R. S. Irwin, J. S. Alport, and M. S. Fink, 1916–22. Boston: Little, Brown and Company.

Gosselin, R. 1978. *A Study of the Interdependence of Medical Specialists in Quebec Teaching Hospitals.* Ph.D. Thesis, McGill University.

Groeger, J. S., M. A. Strosberg, N. S. Halpern, R. C. Raphael, W. Kaye, K. K. Guntupalli, D. L. Bertman, D. Greenbaum, T. P. Clemmer, T. J. Gallagher, L. D. Nelson, A. E. Thompson, F. B. Cerra, and W. R. Davis. 1992. "Descriptive Analysis of Critical Care Units in the United States." *Critical Care Medicine* 20 (6): 846–63.

Iberti, T. J., E. P. Fischer, A. B. Leibowitz, E. A. Panacek, J. H. Silverstein, T. E. Albertson, and the Pulmonary Catheter Study Group. 1990. "A Multicenter Study of Physicians Knowledge of the Pulmonary Artery Catheter." *Journal of the American Medical Association* 264 (22): 2928–32.

Joint Commission on Accreditation of Healthcare Organizations. 1990. *Accreditation Manual for Hospitals, 1991.* Oakbrook Terrace, IL: JCAHO.

Lee, K. P., A. J. Swinburne, A. J. Fedullo, and G. W. Wahl. 1994. "Withdrawing Care: Experience in a Medical Intensive Care Unit." *Journal of the American Medical Association* 271 (17): 1358–61.

Lumb, P. D. 1993. "Management as the Art of Politics." *Critical Care Clinics* 9 (3): 425–36.

Marshall, M. F., K. J. Schwenzer, M. Orsina, J. C. Fletcher, and C. G. Durbin. 1992. "Influence of Political Power, Medical Provincialism, and Economic Incentives on the Rationing of Surgical Intensive Care Unit Beds." *Critical Care Medicine* 20 (3): 387–94.

Mintzberg, H. 1979. *The Structuring of Organizations.* Englewood Cliffs, NJ: Prentice-Hall.

National Institutes of Health. 1983. *Consensus Development Conference on Critical Care Medicine: Summary.* Bethesda, MD: U.S. Public Health Service, National Institutes of Health.

Naylor, C. D., W. J. Sibbald, C. L. Sprung, S. P. Pinfold, J. E. Calvin, and F. B. Cerra. 1993. "Pulmonary Artery Catheterization: Can There Be an Integrated Strategy for Guideline Development and Research Promotion?" *Journal of the American Medical Association* 269 (18): 2407–11.

Pfeffer, J. 1981. *Power in Organizations.* Boston: Pitman.

Robin, E. D. 1987. "Death by Pulmonary Artery Flow-Directed Catheter: Time for a Moratorium?" *Chest* 92 (4): 494–96.

Ruelas, E., and P. Leatt. "The Roles of Physician-Executives in Hospitals: A Framework for Management Education." *Journal of Health Administration Education* 3 (2, Part I): 151–69.

Schneiderman, L. J., and N. S. Jecker. 1993. "Futility in Practice." *Archives of Internal Medicine* 153 (4): 437–41.

Shear, L., J. Steingrub, D. Teres, and L. Shear. 1988. "ICU Patient Triage Ranking: A Flawed Practice?" (Abstract): *Critical Care Medicine* 16 (4): 409.

Simon, H. 1964. "On the Concept of Organizational Goal." *Administrative Science Quarterly* 9 (June): 1–22.

Singer, D. E., P. L. Carr, A. G. Mulley, and G. E. Thibault. 1983. "Rationing Intensive Care: Physician Responses to a Resource Shortage." *New England Journal of Medicine* 309 (19): 1150–60.

Smedira, N. G., B. H. Evans, L. S. Grais, N. H. Cohen, B. Lo, M. Cooke, W. P. Schecter, C. Fink, E. Epstein-Jaffe, C. May, and J. M. Luce. 1990. "Withholding and Withdrawal of Life Support for the Critically Ill." *New England Journal of Medicine* 322 (5): 309–15.

Society of Critical Care Medicine. 1988. "Recommendations for ICU Admission and Discharge." *Critical Care Medicine* 16 (8): 807–08.

Society of Critical Care Medicine. 1994. "Consensus Statement on the Triage of Critically Ill Patients." *Journal of the American Medical Association* 271 (15): 1200–1203.

Society of Critical Care Medicine. 1996. "SCCM Responds to *JAMA*" *Forum* 3 (Fall): 1.

Strauss, M. J., J. P. LoGerfo, J. A. Yeltatzie, M. Temkin, and L. D. Hudson. 1986. "Rationing of Intensive Care Unit Services." *Journal of the American Medical Association* 255 (9): 1143–46.

Strosberg, M. A., D. Teres, I. A. Fein, and R. Linsider. 1990. "Nursing Perception of the Availability of the Intensive Care Unit Medical Director for Triage and Conflict Resolution." *Heart and Lung* 19 (5): 452–55.

Teres, D. 1993. "Civilian Triage in the Intensive Care Unit: The Ritual of the Last Bed." *Critical Care Medicine* 21 (4): 598–606.

Teres, D., and S. L. Turner. 1996. "The Special Care Unit Committee." In *Intensive Care Medicine,* 3rd ed., edited by J. Rippe, R. S. Irwin, M. P. Fink, and F. B. Cerra, 2599–2607. Boston: Little, Brown and Company.

Zussman, R. 1992. *Intensive Care: Medical Ethics and the Medical Profession.* Chicago: University of Chicago Press.

CHAPTER

4

SIX PATIENTS: GATEKEEPING AT ANYWHERE HOSPITAL ICU

MANY PARALLELS exist between managing the patient needing critical care and managing the resources of the ICU. Patient care management can therefore be used as a metaphor for ICU management. Just as the physiological functions of the critically ill patient may fluctuate dramatically, the patient load, case mix, and available staff also may fluctuate widely and unpredictably. Strategies or routines must be developed to cope with and reduce the impact of the fluctuations as much as possible. The goal is to create and maintain a degree of order in a dynamic environment where a great deal of uncertainty occurs (Thompson 1967). Well-established strategies or routines include surrounding the ICU with intermediate care units and step-down units to help smooth the flow of patients into and out of the ICU; maintaining redundant capacity in the recovery room, emergency room, and other units to temporarily absorb peak demand; avoiding block booking of elective cases to minimize the number of days with large numbers of admissions; and using downtime for training periods.

Other strategies, perhaps not as publicized, include disguising troughs in demand to protect against budget and staff cutbacks (i.e., keeping personnel busy all of the time to ensure enough resources for times of peak demand); diluting case mix with patients with less severe illnesses to hold beds open, preserve slack time, and temporarily slow admissions; and showing leniency in supervision of rules during downtime as a way of creating obligations for subordinates to respond energetically to an emergency (Thompson 1967).

In their general application, these routines are certainly not unique to hospital settings. Their effective use is situation dependent and requires the skills of an adept management. Ultimately, however, as with any organization, when demand overwhelms capacity, the ICU must ration services by diluting the level of care provided or by restricting access. In the words of James D. Thompson (1967), "Rationing is an unhappy solution . . . Yet some system of priorities for the allocation of capacity under adverse conditions is essential if a technology is to be instrumentally effective—if action is to be other than random." (p. 23)

The Challenge

The central purpose of this series of case studies is to simulate gatekeeping decision making, to show how decisions in the various "rounds" are interrelated, and to illustrate key resource allocation issues as they unfold over time. In particular, we will provide insight into how and why ICU gatekeeping diverges from the rational model of the organization. To this end, the decision rounds have been rigged, and many variables have been held constant so as not to distract from these key issues. As will be seen, the rounds have been constructed to limit the options of the decision makers. There are no step-down units, intermediate care units, or respiratory care units. Mechanical ventilators are not allowed on the regular floors.

ICU census is subject to fluctuation, the sources of which include random emergency admissions, admissions related to diseases with seasonal variation, and admissions from the operating room. Each of these sources of admissions can be cast as frequency curves. Over time, the net effect of the summation of these curves may produce a condition of empty beds, a high census lasting a relatively short time (a narrow peak), or a prolonged period of high census. Most of the following rounds assume the last condition, necessitating a state of high-level triage where the opportunities of placing overflow patients in the usual spots (e.g., postanesthesia care unit, emergency room, coronary care unit) are severely limited, and most of the patients currently in the ICU are receiving active therapy (Teres 1993).

Readers may wish to view the facts of the cases from the perspectives of the four decision makers (attending physician, triage officer, nurse manager, and hospital administrator) described at the beginning of the previous chapter. In Appendix E, we show how you can role play the rounds to simulate the decision-making process.

It is intended that the decision that is presented at the end of each round will be consistent with the organizational dynamics of Anywhere

Hospital and its ICU. The decision, however, may not be consistent with the guidelines, recommendations, and policies of the various professional societies and associations. The decision of the simulation reflects "what is," not necessarily "what should be," according to various professional society pronouncements. The reasoning of the decision makers, which in some instances can only be inferred, is presented in the rationale section and amplified in the discussion section. The rationale for the decision is more likely to be consistent with the political model of the organization than the rational model.

Conditions at the Beginning of Round 2: Hospital Characteristics, Admissions Policies, and Bed Disposition

Each hospital and ICU operate with a unique set of organizational characteristics and within a unique environment. A different set of characteristics could produce a different decision. Therefore, it is important to understand the organizational context of decision making.

Hospital Characteristics of Anywhere Hospital

Located in a metropolitan area with a population of 750,000, Anywhere Hospital is a 450-bed voluntary community teaching hospital affiliated with a medical school that is located in a distant city. Anywhere Hospital is considered the tertiary hospital of the region. No public (local government) hospitals operate in the area, but several nearby suburban hospitals do compete for patients, especially elective surgery patients. Many of the physicians on Anywhere Hospital's medical staff also are members of the staffs of these other hospitals. Anywhere Hospital has contracts with several HMOs in the region and has built up stable referral patterns.

Anywhere Hospital has a 12-bed medical-surgical ICU serving patients over 17 years of age. In addition, it has a pediatric ICU, neonatal ICU, and a CCU. It has no step-down units. The policy of Anywhere Hospital, based on nursing requirements, is that patients on mechanical ventilation must be cared for in the ICU and not on the regular floors. The exception is for a ventilator patient for whom a DNR order has been written. In such a case, the patient may be transferred to a special bed on one of the floors.

The medical-surgical ICU is jointly managed by medicine and nursing and is overseen by a critical care committee composed of members from the departments of medicine and surgery. The unit has a part-time, paid medical director who is an intensivist and is part of a critical care medicine group that provides coverage of the unit on a consultative basis. The medical director serves as triage officer on a rotating basis along with members of the group and community attending physicians. The organizational arrangements for admission, discharge, and triage decision making can be considered semi-closed (see Exhibit 2.8).

Nursing staff includes a nurse manager, assistant nurse manager, RNs, and a unit secretary. The unit is staffed with nurse-to-patient ratios of 1:2, and on occasion, 1:3. The unit also is served by residents on a critical care medicine rotation. In general, the medical director can be considered a working medical director.

Policies and Guidelines: Admission-Discharge, Triage, Medical Futility

The admissions and discharge policies adopted by the Critical Care Committee of Anywhere Hospital medical staff are presented in Exhibit 4.1. In general, in Anywhere Hospital, any physician can admit a patient provided that the patient meets admission criteria. When the ICU is full, it is the responsibility of the triage officer to decide on admission and discharge. However, the admitting physician remains the primary or personal physician and is principally responsible for directing treatment.

Although not part of the official admissions policies, the Critical Care Committee has made available to the medical staff various guidelines on admission, discharge, and triage (see Appendix A).

It should be pointed out that at least one of these guidelines, SCCM Consensus Statement on the Triage of Critically Ill Patients (1994b), comes with the following disclaimer, "No portion of this statement is offered or intended as legal advice for any of the matters discussed. Competent legal counsel should be consulted as appropriate for specific cases involving these issues." It should also be pointed out that, like many hospitals, Anywhere Hospital has no official policy or definition of medical futility.

Description of Patients and Disposition of Beds at the Beginning of Round 2 (See Exhibit 4.2)

Bed 1. Open for patient admission
Bed 2. Open for patient admission
Beds 3–8. High-benefit patients (good prognosis). The NIH Consensus Development Conference Panel (1983) includes in this category:

> ... the patient with acute reversible disease for whom the probability of survival without ICU intervention is low, but the survival probability with such

> **Exhibit 4.1** Admission and Discharge Criteria
>
> Admission Criteria
>
> *Intensive Care Unit*
> 1. Patients requiring mechanical ventilation for respiratory or ventilatory failure.
> 2. Patients requiring intravascular and/or invasive hemodynamic monitoring.
> 3. Patients with cardiogenic, septic, hypovolemic, or other types of shock.
> 4. Patients who have undergone successful cardiopulmonary resuscitation.
> 5. Patients who must receive intravenous vasoactive medications.
> 6. Patients requiring massive transfusions.
> 7. High-risk surgical patients who require preoperative physiologic assessment and/or management.
> 8. Postoperative patients who require mechanical ventilation, hemodynamic monitoring, intensive nursing care, or surgical monitoring.
> 9. Patients with impending respiratory/ventilatory failure who need intensive medical management to prevent intubation.
> 10. Patients with drug intoxications who either satisfy the above criteria or need intensive medical care for detoxification and/or treatment.
> 11. Patients undergoing diagnostic and therapeutic procedures that, for the individual patient, can logistically only be safely performed in the ICU. These include endoscopy, bronchoscopy, dialysis, continuous arterio-venous ultrafiltration, pacemaker insertion, thrombolytic therapy, etc.
> 12. Patients with metabolic, endocrine, or electrolyte abnormalities requiring close physician and nursing surveillance and care, such as diabetic ketoacidosis, hyperosmolar states, severe dehydration, hypothermia, hyperthermia, etc.
>
> Discharge Criteria
>
> Patients will be discharged from the ICU when the criteria for admission are no longer present (i.e., the patient has improved, or the patient's condition has deteriorated to the extent that he/she has no medically reversible condition). In the latter event, the patient will be transferred to an appropriate floor where comfort care will be continued.

interventions is high. Common clinical examples include that patient with acute reversible respiratory failure due to drug overdose, or with cardiac conduction disturbances resulting in cardiovascular collapse but amenable to pacemaker therapy. Because survival for many of these patients without such life-support interventions is uncommon, the observed high survival rates constitute unequivocal evidence of reduced mortality for this category of ICU patients. These patients clearly benefit from ICU care (NIH 1983, p. 2).

How might these patients be characterized in terms of widely supported admission and discharge criteria? Start with the description, "probability of survival without ICU intervention is low, but the survival probability with such interventions is high." This formulation can be symbolized as P(S/No ICU) is low; P(S/ICU) is high with P indicating probability and S indicating survival at least to hospital discharge (Mulley 1984). For these patients there is also a requirement for immediate action. Life is at stake here; death is imminent without ICU intervention. The criterion of interest is "urgency of need," (i.e., preventing death by treating urgent cases first). Others in less urgent condition can wait until another bed opens up (Kilner 1990).

The patients described above (e.g., a patient with acute reversible respiratory failure due to drug overdose), by virtue of ICU intervention, not only have a high probability or likelihood of survival, they have a high likelihood of benefiting in terms of quality of life and length of life, two additional criteria. The AMA Council of Ethical and Judicial Affairs (1995), in "Ethical Considerations in the Allocation of Organs and Other Scarce Medical Resources Among Patients" recommends that quality of life improvements be measured by comparing functional status with and without intervention. The AMA Council believes that defining quality of life in terms of functional status will allow more objective comparisons between patients competing for the same beds than the use of quality-adjusted life-years (QALYs). On the other hand, duration or length of benefit is more unambiguously measured.

The patients in beds 3 through 8, in whom the potential to benefit is clearly recognized, can be contrasted to a patient where the potential to benefit is very limited (i.e., the patient in bed 9).

Bed 9. Multi-organ failure patient (poor prognosis). Because of the progressive deterioration of organ function, this patient needs the life-sustaining interventions of the ICU. Without them he would die. On the other hand, in terms of leaving the hospital alive: P(S/No ICU) is low; P(S/ICU) is low. Also, the prognosis in terms of improvement in quality of life or in length of life is poor: P(quality of life/No ICU) is low; P(quality of life/ICU) is low, and P(duration of benefit/No ICU) is low, P(duration of benefit/ICU) is low.

Beds 10–11. Monitor patients: potentially high-benefit patients. The NIH Consensus Development Conference (1983) includes in this category:

> ... patients admitted to the ICU, not because they are critically ill, but because they are at risk of becoming critically ill. The purposes of intensive care in these instances are to prevent a serious complication or to allow a prompt response to any complication that may occur. It is presumed that the prompt response to a potentially fatal complication made possible by continuous monitoring plus the concentration of specialized personnel in the ICU increases the probability

of a favorable outcome. The risk of complication may be high (as in the patient with an acute myocardial infarction and complex ventricular ectopy) or low (as in the patient with myocardial infarction suspected because of chest pain in the absence of electrocardiographic abnormalities). Also, the differences in probability of a favorable outcome following a complication inside rather than outside the ICU may be large (as in the patient with postcraniotomy intracranial bleeding) or small (as in the patient with gastrointestinal bleeding). The strength of evidence supporting the effectiveness of the ICU varies with the probability of a complication and with the difference in expected outcome inside and outside the ICU. When the risk of complication is high and the potential gain large, a decrease in mortality is likely. Similarly, when the risk is low and the potential gain is small, an observable decrease in mortality is unlikely. These patients are not likely to benefit from ICU care (p. 3).

For the particular patients in beds 10 and 11, the risk of complication is high and the probability of a favorable outcome by virtue of being in the ICU, as opposed to not being in the ICU, is also high. It should be pointed out that most monitor patients do not go on to have a complication or to need specific ICU therapy.

Bed 12. Closed bed. Although the official ICU bed complement stated on the hospital's operating certificate may be fixed by state regulation, the number of beds actually available for patients may fluctuate. The licensed bed capacity of the ICU is 12 beds, but an administrative decision was made to staff only 11 of these beds. This decision was made because of difficulties in finding a sufficient number of qualified, full-time critical care nurses to staff the beds on a permanent basis.

Round 2: The Smoker Patient

The ICU staff consider:

> . . . an eighty-five-year-old male with a fifty-year history of cigarette smoking and chronic pulmonary disease who has a baseline dyspnea on climbing four or five stairs or on 100 yards of ambulation. Seven days ago he was admitted to the hospital with pneumococcal pneumonia. Since then, despite antibiotics, he has continued to worsen with a persistent cough and progressive hypercapnia. His doctors now believe that he will die without aggressive care including intubation for a period of approximately three weeks. Even if this approach is attempted, his likelihood of survival is only 10 percent. (Blendon et al. 1993, p. 200).

Two beds in the ICU are open (See Exhibit 4.2). *Should the patient be admitted?*

96 *Gatekeeping in the Intensive Care Unit*

Exhibit 4.2 12-Bed Medical/Surgical ICU

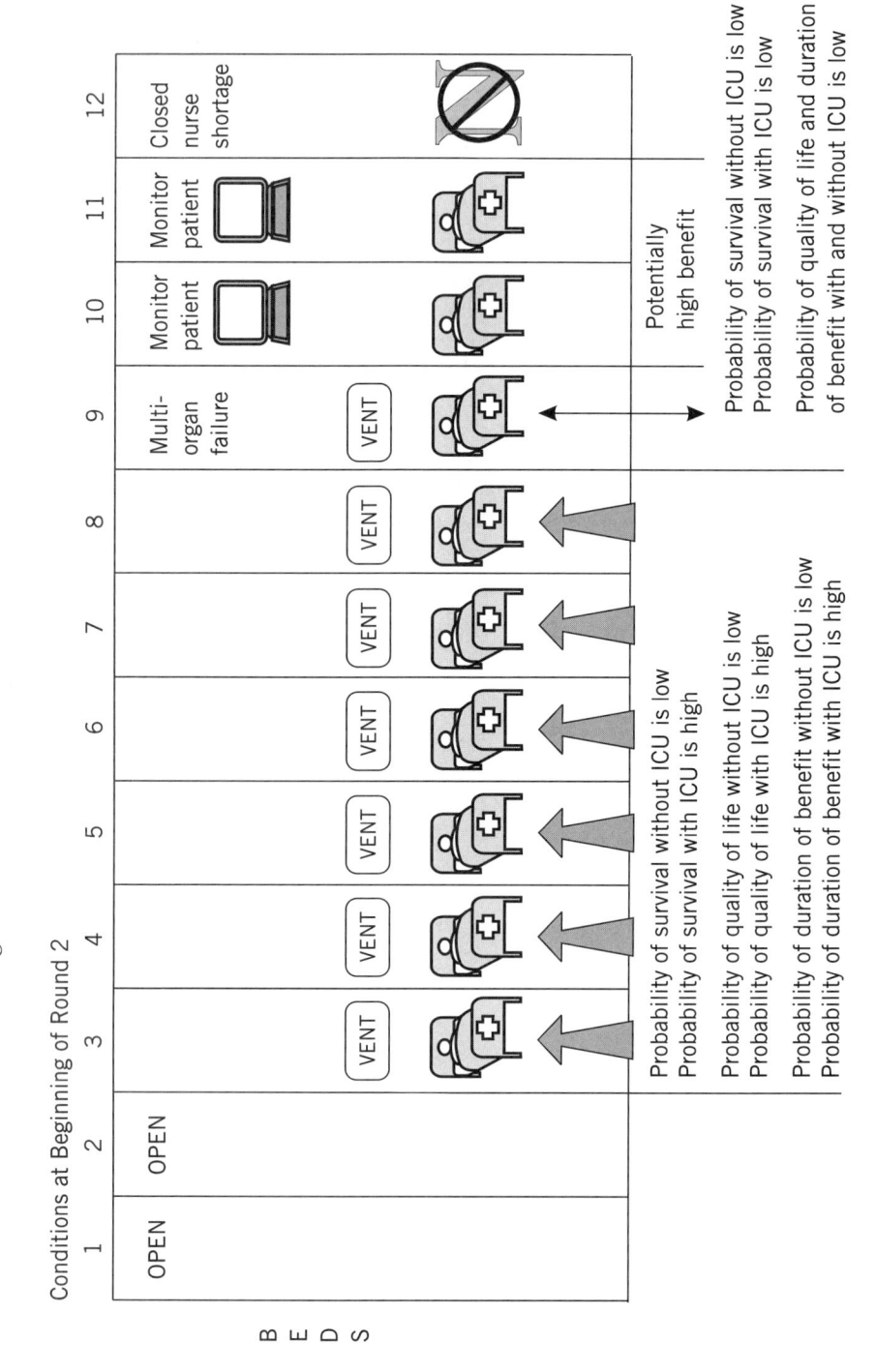

Conditions at Beginning of Round 2

	1	2	3	4	5	6	7	8	9	10	11	12
	OPEN	OPEN	VENT	VENT	VENT	VENT	VENT	VENT	Multi-organ failure VENT	Monitor patient	Monitor patient	Closed nurse shortage

B
E
D
S

Probability of survival without ICU is low
Probability of survival with ICU is high
Probability of quality of life without ICU is low
Probability of quality of life with ICU is high
Probability of duration of benefit without ICU is low
Probability of duration of benefit with ICU is high

Probability of survival without ICU is low
Probability of survival with ICU is low
Probability of quality of life and duration of benefit with and without ICU is low

Potentially high benefit

Round 2 Decision: Admit the Smoker

Rationale
This patient clearly meets the official admission criteria (i.e., admit patients requiring mechanical ventilation for respiratory failure).

Discussion
Although it is highly likely that this patient would be admitted to most United States ICUs, it is not clear that he would be admitted to ICUs in other nations. The vignette described in this round was constructed for use in the "Three Nation Physician Survey" (Blendon et al. 1993) in which physicians were asked to estimate the likelihood of such a patient receiving aggressive care in the hospital where the physician works or where most of his/her patients are hospitalized. The estimates are presented in Exhibit 4.3.

Although the vignette included information on the likelihood of survival (i.e., P(S/No ICU) is low; P(S/ICU) is 10 percent), no information was given on the quality of life or duration of benefit. However, many of these types of patients require long-term ventilation and tracheostomy. Some may not be able to go home to independent living.

It is interesting to speculate on the reasons for national differences. Perhaps U.S. physicians place a different value on a 10 percent chance of survival or on the importance of heeding the patient's or surrogate's wishes. Or perhaps they or their patients place a different value on the length and quality of life assuming survival. Perhaps there is also a strong feeling that age alone should not be a reason for denying admission.

Values may be shaped by the relative supply of ICU beds. Canada, for example, has fewer ICU beds per capita than the United States. Rapoport et al. (1995), in comparing western Massachusetts to Alberta, Canada, found that there were 24 adult ICU beds per 100,000 population in

---

Exhibit 4.3 Likelihood of Admission

Physician Response	United States	Canada	Germany
Very likely	53%	27%	22%
Somewhat likely	26	23	32
Somewhat unlikely	9	15	19
Very unlikely	3	17	5
Not applicable	4	15	8
Not sure	4	4	14

Source: Blendon et al. 1993 (p. 200).

western Massachusetts and 16 per 100,000 population in Alberta. Jacobs and Noseworthy (1990) estimate that ICU utilization in the United States is 2.5 times that of Canada, 108 patient days/1,000 population versus 42 patient days/1,000 population. One difference is that Canadian ICUs do not admit as many elderly, chronically ill patients. However, it is difficult to draw any conclusions regarding the appropriateness of the different utilization rates between the United States and Canada (Jacobs and Noseworthy 1990; Rapoport et al. 1995).

Large variations exist in the supply of certain large-scale technologies whose availability increases the demand for ICU services. For example, the number of open-heart surgery units per million are United States, 3.7; Canada, 1.3; Germany, 0.8. The number of cardiac catheterization units per million are United States, 6.4; Canada, 2.3; Germany, 3.4 (Rublee 1994). Again, it is difficult to draw any conclusions about the appropriateness or inappropriateness of such distributions.

In another international comparison, albeit of limited sample size, Rie examined severity-adjusted mortality data collected by Shabot et al. (1992) comparing patients in a large Los Angeles ICU with patients in several French ICUs. It was found that at higher intensity levels of illness, a significantly higher death rate occurred in the French ICUs. Rie (1995a) attributes the difference to French public expenditure policy, which limits the capacity of hospitals to acquire technology and labor. In France, ICUs are more likely to operate in the triage mode and implicitly ration without benefit of a formal public articulation of the consequences of resource limits. On the other hand, Rie also notes, "The fact that individuals survive to leave an ICU does not mean that they will be alive to benefit from the fruits of a quality of life that would have made such survival worthwhile" (p. 30).

Age, Mechanical Ventilation, and Chance of Survival

In most clinical reports, the age of the patient is given. But what does a patient's age have to do with decision making? While older people, from an actuarial perspective, have a lower life expectancy than younger people, caution must be exercised in using age as a predictor of individual mortality. Most studies show that age alone is not a reliable predictor of outcome for ICU patients. However, age in combination with other factors may provide useful information for decision makers. For example, Cohen, Lambrinos, and Fein (1993) retrospectively studied patients over 80 years of age who spent at least three days on mechanical ventilators in a medical-surgical ICU in Ellis Hospital. Ellis, a 420-bed, tertiary referral, university-affiliated community teaching hospital is located in

Schenectady, NY. The researchers found that when age (A) plus duration in days on the mechanical ventilator (D) was equal to or greater than one hundred [(A + D) = or >100], the chances of survival until discharge from the hospital were less than 10 percent.

This formula or post hoc, rule-of-thumb index is instructive because it shows that patients' probabilities for survival change over time. After a certain point, the number of days on the mechanical ventilator, perhaps associated with decreasing functioning of the respiratory and other organ systems, is inversely related to the chances of survival. As was pointed out in Chapter 2, a small percentage of patients consume a disproportionate amount of resources, which almost always include mechanical ventilation. Rie comments on the bi-modal distribution of resource consumption in the ICU:

> One mode is characterized by short term use of intensive care with physiologic support and monitoring where biologic healing of the host patient is highly probable. These resource allocations tend to be much cheaper per capita than for the second mode. The second mode is characterized by individuals with multiple organ dysfunction and chronic infirmities often associated with advanced age in which there has been an elective decision to perform heroic life-saving procedures which circumscribe and develop the "definition of the need" for intensive care. Once the patient enters the intensive care cycle there is a medical culture rather than a proven outcome assessment of technology usage that compels physicians to apply invasive technology which may then lead to secondary iatrogenic complications. The result in the second mode is a group of individuals who consume many resources over several weeks or months who have statistically poor prognosis that may culminate in death or serious disability (Rie, 1995b, p. 29).

Is the smoker patient about to embark on an ICU stay that would place him in the second mode of intensive care?

Round 3: The Bleeder Patient

Dr. A requests ICU admission for his patient who is in the ER with a diagnosis of acute gastrointestinal (GI) hemorrhage. Although no evidence exists of active hemorrhage, Dr. A wants his patient monitored in the ICU. The patient is at low risk for developing a life-threatening recurrence of GI bleeding. The nurse manager considers the legitimacy of the request marginal at best. What Dr. A is really worried about is the lack of adequate nursing coverage on the floor.

Although Dr. A has valid concerns about the nursing coverage on the floors, and although a case could be made that the patient would meet the admission criteria, he probably would not seek admission if no bed were available. Dr. A is known to "play ball" with the ICU. For example, when occupancy pressure is high, Dr. A can always be counted on to be accommodating during triage; he will quickly move his patients when other physicians might resist.

The patient in this case would probably require low-intensity nursing coverage. The prognosis is P(S/No ICU) is high; P(S/ICU) is high. Should the bleeder patient be admitted to the ICU?

The disposition of beds is presented in Exhibit 4.4.

■　■　■　■　■

Round 3 Decision: Admit the Bleeder Patient

Rationale

The patient took up the last open bed in the ICU. In addition to admitting patients who are critically ill, one of the purposes of critical care medicine is to admit patients who are at risk of becoming critically ill to prevent or minimize serious complication. However, some question remains whether the bleeder patient is really at sufficient risk of developing a life-threatening condition, thus meeting the eligibility criteria for admission. On the other hand, given an open bed, this was an easy decision. Unlike the transfer patient decision in Chapter 1, no pressing need existed for the involvement of the administrator or the triage officer. There was no perceived crisis requiring a task force–like assembly of staff.

The nurse manager saw advantages to admitting the patient. To begin with, the patient would not stretch nursing services. In fact, nurses would get a breather because the admission would bring the ICU up to full capacity, thus blocking the immediate admission of other, perhaps sicker, patients. In effect, the ICU would become closed "de-facto," requiring the automatic involvement of the triage officer in the next admission decision. Also, the newly admitted patient could easily be discharged at any time.

In this round the nurse manager, carrying out a screening function, was not operating in the triage mode of decision making. If there were no beds available, the patient would have been denied admission. Even in the non-triage mode and with bed availability, the nurse, triage officer, or administrator could have made a case for denying admission if there were appropriate criteria. A denial would have sent a signal that gates of the ICU would be defended through strict adherence to the admission criteria. But the nurse manager had different objectives. She wanted to

Six Patients: Gatekeeping At Anywhere Hospital ICU **101**

Exhibit 4.4 12-Bed Medical/Surgical ICU

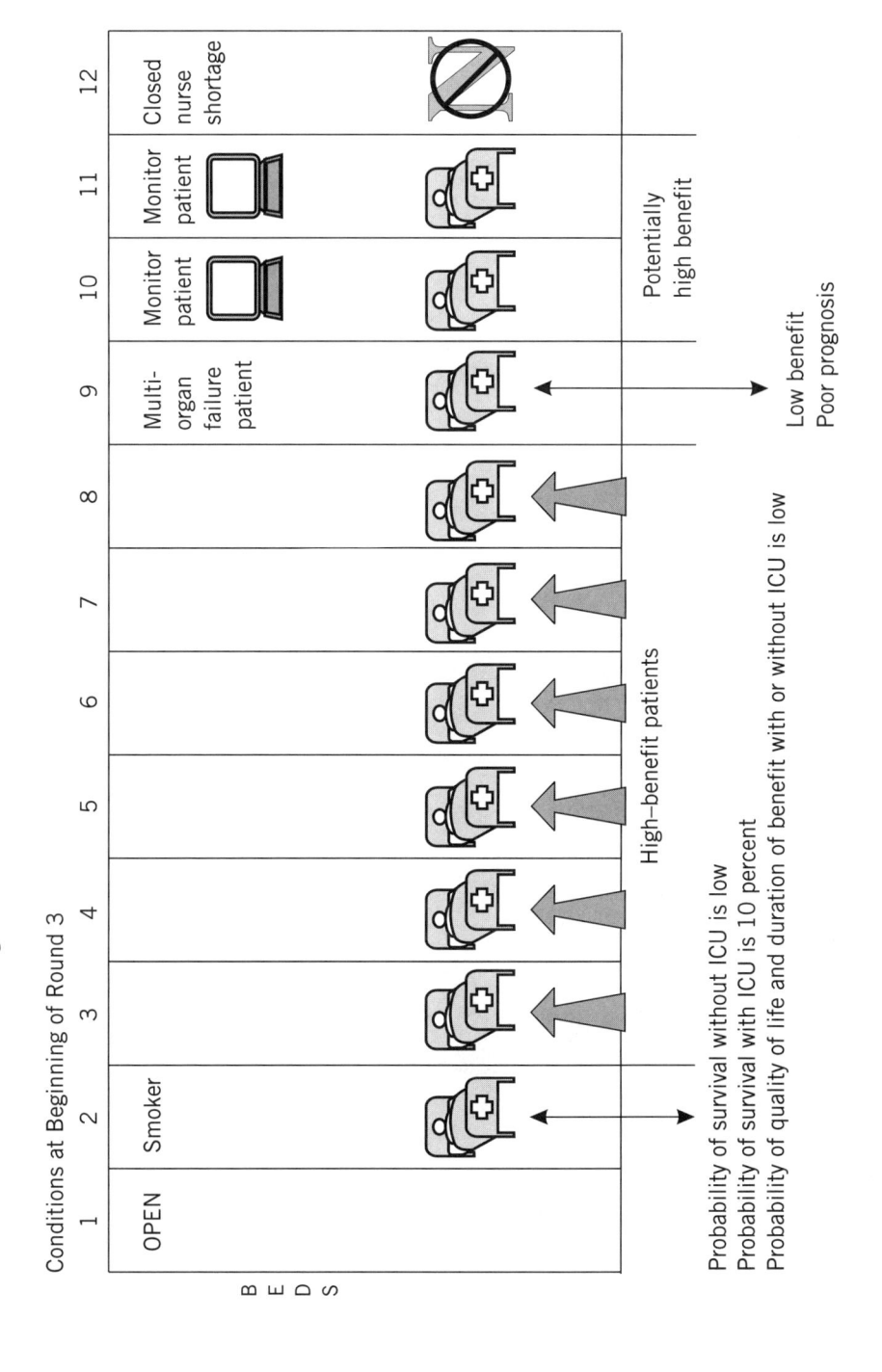

Conditions at Beginning of Round 3

	1	2	3	4	5	6	7	8	9	10	11	12
	OPEN	Smoker							Multi-organ failure patient	Monitor patient	Monitor patient	Closed nurse shortage

B
E
D
S

High-benefit patients (beds 3–8)

Low benefit / Poor prognosis (bed 9)

Potentially high benefit (beds 10–11)

Probability of survival without ICU is low
Probability of survival with ICU is 10 percent
Probability of quality of life and duration of benefit with or without ICU is low

satisfy an accommodating physician who would no doubt return the favor in a timely manner. This arrangement is part of the informal negotiated order of the hospital (Strauss, Schatzman, Ehrlich 1963). Furthermore, she wanted to send a signal to the rest of the hospital that the ICU was now full, and allow the nursing staff a little bit of a breather. With a broader perspective, the administration would have pursued objectives different than the nurse manager's had it known the facts of the case. Perhaps in a managed care plan, administrators and plan sponsors would have a greater incentive to monitor utilization.

Discussion

As opposed to the issues of screening out the "too sick," which were raised in Round 1 (Chapter 1) and to a certain extent in Round 2, the decision in Round 3 involves a patient who may be "too well" to be admitted to the ICU. Rapoport et al. (1995), in comparing the outcomes of patients hospitalized with acute GI hemorrhage in Alberta, Canada, to patients in western Massachusetts, note that 22 percent of the Americans were admitted to the ICU as opposed to 5 percent of the Canadians. There was no difference in survival, indicating that these patients might be safely cared for outside the ICU setting. In Alberta, patients were evaluated and treated in the emergency department where endoscopy could be performed and blood given. Major GI bleeders would go to surgery and to the ICU if still unstable.

Can a prognostic instrument be designed to accurately predict those low-risk patients not likely to benefit from ICU monitoring? Kollef, Canfield, and Zuckerman (1995) suggest that a system of risk stratification applied at the time of admission could be developed to predict the outcomes of patients hospitalized with acute GI hemorrhage. Such a system, if appropriately validated, could be incorporated into ICU admission criteria to help reduce unnecessary admissions.

Round 4A: The Elective Surgery Patient

Dr. B, a surgeon, informs the operating room staff of his intention to perform major elective surgery on his 65-year-old patient and requests time in the operating room schedule. In processing this request and assigning a time slot, the operating room clerk alerts the recovery room, or PACU, and the ICU. The patient will require postoperative care in the ICU. This would be an urgent, although predictable, admission. Postoperatively, the probability of survival with ICU is high and without ICU is moderate. The nurse manager of the ICU informs the clerk that no beds are available in the ICU. Theoretically, the triage officer, with the approval of administration, could require the postponement of elective surgery. Given its competition with other hospitals, administration would like to remain attractive to admitting physicians performing elective surgery. Dr. B admits a large number of patients to the hospital, is a big revenue producer for the hospital, and has the backing of the Department of Surgery. No beds in the ICU are open (see Exhibit 4.5). Should elective surgery be postponed?

■ ■ ■ ■ ■

Round 4A Decision: Do Not Request the Postponement of Elective Surgery

Rationale
Although the triage officer could use his authority to force the administration to officially postpone elective surgery, it would be a very unpopular course of action. Practically speaking, postponement would be very difficult to achieve given the influence of the surgeon and the Department of Surgery. The expectation is that a bed will somehow be made available. After weighing the consequences, the triage officer decides that it is not worthwhile to press for postponement, especially if he knows that the bleeder patient is easily dischargeable.

The triage officer is prepared to stretch the ICU capacity by temporarily keeping the elective surgery patient in the PACU. During this time he will continue to triage.

Discussion
Admission decisions are not made at the gates of the ICU in isolation of other events in the hospital. Many admission decisions are really made "upstream" when it is decided to operate on the patient. There are other examples. In Round 1 (Chapter 1), the admission of the transfer patient to the hospital for cardiac catheterization and almost certain destabilization was tantamount to admitting the patient to the ICU. In cases where patients are intubated in the emergency room or on the regular floors, ICU admission and mechanical ventilation usually follow.

Exhibit 4.5 12-Bed Medical/Surgical ICU

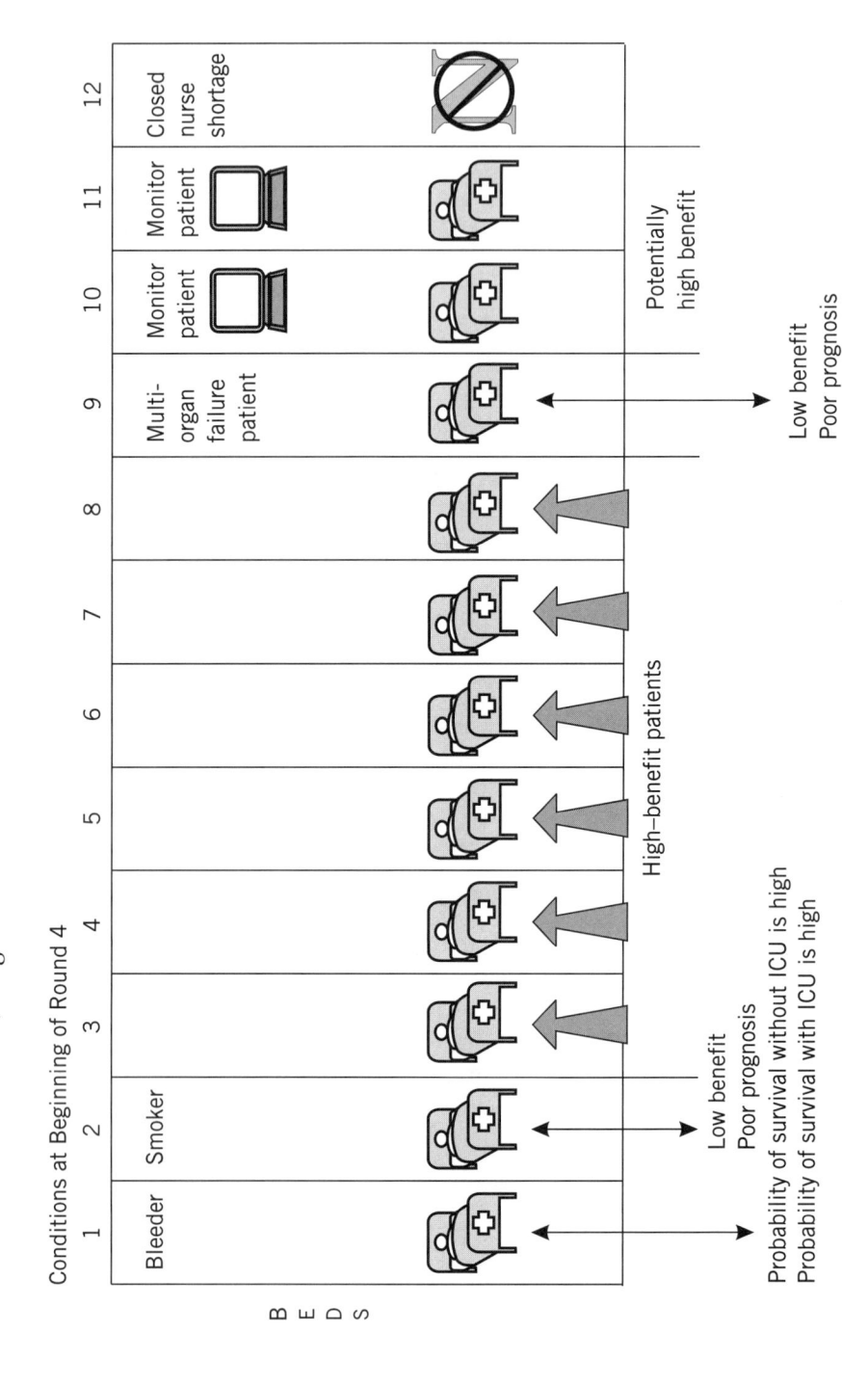

Conditions at Beginning of Round 4

	1	2	3	4	5	6	7	8	9	10	11	12
	Bleeder	Smoker							Multi-organ failure patient	Monitor patient	Monitor patient	Closed nurse shortage

B
E
D
S

← Low benefit, Poor prognosis (beds 1–2)

← High-benefit patients (beds 3–8)

→ Low benefit, Poor prognosis (bed 9)

→ Potentially high benefit (beds 10–11)

Probability of survival without ICU is high
Probability of survival with ICU is high

Round 4B: The Elective Surgery Patient and the Multi-Organ Failure Patient

The staff of PACU is requesting immediate admission to the ICU for the 65-year-old man recovering from an operation. Because the beds are filled, the triage officer has been called to help make the decision.

The PACU staff has informed the nurse manager, the triage officer, and indirectly the administration, that any delay would put the patient at risk for more serious complications. However, according to some of the ICU nurses, the PACU has had a history of "crying wolf." On the other hand, the PACU staff has long suspected the ICU of harboring dischargeable patients and in fact knows about the bleeder patient. The PACU's agenda is different than that of the ICU. The PACU staff is interested in maintaining the operating room schedule and clearing out the PACU.

Prior to the current decision round, the nurse manager had mentioned to the triage officer that the multi-organ failure patient (irreversible dysfunction of at least two organ systems) in bed 9 was severely ill and that he would be a good candidate for a DNR order and a terminal wean off the ventilator (turning down the ventilator setting) and could be moved to a special unit for such patients. The patient, after undergoing surgery to alleviate the acute phase of a chronic condition, was admitted for postoperative care. Over time the patient deteriorated. The patient is an 85-year-old man who has been on the mechanical ventilator for 15 days. The nurse manager said that caring for terminally ill patients like this was demoralizing to the nursing staff.

The triage officer, based on his experience with such patients and based on the literature, believed that the chances of survival to hospital discharge for this patient were negligible, although he could hang on for many days or even weeks. The discharge policies state, "Patients will be discharged from the ICU when the criteria for admission are no longer present (i.e., . . . the patient has deteriorated to the extent that he/she has no medically reversible condition)." However, the surgeon, a frequent admitter to the hospital, told the family that, based on his experience, there was a chance of survival to hospital discharge and not to give up hope. Should the elective surgery patient be admitted and, if so, to which bed?

■   ■   ■   ■   ■

Round 4B Decision: Admit the Elective Surgery Patient

Rationale

It is decided to admit the elective survery patient from the PACU. The bleeder patient is prepared for discharge to the floor. The multi-organ failure patient remained in the ICU. The ICU staff, on the word of the PACU staff that the elective surgery patient required immediate admission, moved quickly to open up a bed by discharging the bleeder patient back to the floor as per the understanding with his physician.

Although the triage officer and the nurse manager agreed that the multi-organ failure patient met the discharge criteria and would never make it out of the ICU alive, their arguments did not prevail nor did they push their position very hard. Once a patient is admitted, it is difficult to discontinue intervention. Furthermore, the lack of agreement by the surgeon (i.e., the attending physician) meant that the patient would remain. As Zussman (1992) points out, the achievement of consensus is often required to produce enough certainty to withdraw treatment. The dissent of a single physician frequently introduces enough uncertainty to block withdrawal.

The nurse manager was concerned about the possible nursing turnover that could result from a demoralized staff. Nevertheless, the surgeon, a frequent admitter to the hospital and in whom the patient's family had faith, prevailed. Because the bleeder patient could be moved out to make way for the elective surgery patient, there was not a great deal of controversy.

Discussion

Patients may have different combinations of organ dysfunction and may progress to the "multiple organ failure syndrome." Beal and Cerra (1994) note that the syndrome is often the final complication of a critical illness. With mortality rates well over 50 percent, it now accounts for most deaths in non-coronary intensive care units. The average length of stay once the syndrome develops is 21 days.

What about the 85-year-old patient on the mechanical ventilator? He was operated on to alleviate the acute phase of a chronic illness. In hindsight, the wisdom of subjecting the patient to a surgical procedure is questionable. Nevertheless, at the time of ICU admission and at the beginning of mechanical ventilation, both the surgeon and the triage officer agreed on a reasonable chance of survival to hospital discharge. Over time chances of survival diminish. In this case, the triage officer and the nurse manager thought the chances had diminished to the point where they would recommend to the family withdrawal of life support or the writing of a DNR order. The surgeon disagreed, however. Why? Perhaps the surgeon was not familiar with the literature or had limited experience with this type of patient. On the other hand, even if there is enough information to establish probabilities and confidence intervals, there is no way of being certain for any single patient, because there is always the possibility of falling outside a statistical confidence limit.

Other possible reasons for the disagreement exist. Perhaps the surgeon placed a different value on what others considered to be only a very small chance of survival and the resulting quality of life. Or perhaps the surgeon was simply reluctant to face the family or himself with the facts.

The surgeon may have been attempting to keep the patient alive for a minimum of 30 days so that a postoperative death (i.e., survival of less than 30 days) would not count on his record. Taking a less cynical view, it is possible that the preoperative surgeon-patient discussion and the resulting informed consent document reflected an understanding that the surgeon would push to get the patient through the postoperative phase, usually defined as up to 30 days. In other words, the patient has agreed not only to the operation but to the postoperative course. The triage officer and the bedside nurse are not always appreciative of these preoperative understandings. The patient may not have bargained for a major complication such as renal failure and dialysis or a stroke. The patient could change his mind, but it may be difficult to override the surgeon's understanding of the preoperative consent. In the long run, the patient could regain kidney function and neurological function.

Theoretically, a potential resolution to the divergence of opinions among providers would be to present the family with a more objective determination of the prognosis and let them decide whether the chance is worth taking. The issue is, of course, how to objectively determine prognosis, especially when a difference exists in clinical opinion, and how to structure the decision so the family can have input. Typically, physicians, as demonstrated by the 1995 Study to Understand Prognoses and Preferences for Outcomes and Risks of Treatments (SUPPORT) and other studies, have not done a good job in communicating with patients about these issues. Even if there is agreement on prognosis, studies have shown wide variability among ICU physicians and nurses in their attitudes and values regarding withdrawal of treatment (Cook et al. 1995), which cannot help but influence patients and surrogates on their treatment options.

Withdrawing Care: The Experience of Two ICUs

Most medical ethicists and physicians agree that life support can be withdrawn when it is unwanted or futile. Lee et al. (1994) describe the interaction between physicians, patients, and families regarding the withdrawal of care in the 16-bed medical ICU (MICU) located in Rochester (NY) General Hospital, a 550-bed community teaching hospital. The unit was supervised by attendings certified in critical care medicine. They distinguished between reasons for withdrawal: (1) when physicians believed that hospital survival was impossible, even if all ICU interventions were continued; and (2) when patients believed that the outcome of ICU intervention would lead to an unacceptable quality of life, even if hospital discharge was possible. They studied 28 patients who agreed (or their families agreed) to withdrawal of care.

Discussions leading to withdrawal of care occurred over a period of about five days. In 21 out of 28 cases, time-limited therapeutic trials were used to see if interventions would be effective. Once life-sustaining interventions were withdrawn, patients stayed about one and one half days in the MICU before being transferred to the general medical floor. Fourteen patients died within 24 hours of the withdrawal of life-sustaining interventions. No patient with a prognosis of "probability of survival-to-discharge = 0" survived to leave the hospital. However, four of the other patients were discharged alive from the hospital, although this was not an outcome desired by patients or family.

Lee et al. concluded that, "finding an accommodation between physician judgments and patient preferences took time and effort but was an effective means of limiting ineffective life-sustaining efforts" (p. 1358). They also stated:

> Although patients' personal physicians usually attended their care in the MICU and often participated in discussions with their patients, in all cases MICU attendings were also involved in the decision-making process. We believed that a process of shared decision making was facilitated by the presence of critical care clinicians who were familiar with and willing to address the ethical and clinical issues in question. Moreover, their availability in the MICU made it possible to hold repeated and often lengthy discussions with patients and families (p. 1360).

In the second study, Campbell and Frank (1997) describe the ten-year experience of a Comprehensive Supportive Care Team established in 1986 at Detroit Receiving Hospital, a 350-bed Level I emergency trauma hospital serving mostly an indigent population. Over 90 percent of the hospital's admissions are through the emergency department. The Comprehensive Supportive Care Team is directed by an Advanced Practice

Nurse in collaborative practice with staff physicians. As an alternative to intensive care for hopelessly ill patients (e.g., patients with severe neurologic dysfunction or with multiple organ failure), the team provides comfort care, also referred to as palliative care, designed to relieve pain and other symptoms. By meeting the physical and psychosocial comfort needs of patients and families, the team cared for patients in private rooms on the general floors with minimal intervention, thus reducing the number of ICU days and the intensity of service (Field, Delvich, and Carlson 1989). The purpose of establishing the team, which takes on primary responsibility for managing the patients until death or to discharge (mostly to hospice care), was to optimize end-of-life care. The team has managed more than 1,400 dying patients and their families. Another purpose, according to Campbell and Frank (1997), "was to promote another triage option for the medical ICU allowing the medical ICU to vacate some beds for the most severely ill who could benefit from a high-intensity therapeutic plan." (p. 199)

Over its ten-year history, the team has seen a dramatic increase in the withdrawal of mechanical ventilation and artificial nourishment for those patients referred to the team receiving these life-sustaining interventions. In 1986, only 10 percent of the patients with mechanical ventilation and no patients with artificial nourishment had these services withdrawn. By 1995, the percentages had increased to 65 percent and 20 percent, respectively.

DNR Orders in the ICU

Cardiopulmonary resuscitation (CPR) is the restoration of heartbeat and/or breathing through medical intervention. It goes without saying that every person experiences cardiac arrest at some point in the dying process. Therefore, decisions about CPR and DNR are potentially relevant for every patient. A DNR order is a medical order issued by a physician to withhold CPR in the event of a cardiopulmonary arrest. In many instances, especially with a frail, elderly hospitalized patient already suffering from underlying chronic illness, the success of CPR in enabling the patient to survive to leave the hospital is minimal. Or it may only partially succeed, leaving the patient brain damaged or otherwise impaired. To some patients, CPR can be a particularly painful procedure. Because of these factors, many patients prefer to forgo CPR and choose to have their physicians write DNR orders. On any given day, according to the SCCM survey, from 6 percent to 12 percent of the patients in ICUs have DNR orders (Groeger et al. 1993).

A DNR order should not be construed to mean "do-not-treat" (i.e., consent to withhold CPR does not imply consent to withhold other life-sustaining interventions). It may be entirely appropriate to continue full therapy or a trial of aggressive treatment on patients for whom DNR orders have been written. It is not unusual, however, for the DNR decision to precede the withdrawal of life-sustaining interventions (e.g., mechanical ventilation, vasopressor for blood pressure support, antibiotics, antiarrhythmic agents, and artificial nutrition and hydration).

Prendergast and Luce (1996) surveyed 126 ICUs associated with teaching programs in critical care medicine or pulmonary-critical care medicine and collected data on 71,513 admissions and 6,110 deaths (9 percent mortality rate). All deaths were classified as following one of five categories of treatment: (1) full ICU care including CPR, 25 percent; (2) full ICU care without CPR, 23 percent; (3) withholding of life support, 13 percent; (4) withdrawal of life support, 33 percent; or (5) declaration of brain death, 6 percent. The authors note considerable nationwide variation among ICUs.

It should be clear that dying in the ICU is not simply a matter of a yes/no decision. It is more realistic to think in terms of degrees of care ranging from "comfort care" to "full aggressive care." For example, in response to a scenario involving a 75-year-old woman in the ICU for ten days admitted with urosepsis who is now ventilator dependent, comatose, and in acute oliguric renal failure, the following options might be considered (Cook et al. 1995):

1. discontinue inotropes and mechanical ventilation but continue comfort measures;
2. discontinue inotropes and other maintenance therapy but continue mechanical ventilation and comfort measures;
3. continue with current management but add no new therapeutic intervention;
4. continue with current management, add further inotropes, change antibiotics and the like as needed, but do not start dialysis; or
5. continue with full aggressive management and plan for dialysis if necessary. (p. 704)

Patient and surrogate decision making regarding maximizing comfort versus maximizing life expectancy is influenced by a variety of factors, including religious and moral values. Economics also plays a role. Covinsky et al. (1996) found that a family's economic hardship resulting from the serious illness of a loved one was associated with a preference for comfort care over life-extending care.

Physicians are not always responsive to the wishes of patients and surrogates to limit or forgo treatment. SUPPORT (1995), a two-phase study conducted in five major teaching hospitals and involving more than

9,000 patients, confirmed substantial shortcomings in care for seriously ill hospitalized adults (overall six-month mortality rate approximately 50 percent) with regard to five specific outcomes: physician understanding of patient preferences; incidence and time of documentation of DNR orders; pain; time spent in an ICU, comatose, or receiving mechanical ventilation prior to death; and hospital resource use. The SUPPORT study researchers found:

> Only 47% of physicians knew when their patients preferred to avoid CPR; 46% of do-not-resuscitate (DNR) orders were written within 2 days of death; 38% of patients who died spent at least 10 days in an intensive care unit (ICU); and for 50% of conscious patients who died in the hospital, family members reported moderate to severe pain at least half the time (p. 159).

One interpretation of the findings is that patients receive more aggressive treatment than they desire (Annas 1995). Nurses may be placed in an untenable situation. In a survey by Asch (1996) of attitudes and practices toward care at the end of life, critical care nurses commented on the lack of physician responsiveness. One nurse stated:

> I have experienced tremendous frustration and anger with physicians who either stress the possibility of a good prognosis, giving false hope—or place their belief system above that of their patients. The physician spends 5 to 10 minutes each day with the patient and then leaves me to carry out his orders and deal with the patient and his/her family for 8 to 12 hours. I'm left with the dilemma of carrying out orders that I believe—and sometimes know—are not in the patient's best interest or what the patient or family has expressed as their desires (Asch 1996, pp. 1337–38).

In the second phase of the SUPPORT study, the researchers, guided by the hypothesis that better communication would improve decision making at the end of life, designed an intervention to overcome shortcomings in communications. The intervention called on specially trained nurses to make multiple contacts with the patient, family, physician, and hospital staff "to elicit preference, improve understanding of outcomes, encourage attention to pain control, and facilitate advance care planning and patient-physician communication." As part of the intervention, physicians received prognostic estimates on six-month survival, functional disability at two months, and outcomes of CPR. The researchers concluded that the intervention failed to improve care or patient outcomes. No improvement occurred in patient-physician communications; in the incidence or timing of written DNR orders; in physicians' knowledge of their patients' preferences not to be resuscitated; in the number of days spent in an ICU, receiving mechanical ventilation, or comatose before death; or in the levels of reported pain. There was also no reduction in the use of hospital resources.

Contrary to original expectations, the structured feedback of prognostic information coupled with the systematic encouragement of physician-patient communication proved insufficient to promote change in physician behavior and decision making at the end of life. Apparently more profound change must occur in organizational structure and culture. We will return to this topic in Chapters 5 and 6.

The Elective Surgery Patient: Boundaries and Interunit Coordination

Because they operate under different constraints, the PACU and the ICU have different perspectives and pursue different objectives even though they are system-linked but physically separate. The PACU, in addition to its concern about quality of care, is also interested in maintaining the operating room schedule. The ICU, in addition to its concern about quality of care, is interested in smoothing the flow of admissions. Obviously, there is some strategic misrepresentation of information on the urgency of admission and the real capacity of the ICU.

The image of crashing and defending boundaries is germane here. One could imagine the PACU nurse and the anesthesiologist probing broadly and repeatedly for weaknesses in the ICU gates and the ICU nurse director calling the Medical Director for defensive backup. Under barrages such as this it might be easier and less time consuming to admit the patient and discharge another one. In the Round 4 case, the bleeder patient was easily dischargeable. But what if an easily dischargeable patient were not available? Would a patient currently in the ICU, in greater need, be discharged? Would the hospital somehow care for all the patients including the newly admitted one with an overstretched staff? Or would enough slack exist in the system to comfortably handle everyone at least in the short term? These questions will be addressed in Rounds 5 and 6.

Other parts of the hospital can also play the same game. For example, in a tertiary hospital, it is not unusual for the emergency room to find out how many beds have been saved in the ICU for elective surgery (sometimes a closely guarded piece of information). Normally these beds have been recently or are about to be vacated (the previous day's elective surgery patients will be extubated and transferred in time for the new elective cases), but they are committed to bodies in the operating room or soon to be in the ICU. With the discovery of empty beds in the ICU, the ER may admit patients whom they would ordinarily send to other hospitals because of lack of ICU beds. Needless to say, the elective surgery schedule is vulnerable to disruption.

Out of necessity, ICU personnel (e.g., charge nurses, staff nurses, house officers) are involved in boundary maintenance and defense: gathering organizational intelligence about other units, negotiating patient transfers, making side deals, defining and regularizing relationships among units. In the triage mode, these same personnel intensify their activities. In this setting, we are a long way from realizing the air traffic controller model of the triage officer.

A variety of ways exist to improve interunit coordination. One approach is to rotate members among the various units to change attitudes and behaviors. Another way is to emphasize superordinate institutional goals that overarch and overcome parochial interests (e.g., each unit is "pulling the oars for the same boat"). Instituting cross-cutting teams and other organizational development (OD) exercises may facilitate this emphasis. Total quality management offers a third approach for breaking down some of the boundaries between units by emphasizing and analyzing the processes that transcend boundaries.

Interunit nursing coordination problems can also be referred up the nursing chain of command to the point in the hierarchy that includes both the ICU and the PACU (e.g., the director of Special Care Units or the vice president for Nursing Services). At this point decisions can be made on the safe disposition of patients among the various hospital units. However, not unlike viewing the seemingly smooth flow of traffic from the top of a tall skyscraper, high-level administrators may not fully appreciate the amount of friction involved in transferring patients in and out of units.

Round 5: The AIDS Patient

A resident suggests that an AIDS patient in the ER with a second episode of Pneumocystis carinii pneumonia (PCP) in respiratory failure be admitted to the ICU. The patient, who is mentally incapacitated but not unconscious, is an IV drug abuser. Because he did not have a regular private physician, he was assigned to an attending physician as a "service patient." However, the resident remains primarily in charge of care.

The nurse manager calls the triage officer to make the decision because the beds are fully occupied. She says that staffing levels are very stretched because several nurses have called in sick.

The triage officer, by phone, consults with the resident. In conversation with the resident, the triage officer said that the literature shows that AIDS patients with a second episode of PCP in respiratory failure almost never survive to leave the hospital. Therefore, the patient should be denied admission to the ICU.

The resident tells the triage officer of an article he recently read in the *Journal of the American Medical Association* entitled "Critical Care of Patients with AIDS" by R. M. Wachter, J. M. Luce, and P. C. Hopewell (1992). The article reviews research findings that show an improving survival rate among AIDS patients with PCP/respiratory failure; some of these patients do survive to go home.

The triage officer responds by saying that in Anywhere Hospital, which treats very few AIDS patients, the chance of survival would be negligible, and even if survival to hospital discharge were possible, length and quality of life would be minimal.

The resident suggests that the patient be given a trial. He reads a passage of the *Journal of the American Medical Association* article:

> Patients or clinicians, knowing that withholding support is ethically and legally no different than not initiating it, may opt for critical care at first, reassessing the benefits and burdens over time. Such a strategy is perfectly reasonable. However, all parties involved in such decisions should understand that, with the exception of patients who deteriorate soon after bronchoscopy, an ICU stay of less than 10 days is probably inadequate to predict the outcome of mechanical ventilation for PCP and respiratory failure. If the decision is made to discontinue mechanical ventilation, the patient's comfort becomes the overriding concern. In these cases, abandonment, pain, and dyspnea must be combated as aggressively as was PCP before the choice was made to withdraw life-sustaining support (p. 545).

The article also states that the average hospitalization for an AIDS patient that includes one day in the ICU costs $23,360 (1984 dollars).

An administrator, who happened to hear about the case, wondered about the broader implications for hospital policy if new but expensive courses of treatment could be adopted on the basis of a single journal article.

Because the patient is mentally incapacitated (due to the pneumonia), preferences with regard to life-sustaining treatment are unknown. The resident consulted a relative of the AIDS patient, but the relative was not aware of the patient's wishes.

The disposition of beds is presented in Exhibit 4.6. Should the AIDS patient be admitted and, if so, to which bed?

■   ■   ■   ■   ■

Six Patients: Gatekeeping At Anywhere Hospital ICU **115**

Exhibit 4.6 12-Bed Medical/Surgical ICU

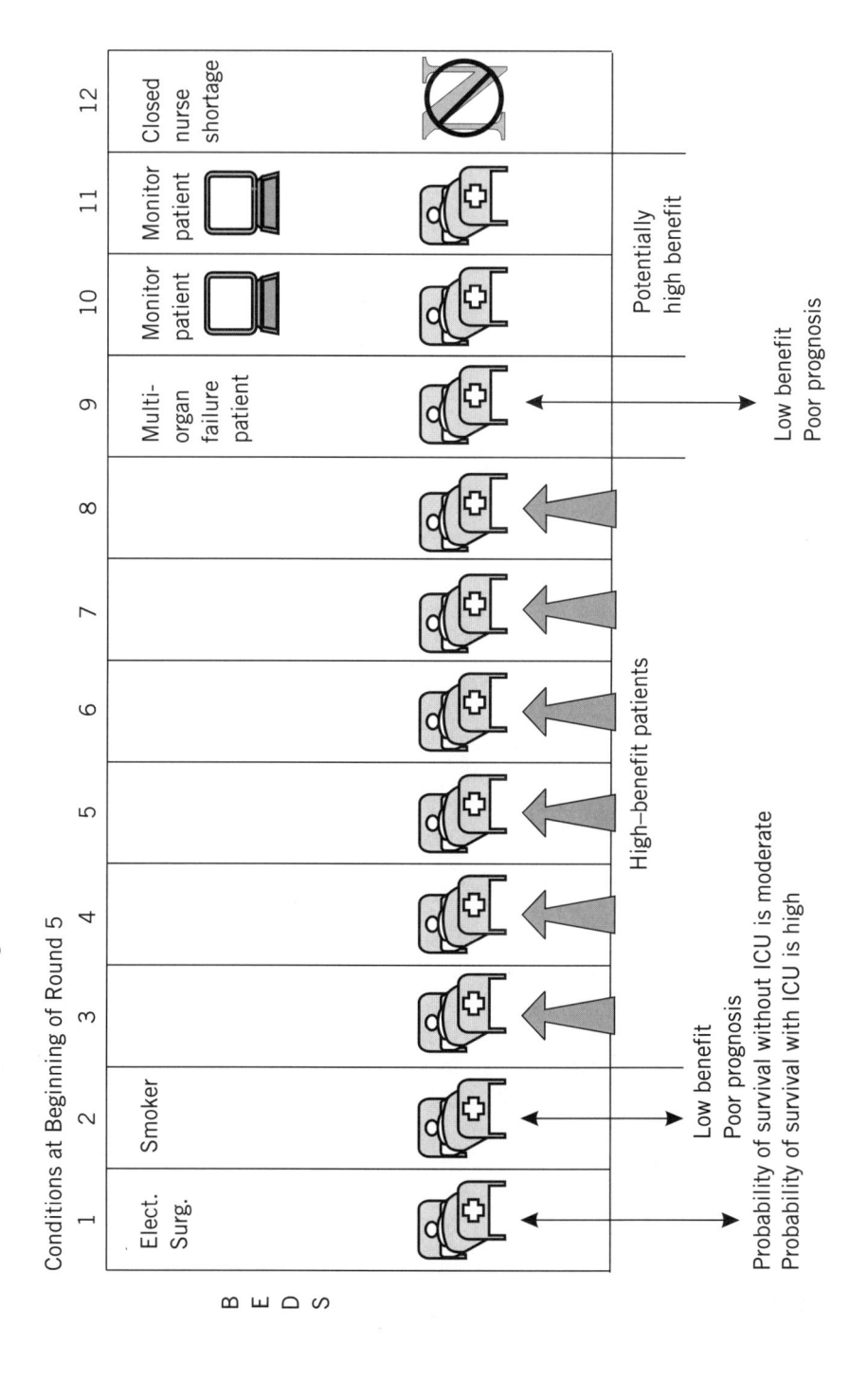

Conditions at Beginning of Round 5

	1	2	3	4	5	6	7	8	9	10	11	12
	Elect. Surg.	Smoker							Multi-organ failure patient	Monitor patient	Monitor patient	Closed nurse shortage

B
E
D
S

← High-benefit patients (beds 3–8)

Low benefit / Poor prognosis (beds 2 and 1)

Multi-organ failure patient: Low benefit, Poor prognosis

Monitor patients (10, 11): Potentially high benefit

Probability of survival without ICU is moderate
Probability of survival with ICU is high

Round 5 Decision: Deny Admission

Rationale
The triage officer excluded the AIDS patient because, in his judgment, the patient's chance of survival was negligible, and even if survival to hospital discharge were possible, the patient's length and quality of life would be minimal. The triage officer determined ICU intervention to be medically futile, even though the resident disagreed. The preferences of the AIDS patient were not known. The relative was told about the decision and did not disagree.

The Outcome
The AIDS patient was placed on the general medical floor and was given aggressive antibiotic therapy and high-flow oxygen. He soon deteriorated and was treated in a comfort care mode with a morphine drip until his death.

Discussion
Is ICU intervention for the AIDS patient medically futile? The concept of medical futility is controversial. Its definition and applicability to medical decision making frequently is debated in the bioethical literature. Nevertheless, its currency as a basis for making decisions is reinforced in statutes, regulations, and guidelines.

Even when the concept of futility is clearly defined by statute, it remains controversial. For example, the New York state DNR law (1987) defined medically futile CPR in statute: "cardiopulmonary resuscitation will be unsuccessful in restoring cardiac and respiratory function or the patient will experience repeated arrest in a short time period before death occurs." At least in New York state, where DNR orders are regulated by a complex statute, physicians feel vulnerable to lawsuit if they do not have a properly executed DNR order, prior to deciding not to give futile CPR. In some instances they feel compelled to go through with CPR or at least the motions (Strosberg 1995). The reason for this is the underlying logic of DNR policies. Physicians have been forced to invert the standard consent process; instead of seeking consent before treatment, they typically presume that consent is necessary only when deciding to forgo intervention—most notably when seeking consent not to resuscitate, that is, to issue DNR orders. Conceptually, such activities as cardiopulmonary resuscitation, mechanical ventilation, and nasogastic feeding are interventions equivalent to any other kind of therapy. One should not require consent not to give a therapy (Baker et al. 1995).

Youngner (1988) delineates futility in terms of the potential goals of the medical intervention in question. Included are physiological goals (e.g., raising blood pressure, restoring the heartbeat). Will vasoactive agents raise blood pressure? Will CPR restore the heartbeat? There is the goal of postponing death. Will physiological intervention, if successful, postpone death? There are also quality and length of life goals. Will the intervention lengthen the duration of life so that the patient can accomplish certain goals before death?

The Council on Ethical and Judicial Affairs of the American Medical Association (1995b) defines futility in terms of physiological goals and benefit. In its statement on the allocation of scarce medical resources, it asserts that " . . . care that has a low likelihood of benefiting the patient must be distinguished from care that is truly futile (e.g., care that cannot be expected to have any physiologic benefit for the patient). Patients who do have some chance of benefiting, in whatever degree cannot be ruled out in advance as inappropriate candidate for treatment" (p. 30). In this regard, some AIDS patients would argue that the chance of going home, for even a short period of time, would be worth the effort.

According to the AMA's position, ICU intervention for the AIDS patient could not be defined as futile. The triage officer, however, defined futility in terms of probability of survival and quality and length of life goals. It must be reemphasized that the patient did not have an ongoing relationship with a primary care physician. No physician really knew the patient's preferences or goals. Therefore, in this case, physician value judgments entered the futility determination. To a large extent, the decision was made unilaterally, with little participation by the relative. Unilateral determination of medical futility, as will be discussed in more detail in Chapter 6, can be highly controversial.

How can family members or close friends participate in the decision? If the patient had a surrogate or proxy (e.g., a family member or close friend) empowered to make decisions on the patient's behalf, then that person could have made a decision based on substituted judgment, in other words, what the patient would have wanted under the circumstances. If the surrogate or proxy did not have a clear understanding of the patient's wishes, then he or she could have made the decision based on the best interests of the patient. Best interests determination involves weighing the benefits and burdens of treatment and may lead to a decision to forego life-prolonging therapy. In cases where no surrogate is available, physicians can make the decision to deny ICU admission based on the best interests of the patient (Civetta 1996).

Inappropriate Criteria

It is generally accepted that criteria such as social worth (patient contributions to society), ability to pay, perceived obstacles to treatment (special circumstances such as alcohol and drug abuse, which diminish chances of successful treatment), and patient contribution to disease (due to past behavior and lifestyles) are inappropriate reasons for allocating scarce ICU resources (AMA Council on Ethical and Judicial Affairs, 1995b).

Most experts also agree that futility-based judgments should not be made to mask resource-allocation or rationing decisions made at the bedside. This would have been the case if the triage officer had covertly made the futility judgment based on comparative entitlement or cost considerations. One wonders how the AIDS patient, who was denied admission on the basis of medical futility and not comparative entitlement, compares to the transfer patient (Round 1) who was admitted with the slightest chance of benefit or to the smoker patient (Round 2) who had a 10 percent chance of survival. Would the decision have been different if there had been open beds or a different illness? Do patients with similar prognoses but different diseases receive similar treatments? The principle of justice requires that equals be treated equally and unequals unequally. Wachter et al. (1989), to determine whether resuscitation decisions are made equitably, analyzed the frequency of DNR orders among AIDS patients and three other groups with different diseases but similar long-term prognoses (lung cancer, cirrhosis, and severe congestive heart failure with coronary artery disease). Controlling for severity, they found AIDS and lung cancer patients are much more likely to receive DNR orders than cirrhosis and heart failure patients. Wachter et al. could not determine whether the AIDS and lung cancer patients received too many DNR orders or the cirrhosis and heart failure patients, too few.

Would the decision have been any different if the AIDS patient had a private physician advocating for him instead of a resident, or had a vocal relative demanding to play the role of surrogate decision maker? Kollef (1996), in a study of 159 consecutive deaths in a medical ICU over a 12-month period, assessed the influence of a patient having a private attending physician on the withdrawal of life-sustaining interventions. Kollef concluded that socioeconomic factors, such as having a private attending, may influence how death occurs in the ICU. He found that patients dying in the ICU without a private attending are more likely to undergo withdrawal of life-sustaining interventions than those with an attending physician. Patients with no private attending physician also incur less cost and have a shorter duration on the mechanical ventilator.

Kollef offers some possible explanations for these differences. Private attendings may:

1. desire not to give up because of a long-established doctor-patient relationship;
2. fear litigation and therefore allow patients to die with life-sustaining interventions in place;
3. not understand the clinical limitations of life-sustaining interventions;
4. lack precise prognostic information; or
5. benefit financially from prolonged ICU stays, assuming that the patients are not under capitation.

An important question raised by the findings is whether patients who have the advantage of a private attending receive prolonged and perhaps unnecessary care, or whether patients who are not so advantaged receive undertreatment and a lower quality of care. Kollef recommends further study to answer this question.

Withholding and Withdrawing Care

Both the AIDS patient and the multi-organ failure patient had poor prognoses. However, the AIDS patient was a candidate for admission while the multi-organ failure patient was already in the ICU receiving treatment. It could be argued that the 15 days spent in the ICU provided ample time for a trial of the effectiveness of the treatment and therefore reduced the uncertainty of the prognosis. The AIDS patient was denied a trial period. On the other hand, withdrawal of treatment from the multi-organ failure patient might have involved a terminal wean off the ventilator. The AIDS patient, in comparison, had yet to come into the ICU and be put on the ventilator. Psychologically, it may be less difficult to withhold treatment than to withdraw treatment, even though ethicists and authoritative bodies consider them to be morally equivalent (SCCM Ethics Committee 1992). In practical terms, physicians may be reluctant to initiate mechanical ventilation knowing that they may have to end life support.

Although there is great controversy over the definition and determination of medical futility, most would agree that there still has to be some basis for withholding or withdrawing worthless or useless interventions. The physician is bound ethically not to offer an intervention that would be harmful or useless to the patient (SCCM Ethics Committee 1994b) or that would be contrary to principles of beneficence or nonmaleficence (Civetta 1996). One central question is, when can physicians morally and legally withhold or withdraw therapy that they deem medically futile even when the patient or the family wants it? Schneiderman and Jecker (1993) contend that futility-based judgments should be made within the context of the evolving professional standards of care. They argue that standards of care, which traditionally apply to the provision of useful treatments, must also be developed for the withholding of useless treatments. "Since such standards of care will serve as guidelines to the court, physicians who decline to use futile treatments, even in the face of demands from patients and families, will be able to make these decisions with ethical and legal support" (p. 437). Most of these standards of care and the accompanying societal consensus have yet to be developed. The physician must fall back on personal judgment and experience. We will reexamine this topic in Chapter 6.

Advance Directives, Surrogates, and Patient Self-determination

In 1991, the federal Patient Self-Determination Act went into effect. The Act requires hospitals, nursing homes, and hospices to advise patients upon admission of their right under state law to accept or refuse medical care and to execute an advance directive. Written advance directives include living wills, where patients leave instructions on end-of-life care should they become mentally incapacitated. The living will might, for example, delineate the circumstances under which they would want treatment withheld or withdrawn. Advance directives also include a durable power of attorney or healthcare proxy appointing someone to decide about treatment. According to the Act, the institution is required to document whether the patient has an advance directive and follow the patient's preferences.

It has been well recognized that the emergency admission to an acute care hospital is not the time or place to discuss end-of-life decisions. Ideally, these discussions should have occurred in the office of the primary care physician or the office of the surgeon prior to high-risk elective surgery. The vast majority of patients, however, have not had these discussions and have not completed a living will. Nor have they appointed a healthcare proxy, another form of advance directive allowed in certain states whereby surrogate decision makers can make decisions on life-sustaining treatments should the patient become mentally incapacitated.

ICU patients frequently enter the hospital through the ER (see Exhibit 2.5). In a study of patients admitted to ICUs from the ER of a 600-bed university hospital, Hanson et al. (1994) document some of the major obstacles patients face in communicating their preferences with regard to treatment decisions. In addition to their lacking an advance directive, these patients often come to the emergency room after an acute illness of brief duration which would limit the time to consider and discuss preferences, or they suffer acute mental status deficiencies (e.g., coma). ICU staff, not knowing the preferences of the patient because of mental incapacity and lack of appropriate documentation, often opt for treatment, fearing legal consequences of acting otherwise. In many instances, ICU staff may turn to a family member or close friend, when present, to help determine the preferences of the patient. Most states recognize the legal standing of family members and close friends to act as surrogate decision makers, even though they have not been officially appointed by the patients though durable power of attorney or health proxy laws.

Campbell and Frank (1997) describe the end-of-life decisions made for 471 patients under the care of the Comprehensive Supportive Care Team at Detroit Receiving Hospital between 1993 and 1995. Seventeen percent of surrogates could provide the patient's advance directive and 12 percent of these advance directives were written. Fifty-six percent of the decisions were made on the basis of substituted judgment and 18 percent were made on the basis of best interests. Only 9 percent of the end-of-life decisions were made by autonomous patients. It should be pointed out that the Detroit Receiving Hospital serves an indigent population with limited access to primary care and other social and community support that might facilitate end-of-life decision making in a non-crisis situation.

In the cases discussed thus far, with the exception of the discharge of the bleeder patient, decision makers have not had to make comparative entitlement decisions, (i.e., choosing among individual patients). Previous decisions were based on general admission criteria in the non-triage mode or on some definition of medical futility.

Round 6: The Asthmatic Patient

The nurse manager receives a request from the ER for the admission of a 25-year-old asthmatic patient with acute respiratory failure. For this particular patient, the probability of survival without ICU is low and the probability of survival with ICU is high. There is a high degree of urgency. Because the ICU beds are filled, the nurse manager calls the triage officer.

The triage officer does not want to consider the possibility of delaying the admission of the asthmatic patient. The choices are discharging either the multi-organ failure patient or the elective surgery patient, who has now been in the ICU for 24 hours. Although postoperative patients with conditions similar to the elective surgery patient typically may stay in the ICU for 48 hours, the triage officer feels that under certain conditions it would be safe to discharge the patient to the surgical floor. However, the surgeon, the attending physician of the elective surgery patient, feels that discharge would be premature and would place his patient, who has underlying chronic obstructive pulmonary disease (COPD), at risk for significant complication. The surgeon feels that not enough respiratory therapy is available at night and the patient will "bounce back" to the ICU with pneumonia. The triage officer tells the surgeon that the elective surgery patient would be placed right next to the nurses' station on the surgical floor to facilitate close observation. He will try to arrange respiratory therapy support and will add a pulse oximiter, a device which can monitor the patient's blood oxygen saturation. Furthermore, the ICU resident will visit the patient before going to late-night snack. There are no open beds in the ICU (see Exhibit 4.7). Should the asthmatic patient be admitted to the ICU and, if so, to which bed?

■ ■ ■ ■ ■

Round 6 Decision: Admit the Asthmatic and Discharge the Elective Surgery Patient to the Surgical Floor

The surgeon, the attending physician of the elective patient, is convinced by the triage officer to move the patient from the ICU to a closely watched bed on the surgical floor fully recognizing that the patient has been put at higher risk for complication. The patient and the family were not asked to consent to the move. The multi-organ failure patient remains in the ICU with a very low probability of survival.

Rationale

The 24-year-old asthmatic patient clearly meets the ICU admissions standards of Anywhere Hospital. He has to be speedily admitted to the ICU. The mechanical ventilator maneuvers are difficult and cannot be handled by the ER staff. He requires an intensivist and/or pulmonologist. His probability of survival with ICU is high and without ICU is low; his expected quality of life and duration of benefit are high.

Should a current patient be discharged to make room for the asthmatic patient? If so, which one—the recently admitted elective patient or

Six Patients: Gatekeeping At Anywhere Hospital ICU 123

Exhibit 4.7 12-Bed Medical/Surgical ICU

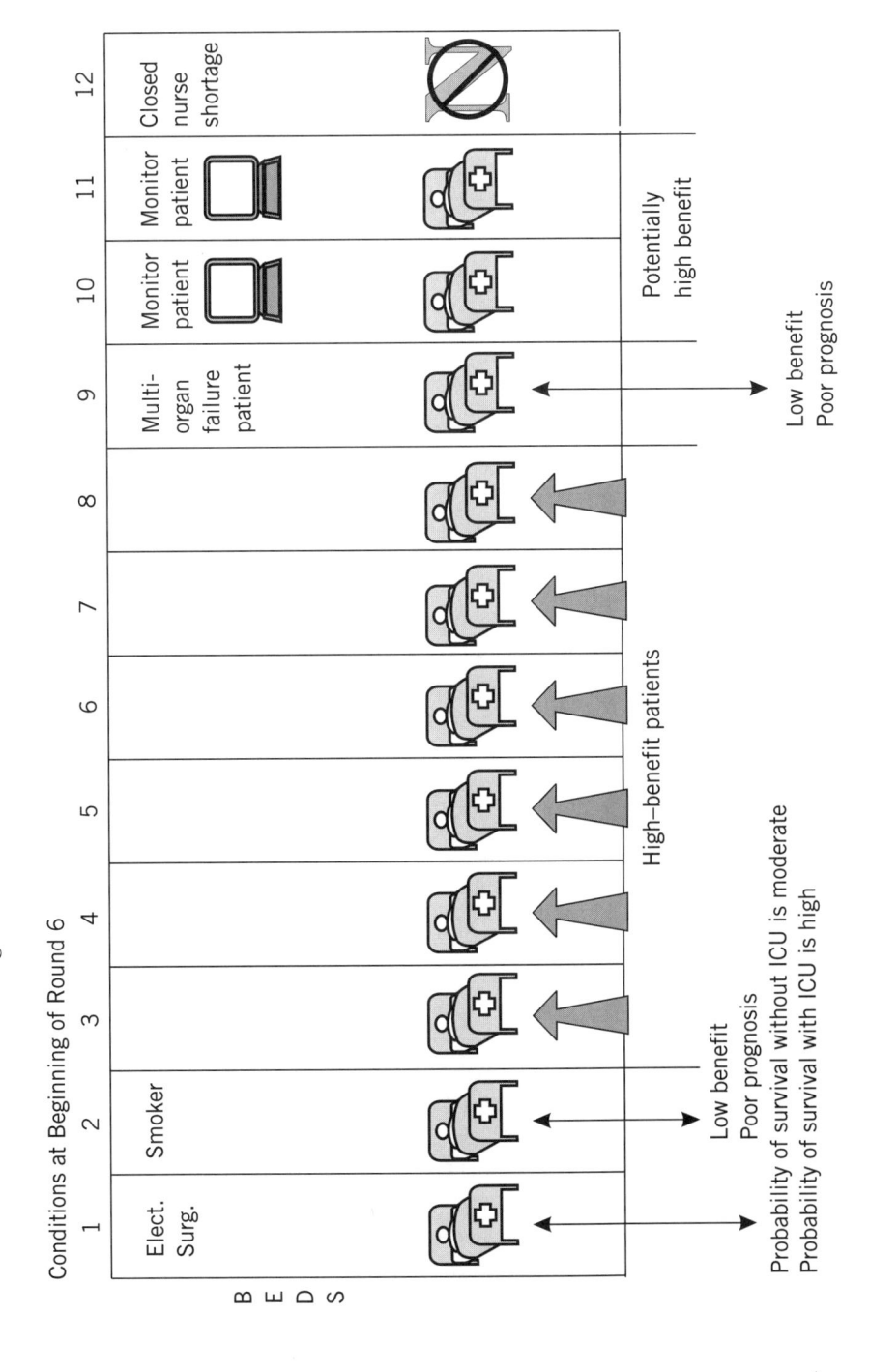

Conditions at Beginning of Round 6

1	2	3	4	5	6	7	8	9	10	11	12
Elect. Surg.	Smoker							Multi-organ failure patient	Monitor patient	Monitor patient	Closed nurse shortage

B
E
D
S

← High-benefit patients

← Potentially high benefit

↔ Low benefit / Poor prognosis

↔ Low benefit / Poor prognosis

Probability of survival without ICU is moderate
Probability of survival with ICU is high

the multi-organ failure patient? The prognosis of the latter is poor. The probability of an improvement in quality of life and of any significant duration of benefit with and without ICU treatment is low, although continued treatment would not be futile according to the surgeon and the patient's family. Even the triage officer and the nurse manager believe that the patient could survive for several more days if not weeks.

With regard to the elective survery patient, the prognosis is good. Without further ICU care (postoperative care), however, there is risk of a complication. In transferring the patient and stretching the ICU, the potential exists to damage his condition. All parties (not including the patient) recognize this fact but are willing to take the risk.

Discussion

Although the benefit to the asthmatic patient would be substantial, a possibility existed that the elective surgery patient would suffer adverse effects through premature discharge. On the other hand, the decision makers chose not to discharge the multi-organ failure patient, even though AMA and SCCM triage guidelines allow for the exclusion of such patients. If terminal wean were the option, the triage officer would need to engage the attending physician and the family in substantial and perhaps time-consuming discussion.

The elective patient was not asked for permission to be transferred to the floor, even though he was put at risk. The Consensus Statement on Triage, written by the SCCM Ethics Committee (1994b) states:

> Triage policies should be disclosed in advance to the general public and, when feasible, to patients and surrogates on admission. Triage decision may be made without patient or surrogate consent. Disclosure of triage decisions may help to facilitate communication, understanding, and cooperation among patients, surrogates, and physicians (p. 1201).

The degree of compliance with this disclosure policy is not known. But it is not likely to be high. (ICU gatekeepers do seek permission from attending physicians, provided of course the ICU is not a fully closed unit). Some ICUs, however, tell patients or families that they can stay an extra night unless the bed is needed for a much sicker patient. For example, a patient might be told, "Once off the ventilator you will generally stay one more day, unless the bed is needed."

In justification of their action of stretching intensive care, decision makers will claim that both the elective patient and the multi-organ failure patient remain alive, albeit the prospects for survival to hospital discharge of the multi-organ failure patient, not to mention the quality and length of life, are minimal. This claim reveals: (1) their rationale, maximize the total number of lives sustained; and (2) basis for prioritization, urgency of need or risk of death or morbidity takes precedence over ability to benefit measured in terms of quality of life and duration of benefit. It should be pointed out that triage guidelines from the AMA and SCCM support the primacy of maximizing the number of lives saved but not if those lives would be of poor quality or short duration. According to the "Ethical Considerations in the Allocation of Organs and Other Scarce Medical Resources Among Patients" (AMA Council on Ethical and Judicial Affairs 1995b):

> Prioritizing patients according to how long they can survive without treatment can help achieve the goal of maximizing the number of lives saved, depending on the kind of resource involved. For instance, since spaces in an ICU are ordinarily scarce only intermittently, giving priority to urgent cases is generally justifiable because less urgent cases can still gain timely access to the ICU once the scarcity subsides. With heart or liver transplants, however, the persistent scarcity of organs entails that some patients on the waiting list will die before an organ becomes available for them. With cases of persistent rather than temporary scarcity, then, urgency of need should be given less consideration because it would determine merely *who* will survive, rather than maximize the *number* of survivors. Furthermore, an urgency criterion can detract from length and quality of benefit. If patients with a less urgent need are set aside until their condition deteriorates to the point of dire emergency, treatment may not be as beneficial as it would have been had it been begun much earlier.
>
> In sum, while urgency is an important criterion, it must be tempered with other considerations, including likelihood of benefit, the persistent or temporary scarcity of the resource involved, and the length of time other patients can survive without causing them irreparable harm. Preventing death (by treating urgent cases first) should generally be given priority in allocation decisions, but not if the life saved would be of extremely poor quality or extremely short duration. Also, an urgency criterion should not be used to deny resources to current patients in the expectation that others with more need may soon present themselves (p. 31).

The urgency of need criteria is one of five, including the likelihood of benefit to the patient, the impact of treatment in improving the quality of the patient's life, the duration of benefit, and, in some cases, the amount of resources required for successful treatment. This last criteria refers mainly to the allocation of organs, in particular to patients requiring two organs. For example, given two heart transplant candidates, one of whom also needs a liver transplant, all things being equal, the heart transplant-only candidate should be given priority because two lives could be saved instead of one (i.e., the heart transplant patient and another patient who requires only a liver).

Gatekeeping in the Intensive Care Unit

The AMA Council provides guidance on the application of these criteria:

> Once all the potential recipients have been studied, decision makers should allocate resources to maximize the number, length, and quality of lives saved. Because each of the five ethical criteria contribute to this goal in different ways, none is inherently more important than the others. However, because of the intrinsic worth of all persons, maximizing the number of lives saved should generally take priority over other goals, as long as the patients saved would not suffer an extremely poor quality of life or extremely short duration of benefit. For instance, it is better to save two patients who could each live 5 years than to save one patient who could live 10 years. In addition, preventing extremely poor outcomes should take precedence over other efforts to enhance quality of life or duration of benefit. A patient who can go from 0% (i.e., death) to 50% of full functioning, for example, should be preferred over a patient who can go from 25% to 75% of full functioning (p. 33).

The guidelines of the AMA Council would clearly support the discharge of the elective patient to make room for the asthmatic patient. But they would just as clearly justify the discharge of the multi-organ failure patient as "a patient who will suffer an extremely poor quality of life or extremely short duration of benefit."

The SCCM guidelines also would allow the discharge of the multi-organ failure patient in a comparative entitlement decision: "Patients with little or no anticipated benefit from further ICU treatment may be discharged or transferred from the ICU . . . The decision to exclude or discharge a patient from the ICU may appropriately be made despite the anticipation of an untoward outcome [i.e., death]" (p. 1202). Yet, the decision makers retained the multi-organ failure patient, perhaps to the detriment of the elective surgery patient. To understand the reasons for and the implications of making this kind of tradeoff, we reintroduce the concept of QALY, discussed in Chapter 2. Consider the following:

Patient A and Patient B both require ICU intervention. However, ICU intervention if devoted exclusively to A would yield an additional QALY of 0.2 years (e.g., by treating a terminally ill patient with an acute reversible condition) and if devoted exclusively to B an additional QALY of 5. Under conditions of resource availability both A & B would be treated.

However, resources are scarce. How should they be allocated?

Option 1). Maximize total benefit, in other words, QALYs: Use all the resources to treat Patient B which would yield 5 additional QALYs.

Option 2). Maximize total number of lives sustained: Use resources to treat both patients. However, in stretching the ICU by using less resources per patient, the additional QALYs are diminished to each patient, for example, Patient A receives 0.1 and Patient B receives 4.5, for a total of 4.6 additional QALYs.

The Paradox

Most ICU professionals have stated that when push comes to shove, everybody who really needs an ICU bed will get one. Somehow, the ICU will be stretched to safely accommodate everybody; nobody will be denied beneficial care. Theoretically, the rubber band of ICU resources cannot be stretched indefinitely. There must be some breaking point. Do some breaking points go unrecognized?

In choosing the second option, professionals are signifying that when they say they are not denying beneficial services, they are only referring to services that are immediately life sustaining. They do not recognize, or fail to recognize, the denial of services that offer less immediate or dramatic benefit. However, in our example, Patient B would be denied the benefit of 0.5 QALY (as the additional QALY is lowered from 5.0 to 4.5).

With some notable exceptions (e.g., Shoemaker et al. 1992), we rarely hear about the denial of beneficial services as the result of stretching the rubber band of ICU resources. Perhaps we are not measuring the right things. ICUs do not have the technical ability to discern a diminishment in Patient B's benefit by 0.5 QALY. Perhaps we are reluctant to measure the right things. The decrease in QALY for Patient B is a diminishment in the community standard of care with implications for malpractice litigation.

On the other hand, if the first option were chosen, there would be no diminishment in Patient B's benefit, but Patient A's remaining days would be spent receiving comfort care. How do decision makers cope with this dilemma? One possibility is that decision makers might in fact choose the first option in such a way that they consciously or unconsciously estimate the probability of Patient A's survival to be negligible (i.e., medical futility) or they consciously or unconsciously recalculate the resulting QALY to be below some minimum threshold.

What we are suggesting is that the definition of beneficial may vary according to the extent of resource scarcity, to mask the emotional and legal consequences of denying services. Clearly, some underlying mechanism is at work in this "sliding scale" definition. In their study of the British National Health Service, Aaron and Schwartz (1984) discuss the tendency of physicians to redefine standards of care gradually so that they can "avoid the painful realization that they are doing less than the best for the patient."

The definition of the "best" is often subjective. Taken to an extreme, more can always be done to save lives. If an ICU goes all out for every single patient, no matter what, regardless of pain and suffering, functional outcome, quality-of-life issues, patient and family wishes, then undoubtedly a fair number of patients could be pulled through who would now in many other ICUs be allowed to die. Although few might desire such life-sustaining services, the point is, given uncertainty over prognosis and effectiveness of treatment, maneuvering room is available in this sliding scale definition of benefit.

Historical Notions of Triage

The term triage (French meaning, "to sort") originated with Baron Larrey, Surgeon General of Napoleon's army. It is commonly believed that Larrey's objective in triaging battlefield casualties was to identify and treat first those wounded soldiers who could be speedily returned to the fight. Thus triage, sometimes referred to as military triage, has been interpreted as a utilitarian system of allocation where probability of successful outcomes receives greater priority than severity of illness or urgency of need. Actual triage practice in ICUs, however, frequently reverses this prioritization principle.

Baker and Strosberg (1992), in reexamining the historical record, dispute the utilitarian interpretation of Larrey's prioritization scheme. They found that Larrey's principle was "treat first those most likely to die or become disabled provided that treatment can make a difference." This principle was promulgated in reaction to the commonly used principles at the time: "treat officers before ordinary soldiers," and "first come, first served," which resulted in great loss of life. The evidence shows that Larrey's objective was not to return wounded soldiers speedily to the battlefield, but to maximize their opportunities of survival. Presumably the soldiers, if deciding beforehand, would voluntarily choose to support this principle. Even the less seriously wounded, at the time of triage, would recognize their potential to become severely wounded in some future battle. Baker and Strosberg argue that Larrey's concept of triage was more egalitarian than utilitarian.

The modern equivalent of a utilitarian interpretation of Larrey's principle is to "produce the most benefit per unit of investment." In terms of the QALY example, this principle would have us maximize the total QALYs as per Option 1. ICU triage, however, seems to embody a "maximin" strategy: minimize the worst outcome. If one assumes that nonsurvival is the worst possible outcome, the logic of maximin dictates that patients in greater danger of dying because of a lack of medical treatment have the highest priority for treatment. In terms of Round 6, the surgeon would argue that the multi-organ failure patient does not fall below the minimum threshold. On the other hand, others would raise the threshold of the basic minimum.

Many nationally recognized ICU admissions and treatment policies have equated survival with conscious survival and, therefore, exclude patients in a persistent vegetative state. PVS is a condition of patients with severe brain damage in whom coma has progressed to a state of wakefulness without detectable awareness (Jennett and Plum 1972). It can be distinguished clinically from other forms of permanent unconsciousness, and the diagnostic factors have been delineated (Multi-Society Task Force on PVS 1994). Perhaps the most famous patient with PVS was Karen Ann Quinlan. In 1975 she suffered a cardiopulmonary arrest and died ten years later having never regained consciousness.

In spite of the wide-ranging debate surrounding PVS, the SCCM's (1994a) 1988 survey of attitudes of critical care medicine professionals showed that 43 percent would admit a patient who was in persistent vegetative state. In addition, 54 percent would admit a patient who had no hope of surviving more than a few weeks. How can this be explained? One reason is pressure to admit the patient from the family, primary physician, ER, and from nursing who cannot take care of patients on mechanical ventilators on the regular floors. Presumably they also believed that the patients were alive and hence deserved care.

Admission Candidates versus "Squatters"

What about the option of delaying the admission of the asthmatic patient? Like the AMA guidelines, the framework of the SCCM triage guidelines are based on the principle that access to intensive care should be prioritized on the basis of expected outcome in terms of survival and function. However, as opposed to the AMA guidelines, this principle, which is used for judging comparative entitlement among candidates for admission, is not applied by the SCCM when comparing candidates for admissions to patients already in the ICU:

> As a general rule, obligations to patients already hospitalized in an ICU who continue to warrant ICU care outweigh obligations to accept new patients. There may be circumstances, however, when it is justified to discharge a patient from the ICU in order to admit another patient. If admission of a new patient is likely to adversely affect the outcomes of patients already under care, then that admission is ordinarily justified only if the benefit to the new admission is significant and quite likely and the adverse effects on the present ICU patients are either conjectural or unlikely to be significant (SCCM 1994b, p. 1201).

In contrast, Englehardt and Rie (1986) have advocated applying the "ability to benefit" principle across the critical care continuum which, as was mentioned in Chapter 1, mandates the discharge of a patient to make way for a newcomer who can derive more benefit.

The SCCM triage guidelines clearly allow the discharge or transfer of patients with "little or no anticipated benefit," which includes patients with little or no chance of survival. The SCCM triage guidelines, however, are reluctant to define benefit and futility because they are "subjective, value-laden terms for which there is no agreement."

Why does the SCCM Ethics Committee enshrine the principle of "squatters rights"? Perhaps the triage guidelines reflect prevailing beliefs and norms: physicians do not have a contract with and obligation to the candidate for admission as opposed to the patient already in the bed; lowering the level of intensive care is, therefore, ethically less desirable than never providing it. Or, physicians may believe that appropriate intensive care can be found in another setting or in another hospital (SCCM 1994a).

The precedence given to current ICU patients over candidates for admission is not at odds with prevailing attitudes of critical care medicine professionals. The SCCM Ethics Committee (1994a), in a 1988 survey of intensivists' attitudes, asked respondents what conditions would warrant discharge of an ICU patient in order to admit a 25-year-old asthmatic patient with acute respiratory failure requiring intensive care. At least 50 percent of the respondents would not discharge patients such as those described in the following scenarios:

> A 20-yr.-old man with a massive subarachnoid hemorrhage who remains in a coma 2 weeks after admission and who breathes spontaneously but receives ventilator support which is usually not provided on the general ward.
>
> A 45-yr.-old woman with multiple organ failure in the ICU for 8 weeks who receives moderate doses of dopamine and moderate levels of positive end-expiratory pressure.
>
> A 6-yr.-old brain dead child who is a potential organ transplant.
>
> A 40-yr.-old woman who tried to commit suicide by driving her car into a pole. She is postoperative after repair of her traumatic injuries, requires a ventilator, and requests that everything be removed so she can die in peace (p. 361).

On the other hand, for the AMA Council on Ethical and Judicial Affairs, "The 'first-come first-served' method should not be used to abdicate responsibility for making decisions when appropriate criteria can give a sound basis for preferring some patients over others." The AMA suggests that first-come first-served be used only when uncertainty is too great or the differences among candidates too close to call.

The SCCM position places the triage officer, who is charged with making comparative entitlement decisions explicitly and fairly for all patients in the hospital, in a tenuous situation, thus constraining the full application of the five ethical criteria (see p. 218). The structure of explicit criteria that are supposed to minimize the need of the triage officer to make ad hoc decisions for individual patients dissolves when those patients pass through the gates of the ICU. This is ironic because the prognostic uncertainty that characterizes most critical care decisions is reduced when a patient enters the ICU and is given a trial.

In most instances, the expanding rubber band of critical care services submerges the contradiction between the two positions. Usually patients can be safely accommodated in the ER, PACU, or at other hospitals. But cases such as the King-Drew Medical Center in Los Angeles, referred to in Chapter 1, will not be so rare as managed care becomes more widespread. In such cases, where a contradiction in expectations occurs, or where rules fail to explicitly guide triage officers, and against the backdrop of legal uncertainty, triage officers are forced to exercise discretion and make hard choices.

The decision makers in Round 6 chose to dislodge the elective surgery patient in favor of the asthmatic patient. The elective patient was more easily and quickly moved than the multi-organ failure patient. Would they have made this tradeoff if the choice was only between the asthmatic and the multi-organ failure patient or the other types of patients mentioned above? In studies of rationing arising when ICU beds were temporarily closed, Singer et al. (1983) and Strauss et al. (1986) found that physicians admitted sicker patients and decreased length of stay but with no acceleration of withdrawal of care from the terminally ill patients or transfer of patients deemed hopeless.

Round 7: The "Bounce Back" of the Elective Surgery Patient

The surgeon of the recently transferred elective surgery patient believes that his patient is becoming unstable on the surgical floor and requests readmission for his patient. The triage officer again discusses the prospects for the multi-organ failure patient with the patient's surgeon. The surgeon of the multi-organ failure patient now agrees that further treatment would be futile in terms of contributing to the patient's chances of leaving the hospital alive, and the ventilator should be withdrawn. At the surgeon's request, the triage officer agrees to discuss the situation with the family. He explains to the family that the chances of leaving the hospital alive (the family's original goal) were negligible. The triage officer fully expected that the family would consent to the withdrawal of treatment. However, the family refused the recommendation of the triage officer and demanded continuance of aggressive care. The family is known to be litigious. The triage officer received the following letter from the attorney: "In the event that the patient is removed from the ICU or from support systems without written consent, the family has authorized me to proceed as vigorously as the law will require to compensate the family for any and all damages which result from your actions."

The decision makers discuss the advisability of removing the patient from the ventilator against the wishes of the family or triaging the patient to the floor (where the staff are not equipped to take care of a ventilator patient and maintain aggressive care). The hospital attorney advises against these options. The triage officer, nurse manager, and administrator consider opening up the 12th bed, realizing that there might be an initial dilution of the quality of care to the other patients as existing nursing staff is stretched. A heated discussion takes place about this last option. See Exhibit 4.8 for disposition of beds. Should the elective surgery patient be readmitted to the ICU and, if so, to which bed?

■   ■   ■   ■   ■

Round 7 Decision: Retain Multi-Organ Failure Patient, Readmit Elective Surgery Patient, Open 12th Bed, Stretch Existing Nursing Staff

Rationale

Ostensibly, the determination of medical futility (defined as a negligible chance of surviving hospital stay) is the rationale for the decision to approach the family about withdrawal of treatment, although the necessity to triage is an underlying factor. The decision makers agree that the patient is too sick to benefit. If the determination of medical futility were considered to be solely a professional decision, the preferences of the patient or family would not be an important consideration. But given the "bioethical revolution of the 1970s" and the movement away from medical paternalism and toward the patient's right to autonomy and self-determination, many physicians would be reluctant to make a unilateral judgment (Baker and Strosberg 1993). In extreme cases, these rights have sometimes included not only the right to accept or reject a

Six Patients: Gatekeeping At Anywhere Hospital ICU **133**

Exhibit 4.8 12-Bed Medical/Surgical ICU

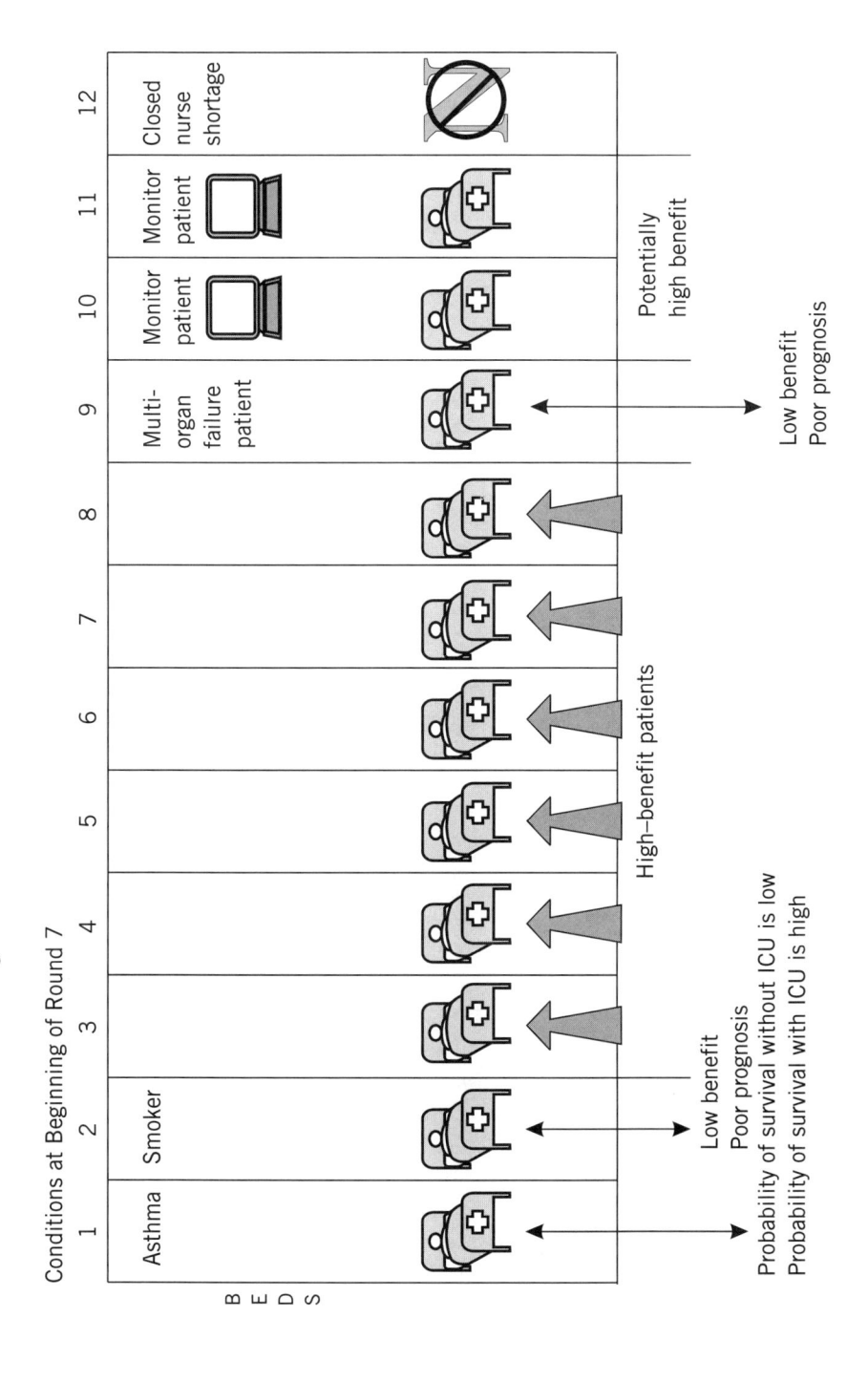

Conditions at Beginning of Round 7

	1	2	3	4	5	6	7	8	9	10	11	12
	Asthma	Smoker							Multi-organ failure patient	Monitor patient	Monitor patient	Closed nurse shortage

B
E
D
S

← High-benefit patients →

↔ Low benefit / Poor prognosis

↔ Potentially high benefit

↔ Low benefit / Poor prognosis

Probability of survival without ICU is low
Probability of survival with ICU is high

proposed treatment but also the right to demand and receive any life-sustaining treatment. Many feel that the revolution has gone too far and that physicians should not be obligated to give in to family demands for continued life-prolonging treatments when the physician believes it to be beyond well-established medical criteria (Paris et al. 1993). The SCCM Task Force on Guidelines (1988) also supports this position. However, as Zussman (1992) points out, most ICU decision makers will accede to family requests even if to make "end stage gestures" (Fiel 1991). Furthermore, concern now exists that the family will argue in court that the withdrawal of the ventilator and subsequent death would be a diminishment of benefit, however marginal.

Discussion

The influence of patient autonomy on decision-making processes is felt more in the United States than any place in the world. In contrast, consider the "benign paternalism" that characterizes the intensivists of the ICUs of New Zealand (Streat and Judson 1994):

> In general, families are not asked to make life-and-death decisions, or even to participate in these decisions, because clinicians consider these decisions our medical responsibility. However, the family are informed of medical opinions and are asked for their agreement to withdraw therapy. We seek the family's consensus rather than their permission. Usually the family agrees, but families may require more time to come to terms with our decisions or to see the patient's deterioration for themselves. While patients and families have the right to refuse medical treatment, New Zealand culture and the country's legal system do not require physicians to provide treatment that will not be beneficial. We do not feel constrained by consensus about patient autonomy in situations where therapy is not indicated on medical grounds (p. 399).

In the United States, there is often fear of the legal consequences of withdrawal of life-sustaining treatments without consent and against the wishes of the patient or family. Recent court cases, which will be discussed in Chapter 6, generally substantiate these fears.

What if comparative entitlement rather than medical futility were the underlying motivation for making the decision? Triage has not generally been conceptualized to include individual or family consent (SCCM 1994b). In theory, the triage decision is a technical judgment by a physician weighing the competing claims of two or more patients. But triage may result in one party receiving diminished benefit. If this diminishment constitutes a lowering of the community standard of care, the question arises whether the legal system gives physicians and hospitals the flexibility to use scarcity of resources (lack of beds) as justification for lowering the standard (Morreim 1992). In the previous round, decision makers were willing to take this step by transferring the elective surgery patient to make room for the asthmatic patient. But they are generally not willing to give priority to a new candidate for admissions over an existing ICU patient receiving life-sustaining treatment.

Very few court cases deal with triage or the failure to triage. One such case was that of Susan von Stetina (*von Stetina* versus *Florida Medical Center* 1985), a young woman who had been injured in a car crash and was admitted to the ICU for post-traumatic distress which developed after surgery. While she was in the ICU, her mechanical ventilator malfunctioned causing brain damage. The court found that ICU staff failed to properly monitor the ventilator because the ICU was overcrowded. Patients should have been triaged to relieve the overcrowding, including one patient who was near death. This case, illustrating a rather extreme contrast, deals with the comparative entitlement of a young woman who had an excellent prognosis versus another patient close to brain death, and not even a minimal triage system was in place. As of yet there have been no court cases dealing with a triage case when a patient is prematurely transferred out and must be returned to the ICU. Under these circumstances, it is likely that the triage officer and the hospital would be put on the legal defensive. Their vulnerability would probably stem from a lack of careful documentation proving that, at the time of triage, each patient in the ICU had a better reason for being there than the one who was moved out. Also, the ICU would have to definitively show that it exhausted all opportunities to transfer the patient to reasonably available, comparable hospitals.

Ethics Committees

One step that the physicians and staff in Round 7 might have taken was to call upon the hospital ethics committee to help resolve the differences between the physicians and the family. Ethics committees are multidisciplinary groups composed of physicians, nurses, clergy, social workers, community representatives, and lay people and provide an opportunity for thoughtful consideration of issues involved in end-of-life treatment decision making. Most hospitals have ethics committees. Their functions typically include policymaking (e.g., formulating hospital policies on DNR), education (e.g., sensitizing physicians, nurses, and other staff to ethical concerns; informing the public on the importance of having an advance directive), and in some instances, consulting on individual cases.

What, for example would be the purpose of the ethics committee in regard to the multi-organ failure patient? There are a variety of functions that the committee might have pursued. It could provide an open and nonjudgmental forum for the parties to separately discuss options. For a given set of facts, different conclusions may be drawn depending on the values of the parties involved. The one right answer does not necessarily exist. Ethics committees can serve a purpose by establishing procedures for collecting the facts and clarifying the values of the decision makers. Furthermore, a committee could have facilitated communication among those parties by holding meetings with the family and the medical team. Mediation is another role. For example, the New York State Do-Not-Resuscitate Law mandates that hospitals establish dispute mediation systems to help mediate (not adjudicate) conflicts concerning the issuance of DNR orders. Many hospitals in New York have used their ethics committees to fulfill this role. One idea behind the dispute mediation system is that conflicts are better handled at the hospital than in the courts. The New York law gives the dispute mediation system 72 hours to mediate a resolution before a party to the conflict can seek judicial relief in the courts (New York State Task Force on Life and the Law 1988).

Hoffmann (1993) and many others note potential contradiction as the ethics committee carries out its functions. Should, for example, an ethics consult be focused solely on the interests of the patient in order to assist the family in making an ethically correct decision based on the values of the patient? Should the consult be conducted impartially to assist all interested parties—caregivers, patients, family members, the institution—in resolving differences by taking a balanced approach? With regard to comparative entitlement and the stewardship of societal resources, Veatch (1984) has argued that resource allocation should not be a legitimate concern of an ethics committee because it conflicts with the purpose of protecting individual patients.

In a national survey of ICUs conducted in 1991, 73 percent of the reporting ICUs stated that their hospital had an ethics committee. Of those hospitals, 49 percent of the ethics committees had as a member the ICU medical director or designee, and within a year's period 55 percent of the ICUs had sought the help of their hospital ethics committee at least once (SCCM Task Force for Distribution of ICU Resources in the United States 1993). The survey, however, does not provide information on the purpose of the interaction between the ICU and the ethics committee and the process of the consultation. Most ethics committees hear about cases retrospectively (i.e., the case is presented as a teaching case). Or the case appears very late in the ICU stay when an open conflict exists among family members or between a family member and a member of the healthcare team. In concurrent case reviews, the response generally is slow and the case review discussion of options may not be part of the medical record.

Patient Autonomy: Another Perspective

Thus far we have been discussing patient autonomy in terms of the controversy arising when patients and/or families demand futile or marginally beneficial treatments. What should also be recognized are the violations of autonomy when physicians override patients' wishes and give unwanted interventions. One such case is that of 87-year-old Georgia Hansot, whose story of her five-day stay in an ICU of a major teaching hospital is told by her daughter (Hansot 1996). Although there was clear evidence from Mrs. Hansot and her daughter, her legally designated agent, that she did not want to be kept alive by mechanical ventilation, physicians apparently disregarded that evidence, in the interests of preserving life. It took five days for the daughter to convince the attending pulmonologist and a cadre of cardiologists and neurologists to agree to the withdrawal of the ventilator. In this case, obvious failures occurred in the safeguards protecting patient autonomy. Where was her primary care physician? Where was the ICU medical director? Where were the oversight committees?

The JCAHO, in its *1996 Comprehensive Accreditation Manual,* attempts to address these types of concerns. In the section "Patient Rights and Organization Ethics," it presents standards concerning the rights of patients and families to participate in end-of-life decision making and the expectations of hospitals to support the exercise of those rights through the establishment of policies, procedures, codes of ethics, ethics committees, and ethics consultation services.

In light of the SUPPORT study findings, showing disturbing deficiencies in patient-physician communication, Strosberg and Teres propose the establishment of a Rapid Ethics Evaluation Process (REEP) team, a subset of the ethics committee composed of a physician, a nurse, a chaplain or social worker, and a community member. The latter should have no financial connection with either the hospital or the managed care plan. The process would be carried out on patients who are failing aggressive ICU therapy and/or have developed multi-organ failure. It is proposed that the team meet separately with the patient and the family and with the medical staff to evaluate level of communication, the patient's medical condition, prognosis, and treatment plan. The team will assess such questions as, is there a good understanding of the diagnosis, problems, and prognosis? Is there a need for a formal ethics committee review? Does the physician need counseling or guidance?

Gatekeeping in the Intensive Care Unit

The team will then write up its assessment of the situation and complete the recommendation checklist (see Appendix D for a description of the process and the checklist). As opposed to a formal ethics committee case review, the REEP team would not be expected to resolve serious dilemmas through facilitated communication or mediation, only to flag those cases that should be referred. The authors believe that there is a need for a more open approach to communication than the private discussions between physicians and families and that this process will be better able to delineate various options in a manner that is fair, deliberate, nonthreatening, and of minimal burden to the doctor-patient relationship. The authors hypothesize that a REEP team intervention, by improving communication, may reduce intensive care utilization by patients with a poor prognosis.

There are those who believe that more profound reforms are required to change the high-technology culture of the ICU. Many consider the Oregon Death with Dignity Act of 1994, which would legalize physician-assisted suicide, as a wake-up call to American physicians to improve end-of-life care. Lo (1995) has suggested "developing practice guidelines for intensive care, cutting the supply of intensive care beds and specialists, and placing intensive care physicians at financial risk for the services they provided." The federal Health Care Financing Administration (HCFA), in order to legitimize and encourage the use of palliative care, has established a new diagnostic code recognizing the delivery of palliative care to a dying hospital patient. The new diagnostic code will allow the HCFA to study the feasibility of creating a special DRG, which would allow payment for end-of-life care in hospitals (Cassel and Vladeck 1996). Miller and Fins (1996) propose the establishment of a hospice-like alternative-care unit as a full-fledged partner of the critical care service to be located right next to the ICU to maximize the impact on clinical education and practice routines.

Consequences for the Hospital and Society

While existing staff are stretched to cover the elective surgery patient, thus diluting the care to the other patients, the nurse manager and the administrator attempt to secure the services of agency nurses to staff the 12th bed. The funding will come from an already tight nursing budget, which means that personnel will have to be cut back in other areas of the hospital. The family, of course, does not bear the financial consequences of the decision; Medicare or some other third party payor does. For patients with no insurance, the hospital absorbs the cost.

What are the economic implications of treating patients for conditions where the probability of survival is very small? Cohen, Lambrinos, and Fein (1993) calculated the hospital charges (not including physician fees) that are incurred after patients 80 years of age and older reach the point of "age plus days on the ventilator is equal to or greater than 100" and determined the incremental charges per life saved (i.e., incremental charges for survivors and non-survivors divided by number of survivors) and per year of life saved. They are, in 1992 dollars, $721,895 per life saved and $300,790 per year of life saved.

Round 8: Create Your Own Scenario

Although typical of the experience and actions of many U.S. hospitals, these seven rounds and outcomes represent the organizational responses of one hospital. Based on your own experience, readers may wish to critique the previous scenarios or create new ones. See Appendix E for suggestions.

■   ■   ■   ■   ■

Synopsis and Analysis of Cases and Issues

One way of analyzing the foregoing cases is to array them in terms of their likelihood of a good prognosis with and without ICU treatment and to examine them in terms of the three decision rationales for gatekeeping: (1) non-triage mode (bed availability), (2) triage mode/comparative entitlement, or (3) medical futility.

Good Prognosis With or Without ICU: The Bleeder Patient

With one bed open, this patient was admitted to the unit under a rather loose interpretation of the admissions policies. This is a patient who may have been "too well" to realize much benefit in the ICU. Nevertheless, he was admitted as a part of the negotiated order of the hospital, the informal organizational arrangements that have been worked out over time. As expected, he was easily discharged to make room for the elective surgery patient.

Good Prognosis With ICU and Poor Without ICU: The Asthmatic Patient, the Elective Surgery Patient

The asthmatic patient clearly met even the most stringent criteria for admission to an ICU with an open bed. The asthmatic patient was truly an urgent case. The elective surgery patient could have been kept temporarily in the PACU for a short time and might have been able to bypass the ICU if an intermediate care unit existed. (Although the triage officer could have postponed the elective surgery, he thought twice about alienating powerful economic and political forces in the hospital.) However, the beds were filled. In both cases, other patients were discharged to make room for them.

Poor Prognosis With or Without ICU: The Smoker, the AIDS Patient, the Multi-Organ Failure Patient

With regard to the elderly smoker, the regular admission criteria were applied with two beds open, and he was admitted. The smoker had a 10 percent chance of surviving to hospital discharge. In the United States, compared to other countries, a 10 percent chance might be considered well worth taking. But what about less than a 10 percent chance? We remember the transfer patient in Chapter 1 who was admitted with the slightest chance of survival, considerably less than 10 percent.

The AIDS patient was denied admission on the basis of medical futility determined by the triage officer during a period when no beds were available in the ICU. Medical futility was defined by the triage officer as a slim chance of survival and/or poor quality of life with short duration. The patient and the patient's relative were unable to provide input. The triage officer's definition of futility is different from that of the AMA's triage guidelines. Assuming similar survival chances to the smoker, shouldn't the AIDS patient have been given a trial?

The multi-organ failure patient, on the other hand, was given a lengthy trial. During the course of the trial, decision makers tried a variety of approaches in attempting to discharge him.

First, the ICU discharge criteria were applied: "Patients will be discharged from the ICU when the criteria for admission are no longer present (i.e., the patient has improved or the patient's condition has deteriorated to the extent that he or she has no medically reversible condition). In the latter event, the patient will be transferred to an appropriate floor where comfort care will be continued." The attending physician's assessment that the patient was receiving sufficient benefit in the ICU to warrant continued treatment overruled the triage officer, even though he had official responsibility for enforcing the discharge criteria.

Second, the multi-organ failure patient's entitlement to continued ICU treatment was compared to the elective surgery patient in consideration of the asthmatic patient waiting in the ER. It was the elective surgery patient who was triaged out of the unit to the floor to make way for the asthmatic. The elective patient was not asked to consent to his transfer. Unquestionably, the elective surgery patient was made worse off by the triage decision.

Third, although the multi-organ failure patient's continued entitlement to ICU treatment could have been compared to the elective support patient awaiting readmission, the initial approach taken was to attempt to convince the family that further treatment would be futile in meeting their goal of survival to hospital discharge. Perhaps, given the necessity to readmit the elective surgery patient, they were following advice to try to DNR their way out of a tight situation (see Exhibit 3.6). As opposed to the AIDS patient who had no active surrogate, the family of the multi-organ failure patient asserted their right to share in the determination of medical futility. The decision that was finally reached was to stretch the ICU with the potential of diluting the quality of care for every one in the unit.

The Challenge of the Multi-Organ Failure Patient: Implications for Public Policy

The difficulty in triaging the multi-organ failure patient provides a major challenge to ICU gatekeepers. Against the backdrop of patient autonomy, legal uncertainty, and the unwillingness of the profession or society to explicitly define benefit and futility, it is understandable why decision makers find it difficult to discharge and/or triage from the "too sick" side of the continuum. They must look either to changes in public policy in the form of legislation and judicial opinions, or to changes in professional and community standards of care for resolutions to these difficulties. On the other hand, will changing the incentives—placing physicians and hospitals at financial risk for their decisions—make it more or less difficult for them to consider less aggressive treatment and discharge? In Chapter 6 we will examine trends in public policymaking that attempt to clarify admission, discharge, and triage criteria, to define medical futility; and to prevent conflicts of interest. However, in addition to public policy and ethical issues, the cases raise some important managerial questions, which we now address in Chapter 5.

References

Aaron, H. J., and W. B. Schwartz. 1984. *The Painful Prescription: Rationing Hospital Care.* Washington, D. C.: The Brookings Institution.

American Medical Association Council on Ethical and Judicial Affairs. 1995a. "Ethical Issues in Managed Care." *Journal of the American Medical Association* 273 (4): 330–35.

American Medical Association Council on Ethical and Judicial Affairs. 1995b. "Ethical Considerations in the Allocation of Organs and Other Scarce Medical Resources Among Patients." *Archives of Internal Medicine* 155 (Jan 9): 29–40.

Annas, G. J. 1995. "How We Die." *Hastings Center Report (Special Supplement)*, 12 (6): S12–14.

Asch, D. A. 1996. "The Role of Critical Care Nurses in Euthanasia and Assisted Suicide." *New England Journal of Medicine* 334 (21): 1374–79.

Baker, R. 1995. "The Legitimation and Regulation of DNR Orders." In *Legislating Medical Ethics: A Study of the New York State Do-Not-Resuscitate Law*, edited by R. Baker and M. A. Strosberg, 33–101. Dordrecht: Kluwer Academic Publishers.

Baker, R., and M. A. Strosberg. 1993. "The Bioethical Revolution of 1988: The Future of The Futility Controversy." In *Emerging Issues in Biomedical Policy*, edited by R. H. Blank and A. L. Bonnicksen, 55–76. New York: Columbia University Press.

Baker, R., and M. A. Strosberg. 1992. "Triage and Equality: An Historical Reassessment of Utilitarian Analysis of Triage." *Kennedy Institute of Ethics Journal* 2 (2): 103–23.

Beal, A. L., and F. B. Cerra. 1994. "Multiple Organ Failure Syndrome in the 1990s." *Journal of the American Medical Association* 27 (3): 226–33.

Blendon, R. J., K. Donelan, R. Leitman, A. Epstein, J. C. Cantor, A. B. Cohen, I. Morrison, T. Moloney, and C. Koeck. 1993. "Health Reform Lessons Learned from Physicians in Three Nations." *Health Affairs* 12 (3): 194–203.

Campbell, M. L., and R. R. Frank. 1997. "Experience with an End-of-Life Practice at a University Hospital." *Critical Care Medicine* 25 (1): 197–202.

Cassel, C. K., and B. C. Vladeck. 1996. "ICD-9 Code for Palliative or Terminal Care." *New England Journal of Medicine* 335 (16): 1232–33.

Civetta, J. M. 1996. "A Practical Approach to Futile Care." *Bulletin of the American College of Surgeons* 81 (2): 24–29.

Cohen, I. L., J. Lambrinos, and I. A. Fein. 1993. "Mechanical Ventilation for Elderly Patients in Intensive Care: Incremental Charges and Benefits." *Journal of the American Medical Association* 269 (8): 1025–29.

Cook, D. J., G. H. Guyatt, R. Jaeschke, J. Reeve, A. Spanier, D. King, D. W. Molloy, A. Willan, and D. L. Streiner for the Canadian Critical Care Trials Group. 1995. "Determinants in Canadian Health Care Workers of the Decision to Withdraw Life Support from the Critical Ill." *Journal of the American Medical Association* 273 (9): 703–08.

Covinsky, K. E., S. Landefeld, J. Teno, A. F. Connors, N. Dawson, S. Youngner, N. Desbiens, J. Lynn, W. Fulkerson, D. Reding, R. Oye, and R. S. Phillips for the Support Investigators. 1996. "Is Economic Hardship on the Families of the Seriously Ill Associated with Patient and Surrogate Care Preferences?" *Archives of Internal Medicine* 156 (15): 1737–41.

Engelhardt, H. T., and M. A. Rie. 1986. "Intensive Care Units, Scarce Resources and Conflicting Principles of Justice." *Journal of the American Medical Association* 255 (9): 1159–64.

Fiel, S. B. 1991. "Heart-lung Transplantation for Patients with Cystic Fibrosis: A Test of Clinical Wisdom." *Archives of Internal Medicine* 151 (5): 870–72.

Field, B. E., L. E. Delvich, and R. W. Carlson. 1989. "Impact of a Comprehensive Supportive Care Team on Management of Hopelessly Ill Patients with Multiple Organ Failure." *Chest* 96 (2): 353–56.

Groeger, J.S., K. K. Guntupalli, M. A. Strosberg, N. Halpern, R. C. Raphael, F. Cerra, and W. Kaye. 1993. "Descriptive Analysis of Critical Care Units in the United States: Patient Characteristics and Intensive Care Unit Utilization." *Critical Care Medicine* 21 (2): 279–91.

Hanson, L. C., M. Davis, and S. Laxorick. 1994. "Emergency Triage to Intensive Care: Can We Use Prognosis and Patient Preferences?" *Journal of the American Geriatric Society* 42 (12): 1277–81.

Hansot, E. 1996. "A Letter from a Patient's Daughter." *Annals of Internal Medicine* 125 (2): 149–51.

Hoffmann, D. E. 1993. "Evaluating Ethics Committees: A View from Outside." *The Milbank Quarterly* 71 (4): 677–701.

Houston City-Wide Task Force on Medical Futility. 1996. "A Multi-institution Collaborative Policy on Medical Futility." *Journal of the American Medical Association* 276 (7): 571–74.

Jacobs, P., and T. W. Noseworthy. 1990. "National Estimates of Intensive Care Utilization and Costs: Canada and the United States." *Critical Care Medicine* 18 (1): 1282–85.

Jennett, B., and F. Plum. 1972. "Persistent Vegetative State After Brain Damage: A Syndrome in Search of a Name." *Lancet* 1 (753): 734–37.

Joint Commission on Accreditation of Healthcare Organizations. 1995. *1996 Comprehensive Accreditation Manual.* Oakbrook Terrace, Illinois.

Kilner, J. F. 1990. *Who Lives? Who Dies? Ethical Criteria in Patient Selection.* New Haven: Yale University Press.

Kollef, M. H. 1996. "Private Attending—the Withdrawal of Life-Sustaining Interventions in a Medical Intensive Care Unit Population." *Critical Care Medicine* 24 (6): 968–75.

Kollef, M. H., D. A. Canfield, and G. R. Zuckerman. 1995. "Triage Considerations for Patients with Acute Gastrointestinal Hemorrhage Admitted to a Medical Intensive Care Unit." *Critical Care Medicine* 23 (6): 1048–54.

Lee, K. P., A. J. Swinburne, A. J. Fedullo, and G. W. Wahl. 1994. "Withdrawing Care: Experience in a Medical Intensive Care Unit." *Journal of the American Medical Association* 271 (17): 1358–61.

Lo, B. 1995. "End-of-Life Care After Termination of SUPPORT." Hastings Center Reprot (Nov–Dec) (Special Supplement), S6–S8.

Marshall, M. F., K. J. Schwenzer, M. Orsina, J. C. Fletcher, and C. G. Durbin. 1992. "Influence of Political Power, Medical Provincialism, and Economic Incentives on the Rationing of Surgical Intensive Care Unit Beds." *Critical Care Medicine* 20 (3): 387.

Miller, F. G., and J. J. Fins. 1996. "A Proposal to Restructure Hospital Care For Dying Patients." *New England Journal of Medicine* 334 (26): 1740–42.

Morreim, E. H. 1992. "Rationing and the Law." In *Rationing America's Medical Care: The Oregon Plan and Beyond*, edited by M. A. Strosberg, J. M. Weiner, and R. Baker, 159–84. Washington, D.C.: The Brookings Institution.

Mulley, A. G. 1984. "The Triage Decision." In *The Machine at the Bedside*, edited by S. Reiser and M. Anstar, 221–26. Cambridge: Cambridge University Press.

Multi-Society Task Force on PVS. 1994. "Medical Aspects of the Persistent Vegetative State." *New England Journal of Medicine* 330 (21): 1499–1508.

National Institutes of Health. 1983. *Consensus Development Conference on Critical Care Medicine: Summary.* Bethesda, MD: National Institutes of Health.

New York Public Health Law. 1987. Article 29-B (L. 1987, Ch. 818).

New York State Task Force on Life and the Law. 1988. *Do Not Resuscitate Orders: The Proposed Legislation and Report of the New York State Task Force on Life and the Law,* Second Edition.

Paris, J. J., M. D. Schreiber, M. Statter, R. Arensman, and M. Siegler. 1993. "Beyond Autonomy—Physicians' Refusal to Use Life-Prolonging Extracorporeal Membrane Oxygenation." *New England Journal of Medicine* 329 (5): 354–57.

Prendergast, T. J., and J. M. Luce. 1996. "A National Survey of Withdrawal of Life Support from Critically Ill Patients." (Abstract): *American Journal of Respiratory and Critical Care Medicine* 153 (4): A360.

Rapoport, J., D. Teres, R. Barnett, P. Jacobs, A. Shustack, S. Lemeshow, C. Norris, and S. Hamilton. 1995. "A Comparison of Intensive Care Unit Utilization in Alberta and Western Massachusetts." *Critical Care Medicine* 20 (8): 1336–46.

Rie, M. A. 1995a. "The Oregonian ICU: Multi-Tiered Monetarized Morality in Health Insurance Law." *Journal of Law, Medicine and Ethics* 23 (2): 149–66.

———. 1995b. "Ethical Issues in Intensive Care: Criteria for Treatment within the Creation of a Health Insurance Morality." In *Critical Choices and Critical Care,* edited by K. W. Wildes, 23–56. Kluwer Academic Publishers.

Rublee, D. A. 1994. "Medical Technology in Canada, Germany, and the United States: An Update." *Health Affairs* 13 (4): 113–17.

Schneiderman, L. J., and N. S. Jecker. 1993. "Futility in Practice." *Archives of Internal Medicine* 153 (2): 437–441.

Shabot, M. M., J. S. Bjenke, M. LoBue, et al. 1992. "Quality Assurance and Utilization Assessment: The Major By-products of a Clinical Information-System." In *Proceedings of the XV Symposium on Computer Applications in Medicine.* Bethesda, MD: American Medical Informatics Association, 554–59.

Shoemaker, W., C. B. James, A. W. Fleming, E. Hardin, G. J. Ordog, R. Sterling-Scott, and J. Wasserberger. 1992. "DeFacto Rationing of Emergency Medical Services." In *Rationing America's Medical Care: The Oregon Plan and Beyond,* edited by M. A. Strosberg, J. M. Weiner, R. Baker, and I. A. Fein, 151–56. Washington, D.C.: The Brookings Institution.

Singer, D. E., P. L. Carr, A. G. Mulley, and G. E. Thibault. 1983. "Rationing Intensive Care: Physician Responses to a Resource Shortage." *New England Journal of Medicine* 309 (19): 1150–60.

Society of Critical Care Medicine Coalition of Critical Care Excellence. 1995. *ICU Cost Reduction: Practical Suggestions and Future Considerations.* Anaheim, CA: SCCM.

Society of Critical Care Medicine. 1994a. "Attitudes of Critical Care Medicine Professionals Concerning Distribution of Intensive Care Resources." *Critical Care Medicine* 22 (2): 358–62.

Society of Critical Care Medicine Ethics Committee. 1994b. "Consensus Statement on the Triage of Critically Ill Patients." *Journal of the American Medical Association* 271 (15): 1200–1203.

Society of Critical Care Medicine Ethics Committee. 1992. "Attitudes of Critical Care Medicine Professionals Concerning Forgoing Life-Sustaining Treatments." *Critical Care Medicine* 20 (3): 320–26.

Society of Critical Care Medicine Task Force for Distribution of ICU Resources in the

United States. 1993. "Advanced Directives, Policies for Terminating Life Support and Utilization of Ethics Committees in Intensive Care Units (ICU): of the United States." *Critical Care Medicine* 21 (4): (supplement): S219.

Society of Critical Care Medicine Task Force on Guidelines. 1988. "Recommendations for Intensive Care Unit Admission and Discharge Criteria." *Critical Care Medicine* 16 (8): 807–8.

Strauss, A., L. Schatzman, and D. Ehrlich. 1963. "The Hospital and its Negotiated Order." In *The Hospital in Modern Society*, edited by E. Freidson, 147–169. New York: Free Press of Glencoe.

Strauss, M. J., J. P. Logerfo, J. A. Yeltazie, N. Temkin, and L. D. Hudson. 1986. "Rationing of Intensive Care Unit Services." *Journal of the American Medical Association* 225 (9): 1143–46.

Streat, S., and J. A. Judson. 1994. "New Zealand." *New Horizons* 2 (3): 392–403.

Strosberg, M. A. 1995. "The New York State Do-No-Resuscitate Law: A Story of Public Policy Making." In *Legislating Medical Ethics: A Study of the New York Sate Do-Not-Resuscitate Law*, edited by R. Baker and M. A. Strosberg, 9–31. Durdrecht: Kluwer Academic Publishers.

The SUPPORT Principal Investigators. 1995. "A Controlled Trial to Improve Care for Seriously Ill Hospitalized Patients. The Study to Understand Prognoses and Preferences for Outcomes and Risks of Treatments (SUPPORT)." *Journal of the American Medical Association* 274 (20): 1591–98.

Teres, D. 1993. "Civilian Triage in the Intensive Care Unit: The Ritual of the Last Bed." *Critical Care Medicine* (21) 4: 598–606.

Teres, D. 1994. "A Different Interpretation of Management Scores." *American Journal of Critical Care* 3 (2): 84–86.

Thompson, J. D. 1967. *Organizations in Action*. New York: McGraw-Hill, 23.

Veatch, R. 1986. "The Ethics of Resource Allocation in Critical Care." *Critical Care Clinics*, 2 (1): 73–89.

Veatch, R. M. 1984. "The Ethics of Institutional Ethics Committees." In *Institutional Ethics Committees and Health Care Decision Making*, edited by R. E. Cranford and A. E. Doudera, 33–50. Chicago: Health Administration Press.

Von Stetina v. *Florida Medical Center*. 2 Fla Supp 2d 55 (Fla 17th Cir 1982):, 436 So Rptr 2d 1022 (1983):, 10 Florida Law Weekly 286 (Fla May 24, 1985).

Wachter, R. M., J. M. Luce, N. Hearst, and B. Lo. 1989. "Decisions about Resuscitation: Inequities among Patients with Different Diseases but Similar Prognoses." *Annals of Internal Medicine* 11 (6): 525–31.

Wachter, R. M., J. M. Luce, and P. C. Hopewell. 1992. "Critical Care of Patients with AIDS." *Journal of the American Medical Association* 267 (4): 541–47.

Youngner, S. J. 1988. "Who Defines Futility?" *Journal of the American Medical Association* 260 (14): 2094–95.

Zussman, R. 1992. *Intensive Care: Medical Ethics and the Medical Profession*. Chicago: University of Chicago Press.

CHAPTER 5

MANAGEMENT

Improvement Levers in the ICU

Shortell et al. (1992) present a cause-and-effect diagram (Exhibit 5.1) identifying opportunities for improvement in performance of ICUs (i.e., outcomes of care) measured in terms of risk-adjusted mortality, functional health status, patient/family satisfaction, and efficiency of utilization. The diagram categorizes six characteristics and their corresponding sub-factors: environmental, interorganizational, hospital, unit, provider, and patient. These six characteristics are conceptualized as "improvement levers" that can be adjusted to affect the various outcomes of care, including the efficiency of admission and discharge decision making.

Unit Characteristics and Processes

At the level of the unit or ICU, performance improvement is related to increasing intraunit and interunit coordination through modification of roles and role interrelationships, grouping of roles (positions) into units, and information and control systems (Robey 1982). To be considered are the formal policies governing the ICU, including those that pertain to admissions-discharge-triage and the relative distribution of power between non-ICU based physicians (e.g., community attendings) and ICU-based physicians. These policies include: admitting and procedure privileges; position descriptions of medical directors and triage officers, including arrangements for payment and time allocation; span of control and reporting relationships; and methods of collecting, analyzing, and communicating information. These structural components are part of the overt organization. But many other important variables lie beneath the surface, such as individual role perceptions and value systems; degree of trust, openness, and risk-taking behavior; and patterns of interpersonal, group, and departmental relationships. Together they become part of the negotiated order of the hospital (Strauss, Schatzman, and Ehrlich 1963).

In this connection, researchers have shown that the interpersonal relationships among the caregivers (physicians, nurses, and other staff) have important implications for ICU performance. Shortell et al. examined the interactions among ICU caregivers by measuring such variables as leadership, communication, coordination, and problem solving. They suggest that ICUs exhibiting a "team-oriented culture, with supportive nursing leadership, timely communication, effective coordination, and with collaborative, open problem solving approaches, are significantly more efficient in moving patients in and out of the unit" (Shortell et al. 1992).

Provider Characteristics and Processes

With regard to provider qualifications, as discussed in Chapter 2, leaders of the critical care profession argue that the availability of qualified or

Exhibit 5.1 Cause-and-Effect Diagram for Continuous Improvement in ICUs

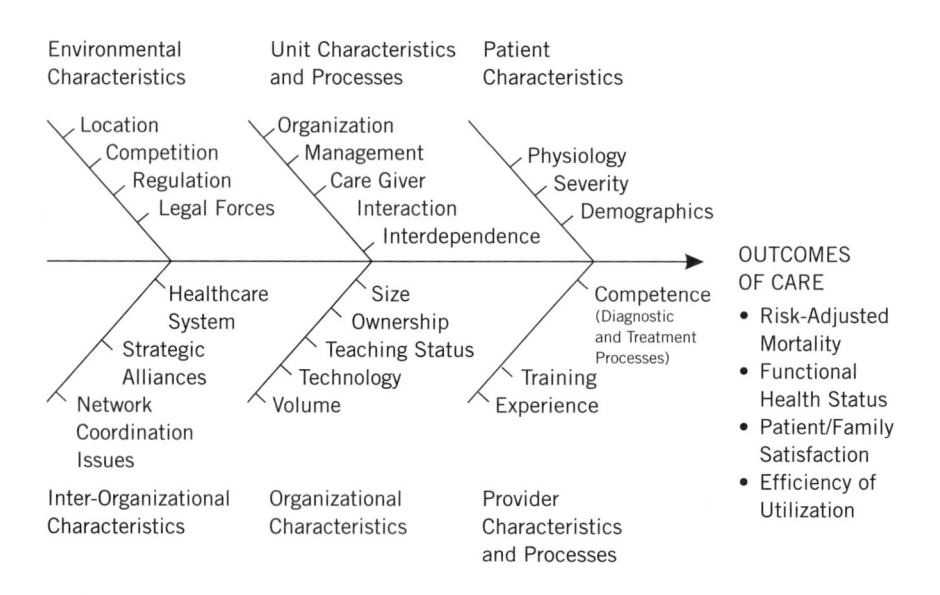

Environmental Characteristics	Unit Characteristics and Processes	Patient Characteristics	
Location	Organization	Physiology	
Competition	Management	Severity	
Regulation	Care Giver	Demographics	
Legal Forces	Interaction		
	Interdependence		**OUTCOMES OF CARE**
Healthcare System	Size	Competence (Diagnostic and Treatment Processes)	• Risk-Adjusted Mortality
Strategic Alliances	Ownership		• Functional Health Status
Network Coordination Issues	Teaching Status Technology Volume	Training Experience	• Patient/Family Satisfaction
			• Efficiency of Utilization
Inter-Organizational Characteristics	Organizational Characteristics	Provider Characteristics and Processes	

Source: S. M. Shortell et al. "Continuously Improving Patient Care" *Quality Review Bulletin* 18: 150–155, May, 1992. Oakbrook Terrace, IL.: Joint Commission on Accreditation of Healthcare Organizations. Reprinted with permission.

certified ICU-based intensivists (i.e., QCCPs) and nurses who provide a coordinated approach to care results in improved outcomes at reduced costs. Later in the chapter we will give some examples illustrating this point.

Environmental Conditions

1) **Location.** The location of the hospital (e.g., inner city, rural, suburban) and patients' socioeconomic backgrounds will influence the types of conditions for which patients are treated. For example, a hospital located in an inner city is likely to serve a lower socioeconomic group, usually with limited access to primary care and with a higher proportion of costly conditions such as diabetes, asthma, hypertension, trauma, and AIDS. For this population, inner-city hospitals are usually hospitals of "last resort." Suburban hospitals may serve a population with a higher proportion of insurance. Rural hospitals, which tend to be smaller, will likely transfer patients with severe conditions to tertiary hospitals.

2) **Market Competition.** Shortell et al. (1992) suggest that the competitiveness of local markets, especially with regard to competition for HMO and managed care contracts, will pressure hospitals to seek efficiencies in the ICU.

3) **Regulation.** State regulatory policy may encourage or discourage competition within a healthcare system. Also, the type of reimbursement system under which the hospitals operate influences ICU treatment and length of stay (Mayer-Oakes et al. 1988).

Interorganizational Characteristics

Increasingly, hospitals, reflecting a national trend toward managed care, are taking part in a variety of interorganizational arrangements designed to preserve and enhance their ability to compete in the market. Managed care brings fundamental shifts in stakeholder interests and incentives. The ICU is not immune from these shifts, as we will soon explain.

Organizational (Hospital) Characteristics

1) **Size.** The number of beds in the hospital is related to a whole host of organizational dimensions: number of different ICUs and special care units, number of beds in those units, occupancy rates, technology, staffing levels, and case mix (Groeger et al. 1992).

2) **Teaching status and mission.** Sociologists have long noted the distinctive cultures of the teaching hospital and the non-teaching hospital (Mumford 1970; Hage 1974). Teaching hospital ICUs, as opposed to non-teaching hospital ICUs, tend to treat more complex cases with a

greater amount of resources, including technology (Zimmerman et al. 1993b). The degree of affiliation with a medical school (community-affiliated teaching hospital versus university or medical center teaching hospital) influences the types of house staff (e.g., residents, fellows) available to the ICU, the role of the primary physician vis-a-vis the house staff, and the relative importance of the patient care mission compared to the teaching and research missions. Whether the hospital is for-profit, voluntary, or governmental (local, state, or Department of Veterans Affairs) also plays a part in determining mission.

Patient Characteristics

Shortell et al. (1992) note that in considering the previous five characteristics and their relationship to outcomes:

> ... it is important to ensure that the observed deviations from desired outcomes are not due to differences in patients—their physiology, severity of illness, or demographic characteristics. Once these factors are taken into account, the remaining deviations and consequent opportunities for improvement are most likely to center on providers, treatment units, and organizational characteristics and processes (p. 151).

Nevertheless, it should be clear that the five other factors have an impact on the types of patients who arrive at the ICU gates, not only in terms of their physiology and severity of illness, but in terms of their socio-economic status, insurance coverage, and relationship with a primary care physician.

Improvement Over Traditional Practice

> ... the traditional practice of individual physicians attending individual patients in individual ICU beds results in regimens of care that vary markedly despite similar disease states from bed to bed. Standardization of protocols is nearly impossible in this environment. Physicians are not immediately available for emergencies. Care is often determined over the phone. Multiple consultants become involved, leading to multiple sets of orders, and often multiple conflicting orders. Formalized rounds on all ICU patients do not occur, since each patient has a different physician, each of whom may be in the unit at different times during the day. The nurses are told to call various doctors for various problems, depending on the organ system involved. During off-hours and weekends, someone who does not know the patient covers for each of the doctors. All too often, there is no one physician coordinating the care of the patient. The nurse is left to sort out conflicting orders and plans requiring multiple calls and explanations to various physicians, at best an inefficient process of care, at worst, chaos (Rainey 1994, p. 1036).

The two levers that most immediately provide the potential to change the practices described above and to improve performance are provider characteristics and processes and unit characteristics and processes. The shift to managed care and the changes generated by interorganizational, organizational, and environmental characteristics will, to a large extent, determine the degree to which the two primary levers are engaged. We will return to this important theme in a later section. But we now focus on the topic of improving traditional practice by changing provider characteristics and processes and unit characteristics and processes. We examine these changes at two levels of aggregation: (1) management of the critical illnesses of the individual patient, and (2) management of the resources allocated to all the patients in the unit.

Management of the Patient: Claims for the QCCP

Not only does the SCCM (1992) claim that critical care delivered by the qualified critical care physician (QCCP) is the most effective method of treating the complications of the critically ill, it also claims that it is the most efficient:

> The immediate availability of the qualified critical care physician, who provides a coordinated and collaborative approach to care for gravely ill patients, results in strongly improved outcomes at reduced cost . . . By medical training and practice, the QCCP can best help patients and their families measure the benefits of current and future therapies, make appropriate choices and preserve costly resources for those who can benefit (p. iii).

According to this definition, the physicians treating Mrs. Hansot (Chapter 4), and the ICU medical director, even if certified in critical care medicine, have not adequately met SCCM's expectations for the role of the QCCP.

The empirical research base upon which the SCCM stakes its claims for the QCCP is still small and is mostly composed of studies of single or a small number of institutions (Reynolds et al. 1988; Pollack et al. 1988; Brown et al. 1989; Shoemaker et al. 1988; Berlauk et al. 1991; Li et al. 1984). However, there are a growing number of multi-institutional studies that lend support to SCCM claims (Shortell-HCFA 1991; Zimmerman et al. 1993a; Malick et al. 1995).

How does the SCCM (1992) envision the QCCP carrying out his or her role? The SCCM describes the role by illustrating the care of an ICU patient under two different scenarios:
Scenario One.

152 *Gatekeeping in the Intensive Care Unit*

>A urologist operated on a 53-year-old male patient to remove a stone from his left ureter. The patient developed an infection of his left kidney postoperatively, a common complication. Upon recognition of infection, the urologist chose to give an appropriate antibiotic. Unfortunately, the infection spread to the patient's bloodstream, precipitating a series of serious problems. Toxins in the blood from bacteria disturbed the integrity of blood vessels, weakened the heart, injured the lungs, interfered with the gastrointestinal tract so that food could not be absorbed and threatened the viability of the kidneys. Rapid interventions to treat or avoid serious complications were required. At that point, the urologist transferred that patient to the ICU (p. 6).

In this first scenario:

>Large quantities of intravenous fluids were ordered to restore a decreasing blood pressure. However, the heart muscle was weakened by arteriosclerotic heart disease and has been further damaged by bacterial toxins; it could not pump adequately to handle the additional fluid. The heart was failing. The urologist requested consultation from a cardiologist. Unfortunately, the lungs were also damaged by toxins, causing respiratory failure. The patient required a mechanical ventilator to support oxygenation. The urologist requested consultation from a pulmonary specialist to help manage the respiratory failure. Meanwhile, the patient's bowel function may have become immobilized by toxins. The kidneys also have been jeopardized by the failing heart and continued infection. The urologist would summon a nephrologist to assess kidney function and to assist with fluid management. An infectious disease specialist would be consulted to monitor antibiotic administration (p .6).

The SCCM interprets this scenario in the following way:

>This complex series of rapidly developing physiologic derangement place the patient at risk of imminent death. The urologist relied on a series of specialists to help manage the deteriorating situation, but they are usually not immediately available in the ICU. Physicians must be summoned from offices, research laboratories or other locations for consultations. In addition, their advice tends to be focused and limited to their area of expertise. The urologists need someone to organize treatment into a coherent plan (p. 7).

If, however, a QCCP were available in the ICU, another course of events might have transpired.
In this second scenario:

>As soon as the patient was transferred to the ICU, the QCCP assessed the priorities of organ system and multiple life-threatening conditions. He developed, implemented and directed treatment plans that may have included: intubation of the patient's trachea; mechanical ventilation; regulation of the ventilator to assure acceptable oxygenation and ventilation; treatment of the cardiovascular system with intravenous fluids and the heart with medications to promote blood flow; provision of nutrition customized to the patient's level of stress and tolerance; administration of antibiotic therapy; reduction of fever; sedation

to reduce cellular demands for oxygen; prevention of stress-induced stomach ulceration; and prevention of heart attack in the patient who has evidence of arteriosclerosis of the heart blood vessels.

Working closely with important members of the critical care team such as a nurse, respiratory therapists and nutritionists, the QCCP will usually develop and implement a comprehensive treatment plan that may include needed consultations from other specialists. Communication with other team members is more effective since the QCCP regularly consults with them. During the patient's initial hours in the ICU, the QCCP resuscitates the patient's cardiac, pulmonary and tissue perfusion functions. Over the next few days care will be planned to prevent or treat additional complications. The full-time presence of a QCCP in the ICU permits moment-to-moment assessments and adjustments of therapy as well as reduction of medications and mechanical support as the patient regains normal organ function. The QCCP may also assist the specialist in talking with the patient's family relative to prognosis and complex treatment issues. The QCCP serves as source of information about the critical illness for the family instead of a series of physicians, each confining their involvement to a single aspect of the illness (p. 7).

As was mentioned in Chapter 2, there are many subspecialty contenders for the mantle of QCCP. They all could serve as QCCPs provided that they fulfill managerial roles discussed in the next section.

Management of the Unit

In addition to claims for the effectiveness and efficiency resulting from involvement of the QCCP in the management of individual patients, the SCCM also stakes out a role for the QCCP as manager of the resources of the ICU and its patients. The SCCM (1991) states in its "Guidelines on the Definition of an Intensivist and Practice of Critical Care Medicine":

> The intensivist participates actively in daily unit management activities necessarily for the efficient, timely, and consistent delivery of ICU services to the patients of the hospital. These activities include but are not limited to: (a) triage and bed allocation, discharge planning (b) supervision of the application of unit policies (c) participation in ongoing quality improvement activities including supervision of data collection (d) interaction with other departments as necessary to facilitate the smooth operation of the ICU. To provide these services, the intensivist must be physically present in the unit or hospital and free from competing obligations such as operating room or office responsibilities (p. 2).

Significantly, for both the management of the critically ill patient and the management of the unit, the SCCM considers the defining characteristic of the QCCP as the physical presence or availability on a 24-hour basis to make decisions either for the individual patient or, in the case of triage, all patients in the unit and candidates for entry. In fact, the SCCM leadership claims that without such availability, a high likelihood exists that care will be suboptimal (Weil, Shoemaker, and Rackow 1988). It should be pointed out that many physicians have passed the certifying exam or are otherwise qualified to perform the many procedures carried out in the ICU but spend the majority of the time in a non-ICU setting.

In some circumstances, intensivists could collaborate with hospitalists (Wachter and Goldman 1996) to cover all in-hospital patients. Intensivists are experienced at making decisions, at negotiating procedures, and at interacting with a modest number of consultants. Although the daily cost may be high, the length of stay would probably be shortened since the link between critical illness and rehabilitation, including nutrition, is so strong. One advantage to this approach is that the primary care physician and traditional subspecialist can more productively spend their time in the ambulatory/office setting. The disadvantage is that overall continuity of care might suffer.

Impediments to Medical Leadership

At both levels (patient management and unit management) the arguments of the SCCM have not been widely accepted. The model of the full-time, hospital-based intensivist, providing concurrent or primary care, is not the national norm. As was pointed out in Chapters 2 and 3, the SCCM survey and the Strosberg et al. (1990) survey show that ICUs lack medical leadership in many of the important management functions:

- bed allocation and discharge planning;
- development and supervision of the application of unit policies;
- participation in ongoing quality improvement activities, including supervision of data collection;
- interaction with other departments as necessary to facilitate the smooth operation of the ICU;
- resolution of conflict;
- negotiating with families on end-of-life decisions;
- and triage, particularly at night.

It has not been easy to reconcile the non-ICU based physicians with the patient care and managerial roles assigned to the QCCP. To begin with, critically ill patients constitute a significant percentage of hospital practice and generate considerable physician charges. The prevailing U.S. practice pattern consists of physicians maintaining primary responsibility for patients in all aspects of outpatient and inpatient care. Traditional reimbursement arrangements, as well as the failure of critical care to emerge as a primary specialty (in contrast to most other nations), have all contributed to the current practice patterns. With regard to managerial roles, a divergence often occurs between the official duties of the medical director and/or designees as called for in hospital policies and professional society guidelines, and what medical directors actually do.

What are some of the conditions that would enable the medical director and other intensivists to carry out the necessary management roles? First, medical directors must spend time in the ICU. For many medical directors reimbursement is not sufficient to adequately compensate for spending time in management activities not directly related to patient care. Compensation must be available to free the physician-manager from competing obligations in the operating room and the office.

Most importantly, medical directors will need the support of hospital administrators, department chairs, and attending physicians. These groups, especially the last two, have often impeded the medical director in exercising leadership in gatekeeping especially if that decision making is perceived to lead to control over patient care. Physicians often see the emergence of a strong medical director as a threat to their autonomy and their ability to consult and perform procedures in the ICU.

New Financial Incentives for Primary Care Physicians: New Opportunities for Intensitivists?

Will managed care change the financial incentives for primary care physicians so that they will no longer want to take care of patients in ICUs, and will they willingly relinquish control to the intensivist? Rapoport et al. (1992) compared resource utilization among patients in managed care versus traditional insurance, using the same teams composed of faculty intensivists and house staff. They found, after controlling for severity, using the Mortality Probability Model, that patients in managed care plans had lower ICU resource use and shorter lengths of stay with no discernible difference in outcome. What is particularly interesting about this study is that the hospital-based, ICU intensivists were reimbursed on a fee-for-service basis. One plausible interpretation of this finding is that primary care physicians working in managed care settings are more willing to turn over their ICU patients to intensivists for management. In this type of concurrent care relationship, intensivists order fewer consultations from single organ system specialists with fewer concomitant procedures and shorter length of stay. A follow-up study confirmed fewer subspecialty consultations in the MICU-managed care patients. (Steingrub, Teres, and Rapoport 1996). In contrast to Rapoport et al.'s study, however, Angus et al. (1996), in a retrospective analysis of the 1992

Massachusetts hospital discharge database, found that patients admitted to the ICU covered under managed care had similar lengths of stay to those patients covered by traditional commercial insurance or Medicare.

On the other side of the country, a Californian physician foresees a new environment and set of opportunities for critical care physicians:

> As the traditional fee-for-service reimbursement is replaced by either discounted rates, fixed per diem payments, or capitated payments, a significant part of the traditional incentive for involving multiple specialists and non-intensivists will dissolve. The biggest challenge to critical care at this time is to market our ability to serve as gatekeepers for hospitalized patients and by so doing to alter the 'business as usual' approach (Gipe 1995, p. 8).

One way in which critical care physicians might respond to this challenge is for them to accept discounted fees from managed care organizations or from primary care physicians who control at-risk contracts. Dr. Bruce Gipe, the Los Angeles critical care physician quoted above, warns that discounted fee-for-service "can become a downward spiral as others compete with progressively deeper discounts." He suggests that critical care physician groups compete on the basis of capitated risk contracts for critically ill patients. To do so they must calculate a per-member-per month (PMPM) rate for critical care services for a given population.

Understanding Critical Care Outcomes

To what extent capitation will replace fee-for-service reimbursement to critical care physicians remains to be seen. However, it is clear that the traditional approach to practice involving multiple specialists and non-intensivist physicians must change. It is also clear that the trend toward managed care will generate pressure to understand, monitor, and control costs for the hospital's sickest and most expensive patients. For hospital administrators and department chairs, a reasonable response will be to support and enhance the managerial roles of the ICU medical director and the QCCP (Mallick et al. 1995). For the purchasers of healthcare, the issue is how to identify hospitals with high-quality, cost-effective ICUs.

The issue is related to the increasing prominence given outcomes research, appropriateness criteria, and practice guidelines, now championed by the major medical associations, specialty societies, and the federal Agency of Health Care Policy and Research (AHCPR). The intellectual foundation of the above owes much to the work of Dr. John Wennberg, who pioneered what has become known as "small-area variation analysis." Wennberg, who can best be described as a medical care epidemiologist, discovered significant variations in medical care utilization among populations in small, geographically distinct towns in New England as well as in large cities such as Boston and New Haven. While he discerned great variation in utilization of medical resources, there was little difference in outcomes but large differences in expenditures. Wennberg offered small-area variation analysis—research to find the sources of variation—as a solution to the cost-escalation problem. He reasoned that if there were significant variation among populations in their utilization of medical resources, with no discernible difference in outcome, why should third parties, including government, pay for the more expensive practice patterns (Wennberg, McPherson, and Caper 1984)?

This logic, compelling to both the private and public sectors, helped spawn a major research endeavor. Outcomes research, appropriateness criteria, and practice guidelines, aimed at finding and implementing the most cost-effective practice patterns, have become a central plank in an overall cost-containment strategy.

Wide variation in the use of intensive care has long been noted in international comparisons. In response, the critical care community has advocated outcomes research to identify which patients could best benefit from ICU intervention. The 1983 NIH Consensus Development Conference (1983) included a plea for outcomes research. While the majority of the participants at the conference were clinicians and scientists, there are now more customers and supporters for this research, including third party payors and managed care organizations.

The Emergence of Managed Care

In Chapter 1, we briefly discussed the ramifications of a paradigm shift initiated by the managed care revolution. In this section we extend this discussion and recognize that there are stages to the transition and concomitant responses by providers (i.e., physicians and hospitals). Shactman and Altman (1995) hypothesize that healthcare markets might evolve along the following lines:

Stage 1. Managed care plans enter markets with limited competition, especially those with high prices and excess acute care beds and medical specialists. Through selective contracting, the plans reduce prices and still produce large profits.

Stage 2. Providers, in response to diminished profits, try to maintain competitiveness by downsizing, improving operating efficiency, and collaborating with others through mergers and joint ventures. Managed care plans continue developing their provider networks, decreasing utilization, and negotiating lower prices.

Stage 3. Providers, in response to lower utilization and reimbursement, join integrated delivery systems. Industry-wide shakeout leads to fewer systems serving a larger proportion of population.

Stage 4. In relatively mature market, some managed care plans provide high quality, cost-effective services that make a profit. Other plans raise prices without maintaining quality.

The above stages, admittedly a set of untested hypotheses, may not adequately portray the amount of turbulence that some fear the managed care marketplace is bringing to nurses, physicians, and hospitals as payors (business and government) aggressively seek greater value for their health insurance dollar through selective contracting and the promotion of price competition. Uwe Reinhardt (1987) warned several years ago:

> If the American business community ever bestirred itself to exercise fully the market power it potentially has in the emerging buyer's market for health care, the nation's physicians and hospitals may yet come to appreciate that the free market so many of them dreamed of in the 1970s is actually a tortuous instrument designed to visit on them daily uncertainty, step-by step monitoring of their clinical decisions by external boards, and morally vexing tradeoffs between economic security and their professional code of ethics (p. 111).

Today it is not uncommon to hear about multi-billion dollar mega-mergers among not-for-profit and for-profit HMOs and other types of managed care organizations, insurance companies, and hospital systems, encompassing millions of covered lives. What will be the impact of managed care on critical care? Prediction is fraught with difficulty. Nevertheless, accepting the general outline and direction of the hypothesized stages with regard to consolidation, downsizing, and integration, we foresee change in the organizational arrangements associated with traditional practice. Most, but not all, of these changes will bring improvement in both efficiency and quality.

ICU Organizational Changes: One View of the Future

Cost-conscious practice styles standardized by practice guidelines and care maps will be part of the future. By far the largest component of the cost of critical care is labor, especially nursing labor. One strategy for reducing labor costs while maintaining or improving quality is the creation of flexible personnel roles (e.g., multitask nurses and technicians) and the redesign of the processes of care.

Leaders of critical care medicine, following the example of business and industry, are now seriously discussing reengineering (SCCM 1995). Reengineering is "the fundamental rethinking and radical redesign of business processes to achieve dramatic improvements in critical, contemporary measures of performance, such as cost, quality, service, and speed" (Hammer and Champy 1993).

Market forces will favor assembly-line processes and high-volume facilities. In high-volume facilities, not only do mortality and complication rates for many surgical procedures decline because of the increased volume, but also the unit cost may be lower with standardization of equipment and with protocols geared to shorten ICU and hospital stay. Already we are seeing the emergence of the large hospital or small specialty hospital with surgical teams performing high-volume surgery (e.g., more than 2,000 open-heart procedures per year). One example of assembly-line protocol-driven care is "fast-track extubation" (a rapid wean from ventilator and removal of the endotracheal tube) for open-heart procedures. It is based in part on advances in anesthesia providing not only cardiac protection and preservation during the operation but also a more rapid post-procedure wake-up (Engelman et al. 1994). For high-volume hospitals doing aortic vascular procedures, the improvements may even mean that many patients can safely bypass the ICU altogether. PACUs or recovery rooms and step-down or intermediate care units can substitute for ICUs.

In hospitals, regardless of size or volume, a new language and set of techniques are being developed to describe, understand, and improve aspects of care processes, including time on a ventilator, time in the ICU, medications for antibiotics, pain, sedation, hypertension, and hypotension. Schriefer (1993), for example, describes the success of an interdepartmental and interdisciplinary quality improvement team, composed of respiratory therapists, nurses, pharmacists, thoracic surgeons, anesthesiologists, and ICU-based intensivists, in reducing the surgical intensive care unit length of stay for postoperative open-heart patients by more quickly weaning patients off mechanical ventilation. This new language and set of techniques is associated with improvement knowledge, which draws upon an understanding of systems, variation, psychology, and theories of learning (Batalden and Stoltz 1993). Improvement knowledge underpins TQM or CQI, which is increasingly being applied to critical care. The Institute for Healthcare Improvement, located in Boston, is taking a leadership position in these efforts.

Mid-Level Practitioners

In the interests of optimizing the use of personnel, hospitals will increasingly turn to a variety of mid-level care practitioners, including acute care nurse practitioners and physician assistants who will manage the processes of care. These practitioners, acting as physician extenders (Snyder et al. 1994), perform tasks that have previously been performed by physicians and house staff. For example, the University of Pittsburgh

Medical Center is developing at the Masters level the acute care nurse practitioner (ACNP) who "combines the nurse practitioner's broad orientation to management of common primary care problems with the specialty training required for care of acutely and critically ill patients." The developers believe that the ACNPs may be more amenable than residents and fellows in accepting and promoting standardized care protocols, especially with regard to high-volume surgical procedures (Snyder et al. 1994).

No doubt physicians, fearing encroachment on their clinical turf and diminishment of their reimbursement base, will resist the idea of the mid-level practitioner. However, the resistance will be lessened by the dramatic reduction in number of specialty training programs for residents and fellows, who will be increasingly shifted to ambulatory and out-of-hospital rotations. The typical medical resident spends approximately 20 percent to 25 percent of his or her time in the ICU, coronary care, or emergency room settings. Family practice residents spend even less time in these same settings. In primary care training, less time will be devoted to critical care. Who will fill the mid-level positions when the residents are in clinic or at the ambulatory center? The most common approach, as has been suggested, will be nurse practitioner or physician assistant models, but a variety of other contenders exist. For example, the highly trained critical care doctor of pharmacy (Pharm.D.) could perform an important role in dosing drugs and evaluating drug-drug interactions. Nurses do not possess this advanced training. In addition, some respiratory therapists could expand their role to include a cardiopulmonary technology function.

Alternatively, mid-level practitioners could serve as case managers throughout the hospitalization—not just in the ICU—rather than on the minute to minute titration of care, fostering continuity among providers across all settings in which the patient receives care (SCCM 1995). Among the goals of case management are early discharge and reduced utilization of resources. Case managers need not be based in the ICU. Some case managers are involved in patient assessment prior to hospitalization as well as after. The home and family are assessed, and post-hospital appointments are made according to the care maps and protocols. These approaches are applicable to high-volume elective surgery.

The mid-level practitioners may also take on other important managerial responsibilities in the ICU. The Professionally Advanced Care Team at the Robert Wood Johnson University Hospital, created in 1987, includes the clinical care manager (CCM), a nurse who combines high-quality clinical management with aggressive business management. Using multidisciplinary clinical care protocols to ensure that expected patient outcomes are achieved, the CCM "plans and facilitates patient transfers and coordinates complex diagnostic testing schedules for critically ill patients. The activities of the CCM relieve the primary nurse of interferences that take the nurse away from the bedside" (Walleck 1994).

The activities of bedside nurses will be modified in the face of cost pressures. The 1:2 ICU nurse-to-patient ratio will be difficult to sustain. Hospitals will be looking for ways to minimize the number of expensive RNs, while at the same time maintaining and improving quality. One solution is the delegation of a variety of nursing tasks to non-RN support personnel and nurse extenders (Walleck 1994). A non-licensed, multi-task technician would perform catheter set-ups and monitoring and recording of vital signs.

Managed Care: Concerns for Critical Care

The above examples are indicative of some of the changes that have already taken place or will likely take place in the managed care marketplace. Many of these changes will improve both efficiency and quality. It has been suggested that market forces could provide the right constraints (e.g., cutting back on ICU beds and the number of specialists) and incentives (e.g., placing intensive care physicians at financial risk for the services they provide) to reduce inappropriate interventions (Lo 1995). On the other hand, critics of the managed care marketplace question whether pressure will be exerted to limit care to high-cost patients, and worry that resource constraints may jeopardize quality.

Exhibit 5.2 summarizes the influences that managed care will have on triage-mode decision making. Undoubtedly, managed care, at least in its initial stages, will reduce the frequency of triage because fewer patients will need ICU care. However, with consolidation and downsizing, too many hospitals may close in a given market. If the demand for medical care is slowed temporarily only to be followed by increased demand, a critical shortage of ICU beds may occur. There are periodic peaks in hospital and ICU censuses when the number of emergency cases and elective procedures coincide, resulting in heightened demand. With less flexibility in the rest of the hospital, the rubber band of critical care services will not have as much stretch as in the golden years of the 1970s and 1980s, increasing the pressure on the triage officer. Public, inner-city hospitals are most vulnerable to disruption. Will the example of King-Drew Medical Center of inner-city Los Angeles mentioned in Chapter 1 be replicated in other major metropolitan areas?

Exhibit 5.2 Factors Influencing Frequency of ICU Triage

Factors leading to less frequent triage
1. Increased efficiencies (especially in the early stages of transition to managed care).
2. Greater use of care maps, protocols, and guidelines.
3. Greater number of low-risk monitor patients bypassing the ICU.
4. Greater use of DNR orders and other advance directives, presumably with more rapid decisions to withdraw life-sustaining therapy.
5. Greater number of patients declining ICU therapy trials.

Factors leading to more frequent triage
1. Downsizing of ICU beds.
2. Downsizing of regular beds due to mergers, consolidations, and hospital closures.
3. AIDS viewed as a chronic disease, not necessarily terminal.
4. Increase in infectious disease and organisms resistant to multiple drugs (Tenover and Hughes 1996) and increasing length of stay.
5. Unavailability of step-down, ICU intermediate care beds.
6. Increased patient awareness and demand for ICU care.

Unresolved Issues

In earlier chapters we discussed the roles of the ICU medical director and the triage officer, and the activities that might make up their position descriptions. We also discussed the managerial role conflict that inevitably arises in the fee-for-service environment of the traditional practice of critical care medicine. Much of this role conflict could ultimately be resolved under managed care with the emergence of closed units headed by working medical directors who facilitate communication and coordination and triage officers who have the political independence to make comparative entitlement decisions. Thus far, however, the QCCP model has not emerged as the industry norm. If the industry moves in the direction of integrated delivery systems, the model's chances of adoption will be improved. Capitation, as Berwick (1996) points out, creates the possibilities and the incentives to design the healthcare system to overcome fragmentation and the myriad of organizational and professional categories. On the other hand, some of the newer organizational and financial relationships (e.g., carve outs) among physicians, hospitals, and insurers are leading in the opposite direction, resulting in more fragmentation and diminished oversight and supervision. Under these conditions, it remains to be seen to what extent the attributes of the

QCCP model will be accepted as indicators of efficiency and quality of care. But in any managed care environment, the issues highlighted at the end of Chapter 3 bear repeating. Whether there are open units with decentralized decision making or closed units with centralized decision making, how do we ensure consistency, fairness, and accountability? How do we ensure that like cases are treated alike and filter out arbitrary and capricious behavior? How do we maintain quality? In theory, these concerns of consistency, accountability, and quality could be resolved in the marketplace. Can consumers, empowered by information on price, quality, and other indicators, make intelligent choices? In a competitive environment, plans that cannot attract consumers must either change or be driven out of the marketplace. In practice, this information, especially as it relates to choices relevant to the ICU, is most often not available. And, of course, the uninsured and the underinsured are not in the position to express their preferences in the marketplace.

What could help is the establishment of better rules for gatekeeping that guide resource allocation and provide the means to hold decision makers accountable. In particular we require better criteria for admission and discharge decision making independent of bed availability. We also require better criteria to help rank-order comparative entitlement during triage. To the extent that decisions can be pre-planned or pre-programmed into a set of "if-then" statements which prioritize candidates for admission, discharge, and triage, decision makers can rely on rules to anticipate contingencies and automatically supply them with appropriate responses minimizing the necessity for ad hoc triage decisions in individual cases. Rules save on information processing time. Decision-making discretion would be limited.

Rules in the form of policies and procedures can also be a way to bring a sense of order to what may be a difficult and ethically confusing decision-making process, especially in end-of-life situations. Prognostic models and severity scoring systems may also prove helpful here. However, institutional governing bodies have been reluctant to adopt policies that effectively guide bedside decision making and balance individual and societal claims to resources. Clinicians and hospitals, because of real or imagined fear of legal challenge, have been hesitant to rely on such policies. Resolution lies, in part, in the courts and legislatures.

Another unresolved issue is the quandary of divided loyalty when physicians have to make treatment decisions for their individual patients while at the same time bearing the responsibility for making admission, discharge, and comparative entitlement decisions affecting all ICU patients. The trend toward closed and centralized units will tend to make the intensivist the physician of record as well as the manager of resources. This quandary and ethical conflict will be heightened by financial pressures in managed care organizations. How do we monitor and moderate the subtle influence of economic pressure on physicians with dual demands?

The Impact of Managed Care On Anywhere Hospital: A Speculation

How might the ICU of Anywhere Hospital be restructured under managed care arrangements? How might the ICU gatekeepers have decided the fate of the patients in the Chapter 4 decision rounds? What would be different? Below we describe the changes at Anywhere Hospital as it enters the third stage of its evolution under managed care (as delineated by Shactman and Altman 1995).

Under managed care, Anywhere Hospital has changed its ICU from a semi-closed to a closed unit with a QCCP medical director and intensivist team responsible for managing the patients and for gatekeeping (see Exhibits 2.8 and 2.9). Under this arrangement the intensivists become the patients' primary physicians. Attending physicians play a much less important role in patient management and are less active as players in gatekeeping negotiations.

Anywhere Hospital has reduced its number of beds because of the decrease in both the number of hospitalizations and the length of stay. The medical-surgical ICU has downsized from 12 to 9 beds. However, alternative settings, including respiratory care units (handling ventilators) and other intermediate care and transition care units, have been created. Many ICU processes have been reengineered or fast-tracked. Length of stay has decreased. Exhibit 5.3 presents the bed disposition of the downsized nine-bed ICU as we revisit the decision rounds starting with the decision whether or not to admit the transfer patient (see Chapter 1).

Revisiting the Cases—Six Patients Under Managed Care

Round 1: The Transfer and the Cardiac Arrest Patients

With no available beds, the request to refer to Anywhere Hospital was denied. The patient remained at his home hospital where he died. Also, the patient in cardiac arrest on the medical floor of Anywhere Hospital was allowed because the physician and family agreed to place a DNR order in the chart.

Management   165

Exhibit 5.3 Anywhere Hospital Under Managed Care: A Speculation
9-Bed Medical/Surgical ICU

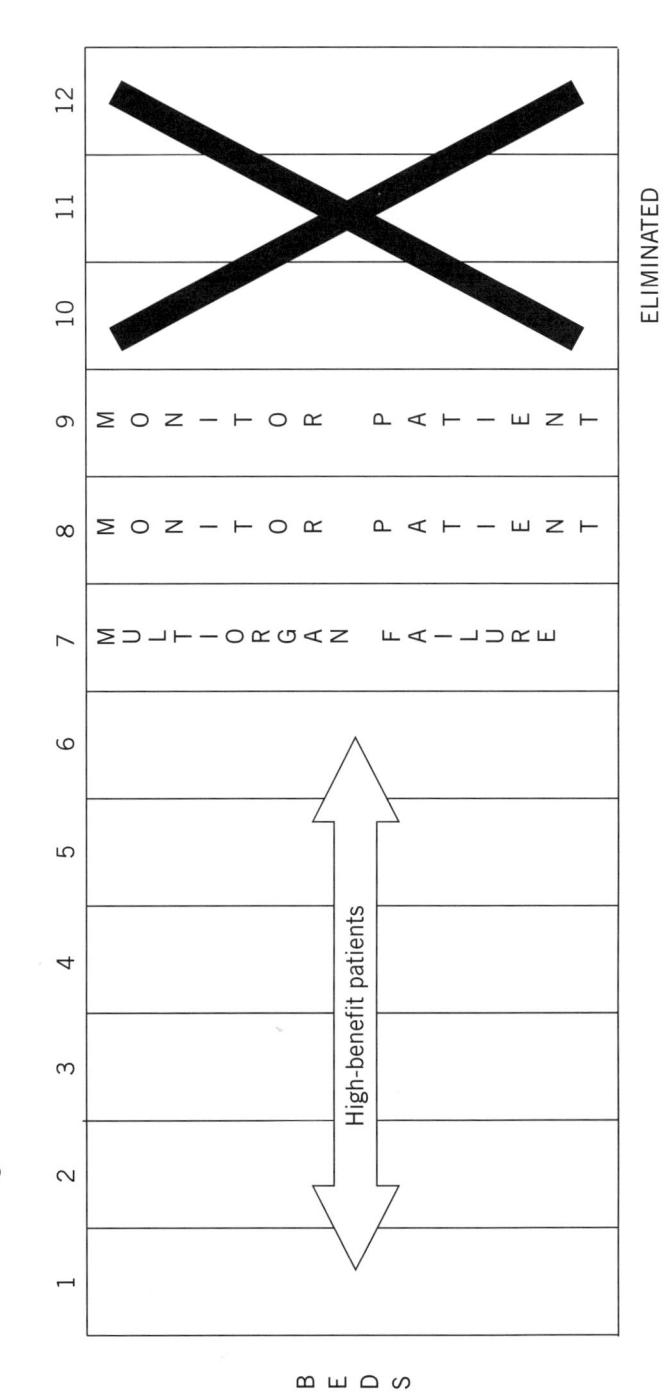

BEDS	1	2	3	4	5	6	7	8	9	10	11	12
				High-benefit patients			Multi-organ failure	Monitor patient	Monitor patient	ELIMINATED		

Round 2: The Smoker Patient

With only a 10 percent chance of survival and poor prognosis, the patient was denied admission to the ICU. He was given comfort care on the floor where he died.

Round 3: The Bleeder Patient

The patient was screened using a risk-stratification instrument designed to predict the probability of acute GI bleeding. Because the patient was found to be low risk, he had endoscopy in the GI suite and then was admitted to intermediate care.

Round 4: The Elective Surgery Patient

Elective surgery was delayed until a bed became available.

Round 5: The AIDS Patient

Because of poor prognosis, the patient was denied admission to the ICU and treated on the floor with comfort care.

Round 6: The Asthmatic and Multi-Organ Failure Patients

The patient was immediately admitted to the ICU. It should be noted that acute episodes like this one are becoming more rare since the managed care plan instituted its disease management protocols for asthma. The multi-organ failure patient, after a five-day trial period, was transferred to hospice care.

Discussion

The rationales for the above decisions can all be justified by the admission and discharge policies of Anywhere Hospital and supported by the consensus statements of various professional societies. The ICU is apparently meeting its performance expectations. But something has changed. The demands of the patients, families, and their physicians who desired aggressive treatment (the smoker, the multi-organ failure patient), postoperative care (the elective surgery patient) or simply admission (the bleeder patient) have been deflected. Does decreased demand have to do with the fact that physicians are now reconsidering the level of treatment for their patients in response to fewer available ICU beds and tighter constraints (and greater likelihood of triage mode decision making)? Does decreased demand have to do with the diminished role of the private attending physicians? Do financial incentives to physicians under managed care provide an inducement not to seek treatments that were formerly thought to be beneficial? Has patient autonomy been diminished in the face of new constraints and incentives, and if so what is the legal recourse? What is the level of societal and patient trust in the ICU medical director and designated triage officer? Many of these questions fall under the rubric of the unresolved issues. They have to be addressed to accommodate the new performance expectations of the renegotiated order of managed care. We will discuss them further in Chapter 6. Before moving on, we conclude this chapter with a discussion of prognostic models and severity scoring systems and their role in management and resource allocation.

Three Potential Uses for Prognostic Models in Gatekeeping, Resource Allocation, and Quality Assurance

1. **To monitor externally and internally the quality of managed care systems in order to detect diminishment of quality and covert rationing.** If cost-containment becomes the single most dominant driving force in the managed care market, there may be an important societal advantage to monitoring the observed and expected mortality and other outcomes within the various plans. As a matter of public policy, externally audited ICU prognostic models could play a pivotal role in providing consumer protection. The plans themselves could use the prognostic models for quality assurance and quality improvement.

2. **To enhance the ability of the triage officer and others to collect, interpret, and disseminate prognostic information.** Is there a way to capture and summarize important prognostic information so that it can be more easily digested, processed, and communicated among primary physicians, consultants, ICU nurses, patients, and families? Because everyone gets involved, the cost of communication is high. But a prognostic instrument linked to a clinical information system may help ameliorate this condition by building a common understanding of the clinical condition.

It is important to emphasize that agreement on prognosis and its associated probabilities does not necessarily mean that agreement also exists on the values that different parties attach to those probabilities or outcomes. For example, to the neurosurgeon, the fact that the patient survived the operation is a good outcome. To the family physician, the fact that this same patient will not work or play golf again is a bad outcome. Also, the availability of prognostic information may not necessarily lead to its use, change in decision making, or an improvement in quality.

The SUPPORT study (1995), carried out at five major medical centers, provided a specially trained nurse with daily probabilities of mortality and poor functional outcome for the purpose of facilitating discussion with physicians and improving the quality of care. However, much to the surprise of the researchers, there was no difference in hospital resource consumption compared to similar patients for whom no prognostic information was provided. The failure of this intervention, as Berwick (1995) points out, illustrates that "systems of care are complex, nonlinear, and difficult to manipulate in simple, cause-and-effect experimental modes" (p. S 21). Changing these systems and improving organizational performance will require a much more sophisticated intervention based on improvement knowledge (Langley et al. 1996).

3. To help clarify and construct criteria that could be used in: (1) admissions and discharge decision making, independent of immediate bed availability; and (2) comparative entitlement decision making during triage (based on rank-ordering criteria). APACHE Medical Systems, Inc. is marketing the "APACHE III Management System." Among the claims for this expensive product is the ability to help decision makers optimize ICU resources:

> ICU resources are valuable and limited. When the physician's desire for intensive care outweighs its availability, physicians are forced to make complex tradeoffs. The APACHE III Management System helps hospital administrators optimize ICU resources by evaluating an individual patient's severity of illness and the likelihood of benefit from ICU services.
>
> Objective, statistically-based assessments of patient risk help determine the best use of ICU resources. On the basis of a widely reviewed methodology, the APACHE III Management System predicts the patient's daily risk of death— Screening patients by APACHE III predictions assists clinicians in making clinical decisions (APACHE Medical Systems, Inc. 1991).

As an aid to clinical decision making, the APACHE III Management System provides an on-line graphic displaying the risk of ICU and hospital death, predicted resource use, and length of stay for all patients.

Knaus (1989) advocates linking admission and discharge criteria for the individual with the probability of benefit from intensive care for the individual patient. He would develop probability assessments for the risk of death and the likelihood that intensive care will lower the risk for those already critically ill, and the risk of developing acute life-threatening problems for patients admitted only for monitoring. Knaus suggests that, since direct observations can be made on patients already in the ICUs, probability assessments are more likely to be useful for making decisions about continued stay, discharge, and withdrawal of life support as opposed to admission decisions.

Thus far there has been much controversy over the claims for APACHE. Although useful for discharging low-risk patients, many question its appropriateness for accelerating DNR or withdrawal of treatment decisions and suggest that severity models in general should be used with caution (Teres and Lemeshow 1994). Nevertheless, for discussions about whom to triage, prognostic models and severity scoring systems can serve as an adjunct to decision making.

While prognostic models are now sufficiently well developed to begin playing a role in quality assurance and improvement, much more needs to be done before they can directly assist gatekeepers. Prognostic modeling is still a very young endeavor. No doubt, continued progress will be made in model building and application. But, as we will see in the next chapter, policy leaders are already anticipating incorporating probabilities into triage, admission, and discharge criteria.

References

Angus, D. C., W. T. Linde-Zwirble, C. A. Sirio, A. J. Rotondi, C. Lakshmipathi, R. C. Newbold, J. R. Lave, and M. R. Pinsky. 1996. "The Effect of Managed Care On ICU Length of Stay: Implications for Medicare." *Journal of the American Medical Association* 276 (13): 1075–82.

APACHE Medical Systems Inc. 1991. *APACHE III Management System: Product Overview*. Washington, D.C.

Batalden, P. B., and P. K. Stoltz. 1993. "A Framework for the Continual Improvement of Health Care: Building and Applying Professional Knowledge to Test Changes in Daily Work." *The Joint Commission Journal on Quality Improvement* 19 (10): 424–52.

Berlauk, J. F. 1991. "Preoperative Optimization of Cardiovascular Hemodynamics Improves Outcomes in Peripheral Vascular Surgery." *Annals of Surgery* 214 (3): 289.

Berwick, D. M. 1995. "The SUPPORT Project: Lessons for Action." *Hastings Center Report* (Special Supplement), 25 (6): S21–S22.

Berwick, D. M. 1996. "Quality of Health Care (Part 5): Payment by Capitation and the Quality of Care." *New England Journal of Medicine* 355 (16): 1227–31.

Brown, J. J., and G. Sullivan. 1989. "Effect on ICU Mortality of a Full-Time Critical Care Specialist." *Chest* 96: 127.

Engelman, R. M., J. A. Rousou, J. E. Flack III, D. W. Deaton, C. B. Humphrey, L. H. Ellison, P. D. Allmendinger, S. G. Owen, and P. S. Pekow. 1994. "Fast-track Recovery of the Coronary Bypass Patient." *Annals of Thoracic Surgery* 58 (6): 1742–46.

Groeger, J. S., M. A. Strosberg, N. S. Halpern, R. C. Raphael, W. Kaye, K. K. Guntupalli, D. L. Bertman, D. Greenbaum, T. P. Clemmer, T. J. Gallagher, L. D. Nelson, A. E. Thompson, F. B. Cerra, and W. R. Davis. 1992. "Descriptive Analysis of Critical Care Units in the United States." *Critical Care Medicine* 20 (6): 846–63.

Hage, J. 1974. *Communication and Organizational Control: Cybernetics in Health and Welfare Settings.* New York: John Wiley and Sons.

Hammer, M., and J. Champy. 1993. *Reengineering the Corporation.* New York: Harper Collins.

Knaus, W. A. 1989. "Criteria for Admissions to Intensive Care Units." In *Rationing of Medical Care for the Critically Ill,* edited by M. A. Strosberg, I. A. Fein, and J. D. Carroll, 44–51. Washington, D.C.: The Brookings Institution.

Langley, G. L., K. M. Nolan, T. W. Nolan, C. L. Norman, et al. 1996. *The Improvement Guide: A Practical Approach to Enhancing Organizational Performance.* San Francisco, CA: Jossey-Bass.

Li, T. C. 1984. "On-site Physician Staffing in a Community Hospital Intensive Care Unit." *Journal of the American Medical Association* 252: 2023.

Lo, B. 1995. "End-of-Life Care after Termination of SUPPORT." *Hastings Center Report* (Special Supplement), 25 (6): S6–S8.

Mallick, R., M. A. Strosberg, J. Lambrinos, and J. Groeger. 1995. "The ICU Medical Director as Manager: Impact on Performance." *Medical Care* 33 (6): 611–24.

Mayer-Oakes, S. A., R. K. Oye, B. Leake, and R. H. Brook. 1988. "The Early Effect of Medicare's Prospective Payment System on the Use of Medical Intensive Care Services in Three Community Hospitals." *Journal of the American Medical Association* 260 (21): 3146–49.

Mumford, E. 1970. *Interns: From Students to Physicians.* Cambridge: Commonwealth Fund Book.

National Institutes of Health. 1983. *Consensus Development Conference on Critical Care Medicine: Summary.* 4 (6). Bethesda, MD: U.S. Public Health Service, National Institutes of Health.

Pollack, M. M., R. W. Katz, and U. E. Kuittiman. "Improving the Outcome and Efficiency of Intensive Care: The Impact of an Intensivist." *Critical Care Medicine* 16 (1): 11–17.

Rainey, T. G. 1994. "Critical Care—Beyond the Ivory Tower: The Presidential Address from the 23rd Educational and Scientific Symposium of the Society of Critical Care Medicine." *Critical Care Medicine* 22 (6): 1035–39.

Rapoport, J., S. Gehlbach, S. Lemeshow, and D. Teres. 1992. "Resource Utilization Among Intensive Care Patients: Managed Care vs. Traditional Insurance." *Archives of Internal Medicine* 152: 2207–12.

Reinhardt, U. E. 1987. "Health Insurance for the Nation's Poor." *Health Affairs* 6 (1): 101–11.

Reynolds, H. N., M. T. Haupt, M. C. Thill-Baharozian. 1988. "Impact of Critical Care Physician Staffing on Patients with Septic Shock in a University Hospital Intensive Care Unit." *Journal of the American Medical Association* 260 (23): 3446–50.

Robey, D. 1982. *Designing Organizations.* Homewood, IL: Richard D. Irwin.

Schriefer, J. 1993. "Quality Connection Storyboard: Reducing the Length of Stay for Post-Operative Open Heart Patients." *Quality* (Spring/Summer): 8–9.

Shactman, D., and S. H. Altman. 1995. *Market Consolidation, Antitrust, and Public Policy in the Health Care Industry: Agenda for Future Research.* Waltham, MA.: Council on the Economic Impact of Health Care Reform, Institute for Health Policy, The Heller School, Brandeis University.

Shortell, S. M., J. E. Zimmerman, R. Gillies, J. Duffy, K. J. Devers, D. M. Rousseau, and

W. A. Knaus. 1992. "Continuously Improving Patient Care: Practical Lessons and an Assessment Tool for the National ICU Study." *Quality Review Bulletin* 18 (5): 150–55.

Shortell, S. M. 1991. Explaining Differences in Treatment Outcomes in Intensive Care Units. Final report submitted to the Health Care Financing Administration. Grant No. 18.

Snyder, J. V., C. A. Sirio, D. C. Angus, M. T. Hravnak, S. N. Kobert, E. H. Sinz, and E. B. Rudy. 1994. "Trial of Nurse Practitioners in Intensive Care." *New Horizons* 2 (3): 296–304.

Society of Critical Care Medicine. 1991. *Guidelines for the Definition of an Intensivist and the Practice of Critical Care Medicine.* Anaheim, CA: SCCM.

Society of Critical Care Medicine. 1992. *Critical Care in the United States: Coordinating Intensive Care Resources for Positive and Cost-Efficient Patient Outcomes.* Anaheim, CA: SCCM.

Society of Critical Care Medicine Coalition of Critical Care Excellence. 1995. *ICU Cost Reduction: Practical Suggestions and Future Considerations.* Anaheim, CA: SCCM.

Steingrub, J. S., D. Teres, and J. Rapoport. 1996. "Importance of Subspecialty Consultation in an ICU: Comparison of Fee-for-Service and Managed Care." (Abstract): *Critical Care Medicine* 24: A56.

Strauss, A., L. Schatzman, and D. Ehrlich. 1963. "The Hospital and its Negotiated Order." In *The Hospital in Modern Society,* edited by E. Freidson, 147–169. New York: Free Press of Glencoe.

Strosberg, M. A., D. Teres, I. A. Fein, and R. Linsider. 1990. "Nursing Perception of the Availability of the Intensive Care Unit Medical Director for Triage and Conflict Resolution." *Heart and Lung* 19 (5.1): 452–55.

The SUPPORT Principal Investigators. 1995. "A Controlled Trial to Improve Care for Seriously Ill Hospitalized Patients. The Study to Understand Prognoses and Preferences for Outcomes and Risks of Treatments (SUPPORT)." *Journal of the American Medical Association* 274 (20): 1591–98.

Teres, D., and S. Lemeshow. 1994. "Why Severity Models Should Be Used with Caution." *Critical Care Clinics* 10 (1): 93–110.

Wachter, R. M., and Goldman. L. 1996. "The Emerging Role of "Hospitalists" in the American Health Care System." *New England Journal of Medicine* 335 (7): 514–17.

Walleck, C. A. 1994. "Nursing and Labor Cost Reduction." *New Horizons* 2 (3): 291–95.

Weil, M. H., W. C. Shoemaker, E. C. Rackow. 1988. "Competent and Continuing Care of the Critically Ill." *Critical Care Medicine* 16 (3): 298.

Wennberg, J. E., K. McPherson, and P. Caper. 1984. "Wall Payment Based on Diagnosis Related Groups Control Hospital Costs?" *New England Journal of Medicine* 311 (5): 295.

Zimmerman, J. E., S. M. Shortell, D. M. Rousseau, J. Duffy, R. R. Gillies, W. A. Knaus, K. Devers, D. P. Wagner, and E. A. Draper. 1993a. "Improving Intensive Care: Observations Based on Organizational Case Studies in Nine Intensive Care Units: A Prospective, Multicenter Study." *Critical Care Medicine* 21 (10): 1443–51.

Zimmerman, J. E., S. M. Shortell, W. A. Knaus, D. M. Rousseau, D. P. Wagner, R. R. Gillies, E. A. Draper, and K. Devers. 1993b. "Value and Cost of Teaching Hospitals: A Prospective, Multicenter, Inception Cohort Study." *Critical Care Medicine* 21 (10): 1432–42.

CHAPTER

6

PUBLIC POLICY FOR CRITICAL CARE GATEKEEPING

Helga Wanglie and Her Legacy of Questions

Mrs. Helga Wanglie, a ventilator-dependent eighty-five-year-old woman in persistent vegetative state, consumed hundreds of thousands of dollars during a stay of several months in a Minneapolis hospital. The hospital physicians, with the backing of the administration, wanted to remove her from the ICU and the life-sustaining ventilator, because they believed that continued care was of no benefit in ending her unconsciousness. Although cost was not an explicit consideration, there was general concern over the "stewardship" of limited societal resources (Miles 1991).

The physicians argued that they were not obligated, on the basis of accepted professional standards of medical practice, to accede to patients' or families' demands (other hospitals also refused to accept her as a transfer patient). Her husband disagreed and demanded continued treatment. The court denied the hospital's request to remove him as her legal guardian with the power to make medical decisions on her behalf. Before the court had a chance to definitively decide the question of whether the physician or the hospital could refuse to provide a requested treatment, Mrs. Wanglie died. Her case raised a series of questions which directly relate to the three rationales for admission-discharge-triage decision making in the ICU (Rie 1991).

1) *Medical futility.* The most obvious question is whether physicians and hospitals have the right to refuse treatment that they deem futile or of little or no benefit but is requested by the patient or family.

2) *Non-triage mode/bed availability.* Assuming that ICU treatment is not futile, is there enough benefit to justify "entitlement" to treatment? This question requires the valuation of burdens and benefits, but resource considerations are also important. From a societal perspective, is there enough marginal benefit to justify the expenditure of several hundred thousand dollars? A related question is, whose insurance premiums increased or became unaffordable because of the additional expenditure?

3) *Triage mode/comparative entitlement.* Assuming that a person such as Mrs. Wanglie were considered an acceptable candidate for ICU admission and continued stay, and assuming that intermittent shortages of ICU beds occurred during a long stay, whose admission to the ICU was denied or delayed because she was occupying a bed? Were there patients who were more entitled to that bed?

All of the above questions were raised in one form or another in Chapter 4. In this chapter we will attempt to address the overarching question: How can individuals and society value the risks, benefits, and costs of critical care and structure a decision-making process that gives expression to those values while at the same time addressing the legal and ethical concerns of patients, physicians, and other professionals? The challenge to public policy implied in this question is amplified in the draft SCCM Consensus Statement on Futile and Other Possibly Inadvisable Treatments (1997), "In general it will not be possible for communities or institutions to set limits on treatments unless there is legal recognition that communities have a legitimate need to allocate resources. Thus when communities develop such policies in consultation with interested parties, the standards established in these policies should be followed by the courts." In short, the legal ambiguities and ethical controversies surrounding the limitation of treatment must be resolved. And patients and surrogates as well as physicians must be assured of a role in decision making. To meet this challenge, society must make some difficult choices. In this chapter, we will explore some options by which communities, institutions, and government can make those choices.

Medical Futility

As was illustrated in the case studies in Chapter 4, futility is a controversial and confusing concept (Truog, Brett, and Frader 1992). Nevertheless, its continuing salience is born out of a serious concern by physicians and nurses that demands for aggressive treatment lead to ICU admissions, which sometimes become an expensive, and often agonizing, preliminary to death—a rite of passage notable more for its rituals than its rationality (Baker et al. 1988; Youngner 1995). Furthermore, the provision of aggressive treatment in the minds of many physicians and nurses and the public violates the ethical principles of beneficence and nonmaleficence. Adherence to these ethical principles requires that a physician, based on his/her professional experience and judgment, possess authority to forgo harmful or useless treatments. However, Youngner questions the validity of such claims to unilateral authority when based primarily on a professional's individual experience and judgment. Great differences among physicians often exist in how they choose to define futility. A study by Curtis et al. (1995) shows the significant variability in thresholds in the application of the concepts of quantitative and qualitative futility to the issuance of DNR orders. In our case studies, we have simulated this difference with regard to the AIDS patient (Round 5) and the multi-organ failure patient (Round 4B), whose surgeon told the family not to give up hope. Youngner also argues that claims to determine futility are weakened when no long-standing physician-patient relationship and concomitant understanding of patient preferences exist or when lack of insurance diminishes access to primary healthcare. We would add to this list when the HMO and physician are at financial risk for the provision of care.

Even with well-accepted and well-communicated professional standards, there is the possibility that a patient or family may reject them; beneficence and nonmaleficence confront patient autonomy. This confrontation is starkly portrayed in the case of Baby K, an anencephalic infant, permanently unconscious, with an extremely poor prognosis. Baby K's mother insisted that everything be done to keep Baby K alive, including mechanical ventilation in the ICU and at home. The hospital argued that aggressive care was futile because it could not end unconsciousness nor significantly prolong life. The courts found in the mother's favor for reasons that will be subsequently discussed.

Morreim (1995) comments on the intractability of the debate between the two positions, "futilitarianism" versus "vitalism":

> On the one side of the question, the hospital, its amici, and many commentaries argue that aggressive care of patients like Baby K is futile. Quantitatively, it is futile because an anencephalic like Baby K will die soon no matter what physicians do. Qualitatively, it is futile because they will never be conscious or enjoy any form of human experience. It is a life so profoundly diminished that it bears little resemblance to human personhood. On this view, which I have decided to call "futilitarianism," physicians need not offer costly, futile care to patients or their families, nor even accede to overt demands for it. There is no significant benefit for the patient, it serves no valid medical goals, it can violate the integrity of the medical profession, and physicians would be poor stewards to waste scarce resources on clearly hopeless causes. A gentler version

of futilitarianism argues that more pressing needs for limited resources must be met before such extraordinary expenditures can be justified.

Opposing futilitarianism is a vitalism holding that all life is infinitely precious, regardless of its quality. On this view, futilitarians are simply wrong to suppose that keeping patients like Baby K alive holds "no benefit." Life is of infinite value, not merely an instrumental value toward some further life goals. Therefore, it is wrong for members of the medical community to impose their definition of "benefit" on others by denying life support to those whose live they personally deem unworthy of living. These patients are fully as human as anyone else, and any attempt to save resources by singling them out is blatant discrimination.

No obvious middle ground can be found between these two positions. However, the definitions in a draft version of SCCM's "Consensus Statement on Futile and Other Possibly Inadvisable Treatments" (1997), which we will refer to as the draft SCCM Futility Guidelines, at least brings some conceptual clarification to the debate:

> Treatments should be defined as futile only when they will not accomplish their intended goal. Conflicts arise when there are disagreements about whether the desired goal is appropriate and whether the probability of success is sufficiently great. For example, some patients and families consider continuation of heartbeat and respiration as appropriate goals, even if the patient is permanently unconscious. In addition, some patients may want to undergo a treatment with a very low likelihood of success, particularly if it is their only chance for survival. Since these conflicts are typically about differences in *values* rather than disagreements about *facts,* clinicians should be very cautious about labeling these therapeutic options as futile. Seen in this context, treatments may be classified into four categories:
> (a) treatments that have no beneficial effect;
> (b) treatments that have beneficial effect but are extremely unlikely to be beneficial;
> (c) treatments that have beneficial effect but are extremely costly;
> (d) treatments that are of uncertain or controversial benefit.

Treatments that fall into the first category, i.e., those that offer no benefit to the patient, should be labeled as *futile*. Treatments that fall into the other three categories may be considered *inappropriate and hence inadvisable*.

The concept of futility is generally not useful in establishing policies to limit treatment. Futile treatments, as we have defined them, are rare, and not usually offered or disputed. They therefore do not account for a substantial fraction of medical expenses. For this reason, policies regarding futile care are not likely to be very useful. On the other hand, there are many treatments that are extremely unlikely, extremely costly, or of extremely marginal benefit, that while not clearly futile, might be considered inappropriate and hence inadvisable to offer.

Unlike inadvisability, futility suggests a unilateral and final determination. Physicians should be under no ethical or legal obligation to provide futile treatment. Decisions based on futility share a characteristic with decisions based on triage criteria; that is, patient preferences are not controlling, and so informed consent is not required, although patients and families should be kept informed. Yet a study of 879 physicians in adult ICUs across the nation (Asch, Hansen-Flaschen, and Lanken 1995), found that 14 percent said they had withheld or withdrawn treatment which they considered futile *without* informing the patient's family. More than 80 percent had withdrawn care against the objections of the family; significantly, many of these treatments would have fallen into categories b, c, and d above.

As a residual category (after excluding b, c, and d), futility should be a noncontroversial concept. However, the controversy is merely transferred to the determination of inadvisable care in categories b, c, and d. Clearly, according to the draft SCCM Futility Guidelines, Mrs. Wanglie's treatment in the ICU was not futile nor would have been the treatment of the AIDS patient in Round 5 had he been admitted to the ICU. Nor would Baby K's. Nor, as we shall soon discuss, would Catherine Gilgunn's. But would the care have been inappropriate or inadvisable? Would it have made any medical sense? Can decisions to withdraw care based on professionally determined standards of appropriateness be unilaterally made by physicians? In the case of Helga Wanglie and Baby K, the courts ordered continued treatment when requested by surrogates.

The court decisions in these cases did not directly address the issues of futility or appropriateness. The decision about Baby K, admitted through the emergency room, was narrowly based on a strict interpretation of the federal Emergency Medical Treatment and Active Labor Act of 1986 (the "anti-dumping statute"), which requires hospitals to stabilize patients who seek treatment or transfer them if absolutely necessary.

Another case, however, has directly engaged the issue of appropriateness. Joan Gilgunn sued the Massachusetts General Hospital and two doctors for refusing to keep alive her 71-year-old mother who was in persistent vegetative state. The attending physician entered a DNR order in Catherine Gilgunn's chart. This decision was supported by the hospital's ethics committee, called the Optimum Care Committee, after extensive deliberation. Two days later she died. The daughter claimed that the DNR order was entered against her wishes and was not what her mother would have wanted. She sued for negligence and the case went before the Suffolk County Superior Court in Boston (Kolata 1995). The jury found that Catherine Gilgunn would have wanted medical care extended, including CPR and mechanical ventilation, but they also found that it would have been futile and of no medical benefit. Therefore, without negligence, the doctors and the hospital were found not guilty.

The Gilgunn case is the first case to address the unilateral withholding of a treatment, CPR. It is important to note that for Catherine Gilgunn, CPR would not have been considered futile according to the draft SCCM Futility Guidelines or under the New York State DNR statute. In a litigious and uncertain environment it will take more than one case to establish a body of law that will assure physicians and hospitals that they can safely refuse requests by families for inappropriate and expensive end-of-life treatments. Physicians, hospitals, and their attorneys will feel secure about unilateral withdrawal only when this practice is accepted as the community standard of care. Important efforts are under way to create these standards of care. One such effort is the Guidelines for the Use of Intensive Care in Denver (GUIDe), a consortium of metropolitan Denver hospitals and healthcare institutions whose goal is to develop guidelines for the use of futile or inappropriate care. GUIDe has structured a process incorporating broad-based community representation to try to reach consensus on these guidelines. The supporters of this approach reason that if the guidelines, crafted in a way that transcends the interests of a single institution or medical staff, were adopted by most of the hospitals with the support of the community, they could in fact become the basis for the community standard of care. The supporters of GUIDe hope that such standards would reduce the risk of litigation and bad public relations (Murphy and Barbour 1994). However, short of well-accepted community standards of care, tested in the courts, providers still face this risk.

As an alternative to a substantive definition of futility, the Houston City-Wide Task Force on Medical Futility (1996) proposed a procedural approach to the definition (See Appendix A). The "Houston approach" structures a fair and open process of a case-by-case review by an institutional interdisciplinary body. The process is designed to balance professional and institutional integrity against patient autonomy. In its deliberations, the institutional body may take the utilization of costly and/or scarce resources into consideration. For example, the treatment of a PVS patient in the ICU might be judged to represent an inappropriate stewardship of resources. The task force acknowledges, however, that the legal standing of the process is still open to question. Resolution awaits action from the courts and/or state legislature.

Paths to Resolution: Policy Formation

The term "policy" is used in a variety of contexts. In a broad context, policy formation means public policy formation. A public policy is what government says and does about matters it wishes to influence. Institutions also have policies, guidelines, and procedures that have been officially adopted by the governing board and its committees, usually at the behest of external bodies such as the JCAHO. The GUIDe approach is aimed at providing hospitals and physicians with legally defensible resource allocation policies that have wide-based community and professional support. The Houston approach establishes procedures for determining on a case-by-case basis inappropriate interventions. A policy is also an insurance contract. An individual subscriber's contract should contain a statement of the plan's policy. As we shall discuss, there are those active in the public policy debate over healthcare who have proposed that the insurance contract be formulated in such a way as to express preferences and values, recognize resource constraints, and minimize litigation. All of the paths to resolution will require changes in public policy emanating from the judicial and legislative arenas.

Inappropriate Care: Valuing the Risks, Benefits, and Costs of ICU Treatment in the Non-Triage Mode

The 1988 SCCM "Recommendations for ICU Admission and Discharge Criteria" stated that patients in persistent vegetative state do not meet routine admission criteria (see Appendix A). The 1994 SCCM "Consensus Statement on the Triage of Critically Ill Patients" (developed after the Helga Wanglie case), added to this recommendation:

> Examples of patients who should be excluded from the ICU, whether beds are available or not, include . . . those in a persistent vegetative or permanently unconscious state. However, religious or moral convictions may legitimately be the basis for the provision of treatment to such patients if the costs are not borne by the general society and the provision of such services does not foreclose the treatment of other patients who would benefit from critical care (p. 1202).

In the above passage, "exclusion" means "do not admit patients with a long-standing diagnosis," but it also means "discharge if the diagnosis is made in the ICU." The former is easier because of the availability of large databases increasing the certainty of diagnosis and because a relationship between the ICU staff and the patient and family has not yet been cemented.

The passage is significant and precedent-setting because it fully recognizes the relevance to gatekeeping of not only risks and benefits (net benefit), but also of costs. Ostensibly the benefits are too small, according to SCCM standards. But implicitly the benefits are also too expensive.

The SCCM criteria excludes PVS or other permanently unconscious patients on the basis of quality of life (a patient in PVS could live on for many years). From an ethical standpoint, the SCCM supports its position by appealing to the principle of distributive justice (i.e., the fair, equitable, and appropriate distribution of medical resources in society) (Luce 1995).

The SCCM passage is much more than a professional society's statement that the ICU treatment of a patient in PVS would yield a net benefit so low that it should be deemed inadvisable or inappropriate. It also recognizes that individuals, for religious or moral reasons, may have different criteria for determining benefit. Therefore, Mr. Wanglie could legitimately decide that further ICU treatment was beneficial for his wife. According to SCCM, however, he, not society, must bear the costs of continued treatment. In this regard, the controversy over futile care and inappropriate care is fueled by resource considerations. There would be little interest in or concern about Baby K, Catherine Gilgunn, or Helga Wanglie if there were no resource considerations.

Medical care at the end of life accounts for 27 percent of the Medicare budget and 10 to 12 percent of all health expenditures (Lubitz et al. 1993). A considerable question arises of just how much society could save by eliminating futile and inappropriate/inadvisable care at the end of life. Teno et al. (1994) estimate the amount of savings that could be produced by eliminating care that would have less than a 1 percent probability of achieving a two-month survival. This threshold, using a quantitative definition, falls into category b of the draft SCCM guidelines, "treatments that are extremely unlikely to be beneficial." In a study of 4,301 very sick patients (i.e., patients with one or more life-threatening diagnoses, such as acute respiratory failure, multiple organ system failure with sepsis, or multi-organ system failure with malignancy) in five academic health centers participating in the SUPPORT study, the researchers found 115 (2.7 percent) ICU patients who fell into this category. If these patients, at a point in time when there was reasonable prognostic certainty, had been prevented by a prognosis-based policy from receiving this care, 199 out of 1,688 hospital days (10.8 percent) would have been eliminated with an estimated savings of $1.2 million in hospital charges. The researchers concluded that the limitation of care with a 1 percent or less chance of producing a two-month survival would yield only modest savings. On the other hand, if a 10 percent or less threshold of survival at two months were used, nearly 25 percent of 1,073 hospital days would have been saved. The researchers emphasize that "this savings would be achieved only if society were willing to accept earlier deaths for 13 patients, nine of whom actually survived for at least the 6-month follow-up period" (p. 1205).

Emanuel and Emanuel (1994) estimated the amount of money that could be saved through wider use of advance directives, hospice care, and curtailment of aggressive end-of-life interventions. Extrapolating from the experience of patients who receive hospice care as opposed to aggressive hospital care, the authors concluded that, at most, 3.3 percent of total national health expenditure could be saved by reducing the use of aggressive, life-saving interventions that yield little benefit. In 1993 this would have been $29.7 billion out of a total expenditure of $900 billion. Part of the reason for the surprisingly low percentage has to do with clinical uncertainty. It is difficult to identify in advance who in fact is going to die. Consequently, resources must be initially expended "until a patient's prognosis becomes clearer and physicians, patients, and the family are sure about either forging ahead with aggressive treatment or withdrawing it" (p. 543). Also, high-quality palliative care offered as an alternative is nearly as costly as aggressive care.

Although the budget impact on society of the potential savings is small in terms of total national health expenditure, it may in fact be significant for a particular hospital or members of a health insurance plan. What about the budget of the HMO to which Mrs. Wanglie belonged? Miles reports that several citizens complained to the hospital treating Mrs. Wanglie that she was receiving care paid by people, "who had not consented to underwrite a level of medical care whose appropriateness was defined by family demand" (Miles 1991, p. 514).

The professionally enunciated policy statement of the SCCM has yet to achieve the status of professional or official institutional policy, let alone of an established public policy. As the cases of Helga Wanglie and Baby K show, unilateral decisions to withdraw or withhold treatment based on determinations of net benefit, with or without cost factored in, do not necessarily withstand legal challenge by patients and families. The public policy challenge posed by the SCCM at the beginning of this chapter bears repeating: "In general it will not be possible for communities or institutions to set limits on treatments unless there is legal recognition that communities have a legitimate need to allocate resources. Thus when communities develop such policies in consultation with interested parties, the standards established in these policies should be followed by the courts." We argue that the Oregon Medicaid Demonstration Project (Oregon Plan), by conferring legitimacy and legal immunity through statute, meets this challenge.

The Oregon Plan: A Public Resource Allocation Methodology

One of the fundamental objectives of President Clinton's proposed Health Security Act was to bring Americans universal access to a basic benefit package of health services. The drafters of the rejected legislation struggled unsuccessfully with the problem of defining what services were to be included and excluded in this basic package. In the end, the determination of medical appropriateness was to be left to a proposed National Health Board.

Public officials face the challenge of trying to define the minimally acceptable basic benefit package whether it is offered in a single payor, egalitarian system like Canada's, or in the multi-tiered, market-driven system that is emerging after the failure of national health reform (Reinhardt 1995). In creating this benefit package, society will no doubt decide not to include all the beneficial services that individuals might prefer. This difference between the beneficial care that is offered and that which is preferred is care that is rationed. Included here are services in categories b, c, and d, mentioned earlier in the draft SCCM Futility Guidelines.

Until recently, rationing was not an issue on the national agenda. There has been no nexus between clinical decision making at the bedside and our political institutions. Representative Willis Gradison (1989) of the House Ways and Means Subcommittee on Health made this assessment at a 1986 Brookings conference on rationing healthcare for the critically ill: "Politicians make choices in ways that will minimize and, if possible, eliminate any public perception that they are rationing care or diminishing its quality." Trimming the fat, yes; cutting to the bone, never. We allocate health resources without much analysis or conscious policy choice. Physicians practice within the resulting resource constraints, that is, they implicitly ration. It is tolerable and politically acceptable. In 1991, in a major watershed in public policy, the state of Oregon, through legislation, adopted a plan that makes politicians and public institutions responsible for an explicit healthcare rationing plan. What has been done in Oregon is to forge a chain of accountability from clinical decision making at the bedside directly to the Oregon state legislature. This chain of accountability enables the healthcare system to: (1) fully recognize the problems of resource scarcity and differential access, and (2) embrace a prioritization method based on cost-effectiveness (Strosberg 1992).

The Oregon Plan expands Medicaid to large numbers of people who currently have no health insurance, but at the price of explicitly deciding not to cover some medical procedures generally accepted as beneficial but of low priority. To accomplish this, a publicly appointed Oregon Health

Service Commission created a rank-ordered list of 709 paired medical conditions and treatments prioritized by clinical effectiveness and social importance. The priority list was submitted to the state legislature which, through its allocation of funds to the Medicaid budget, determined how many of the services on the list could be funded. Those that were too far down on the list were not provided in the basic medical package, even though they might have been beneficial services. In July 1991, the legislature allocated funds that covered services down to 587 on the list of 709. At the bottom of the list were aggressive treatments for extremely small infants and aggressive medical treatments for end-stage cancer and end-stage AIDS.

In the Oregon Plan, treatments for conditions at the bottom of the list would be considered of low marginal benefit and therefore would be excluded from the basic benefit package. However, some (e.g., Mr. Wanglie) would argue that the question of marginal benefit is an individual value judgment. In the Oregon Plan, for the Medicaid population, the individual's value judgment is replaced by a community value judgment made through the political process. In subsequent sections we will show how individual values could be reflected in the insurance contract.

A description of the cost-effectiveness analysis methodology for the ranking is beyond the scope of this chapter, and since 1991 there have been various generations of techniques, approaches, rank-ordered lists, and cutoff points. However, the idea behind it, albeit oversimplified, is illustrated in Englehardt and Rie's ICU Entitlement Index (1986) proposed in a 1986 *Journal of the American Medical Association* article. The calculation of the rank of a particular treatment in the intensive care unit is "*(the probability of successful outcomes)* × *(quality of life)* × *(length of life)* ÷ *(cost)*." Their index, meant primarily to stimulate societal debate, squarely engages the issue of scarce resources by balancing the probability of a successful outcome, the quality of life, and the length of life remaining to a patient against the costs of achieving therapeutic success in the intensive care unit. As the costs increase and the quality and likelihood of success decrease, the reasonableness of the investment diminishes.

The numerator of the formula is a measure of medical effectiveness. It estimates probable outcome from a treatment and places a value on that outcome. In Oregon, the quality-of-well-being (QWB) scale was used as the basis for incorporating QALY-like assessments into the definition of healthcare benefit (Kaplan 1992). Of considerable concern to the Oregon Health Services Commission and to those closely observing the proceeding was the question of where highly beneficial but also very expensive services would rank on the priority list. In a traditional cost-utility analysis, a highly beneficial life-sustaining service could be outweighed by its high cost or by the fact that only a few people will benefit, thus dragging it to the bottom of the list. Departing from a strict use of cost-utility principles, the commissioners adopted an alternative methodology which allowed them first to create a structure of 17 different categories (e.g., acute fatal conditions for which treatment allows full recovery, preventive care for children, comfort care) ranked to reflect community values. The 709 conditions/treatments were placed within one of the 17 categories and then ranked by medical effectiveness. In this approach, they were also able to adjust the list by moving certain life-saving services to a higher, and intuitively more sensible, ranking. At the bottom of the list were aggressive care for end-stage cancer, AIDS, anencephalic babies, and extremely low birth weight babies.

Cost enters the denominator of this "modified cost-effectiveness analysis" (Hadorn 1991) as the amount of funds that the Oregon legislature allocates to Medicaid. In effect the legislature draws a line by appropriating a specific budget that, based on actuarial calculations, will fund down the rank-order list to a cutoff point.

Because Medicaid is a federal-state partnership, Oregon needed approval from Washington to implement its Medicaid experiment. In 1992, The U.S. Department of Health and Human Services under the Bush Administration denied approval, claiming that the use of quality and length of life considerations discriminated against patients with disabilities and would run afoul of the Americans with Disabilities Act. The Department argued that patients with preexisting disabilities would receive a lower rank as compared to those without a particular disability. As an example, the Department singled out the low ranking of extremely low birth weight babies (rank #708) compared to heavier babies (rank #22). In response, Oregon removed quality and duration of life factors from the calculations and based its rankings on probability of survival and other considerations. Oregon reapplied and was given approval by the Clinton Administration. The plan took effect on February 1, 1994.

Discrimination against persons with disabilities was also an issue in the Baby K case. The federal district court, in ruling against the hospital's request to deny mechanical ventilation, argued that denial would violate the Americans with Disabilities Act because it discriminated against Baby K on the basis of her mental handicap. On appeal, the circuit court upheld the decision but on other grounds (violation of the federal Emergency Medical Treatment and Labor Act). Now considerable confusion reigns over the permissible role of the use of medical effectiveness based on quality of life in allocating resources (Orentlicher 1994). Clarification awaits judicial and Congressional action (Peters 1995).

Despite the changes to the original design because of the need to accommodate the perceived requirements of the Americans with Disabilities Act, the Oregon Plan still represents an important model for public resource allocation. The Oregon Plan creates a liability shield by protecting providers against malpractice and professional disciplinary actions when not providing those services that are explicitly excluded from the basic healthcare package. Morreim (1992) emphasizes that this liability shield solves an important jurisprudential dilemma facing physicians: under the current application of the standard of care to malpractice litigation, physicians are required to deliver a roughly unitary level of care to patients regardless of resource constraints and economic considerations.

Standard of Care in Medical Malpractice Litigation: Economic Considerations

Can or should the standard of care be changed to incorporate economic considerations? As cost-control strategies increasingly rely on direct or indirect rewards and penalties to minimize the provision of unnecessary services, there is also the potential to diminish necessary services as well. Hirshfeld (1990) notes that the "standard of care is a powerful inducement against the withholding of needed services" (p. 2004). In applying the standard in individual cases, the court's definitions of needed or necessary care tend to be patient-interest oriented, reflecting the physician's obligation to do all that can benefit the individual patient, not to do what is in the best interests of other patients or society. Managed care organizations expect physicians to weigh the costs and benefits in their clinical decision making. There are those who argue that the courts must recognize that physicians operate under resource constraints and that malpractice standards, which evolved under fee-for-service medicine, must accommodate these new realities (Hall 1987). All beneficial care is not needed or necessary and courts, by making value judgments, are in the best position to exercise leadership in this area. On the other hand, there are those who argue that physicians and courts are not likely to depart from traditional ethical standards and obligations, and it will require legislative action to change the standard of care.

Morreim (1989) proposed dividing the standard of care into two elements—medical expertise and resource use. Under her proposal, the physician is held accountable to the standard of medical expertise for applying a professionally determined level of knowledge, skill, and effort to all patients. The standard of resource use is the level of medical and monetary resources to which the patient is legally entitled. Morreim has suggested that the legal remedies available to patients for breach of the standard of expertise be managed under tort law, upon which malpractice litigation is now based. Breaches of the standard of resource use should be managed under contract law, which requires the parties themselves to decide what is expected of one another and what measures will be taken if expectations are not met. In Oregon, the state legislature assumes explicit responsibility for the standard of resource use for the Medicaid population, in other words, it has created the minimum (basic) benefit package.

Rationing is not uncontroversial. Yet most would agree that, whether the result of conscious policy choice or not, healthcare in America is already being rationed for both the uninsured and the Medicaid population. In times of budgetary pressure, instead of raising taxes, state governments typically respond by reducing Medicaid reimbursement to providers, who will be less likely to treat Medicaid patients, or by dropping coverage of a portion of the poor already on the Medicaid rolls. Such responses ultimately ration care to anonymous people, and the government avoids confronting individuals. In making up the shortfall, hospitals are squeezed, trauma services are cut, ICU nurses are overworked and quit; in short, the conditions described by Shoemaker et al. (1992) at King-Drew Medical Center take place. Thus government is implicitly rationing healthcare resources. Doctors and nurses at the bedside join the ranks of the harassed "street-level bureaucrats" (Lipsky 1980). Society has not given healthcare providers legally or politically defensible allocation rules. But Oregon would.

In Oregon, the debate shifts from whom to cover to what to cover, based on the degree to which health services improve health status. The debate was structured as an open process with a fair amount of public input. If revenues fall short, lawmakers cannot, as they usually do, arbitrarily cut people from the Medicaid rolls, or arbitrarily cut what is paid to medical providers. Their only options are to raise more money or to reduce the service level. If the citizens do not like the level of services (e.g., the 587 cut point), all they have to do is tell their legislators to put more funds into the Medicaid budget. The Oregon Plan and its methodology for the public construction of the basic benefit package ingeniously calls the political question (Kitzhaber 1991).

How well does the Oregon Plan meet the public policy challenge enunciated at the beginning of this section? Based on a recognized need to allocate resources and limit serves, Oregon has created a basic benefit package that confers limited liability when followed by individuals and institutions when not providing care explicitly excluded from the basic benefit package. Major limitations do exist in the applicability of

Oregon's ranking methodology to the range of conditions seen in the ICU. The ranking system is still in its embryonic stages. Many intensivists would point out that the vertical ranking of conditions/treatments lacks a horizontal dimension. They would argue that probabilities should be incorporated into each of the condition/treatment pairs to take into consideration the potential of ICU intervention. For example, as probabilities of survival get worse over time, cutoffs or thresholds for hospice or lower cost options would be available. Clearly, more needs to be done in this area (Hadorn 1994). Nevertheless, the Oregon Plan, by demonstrating the possibilities of a publicly constructed and accountable benefit package, has opened up opportunities for the critical care community to consider the tradeoffs among access, quality, and cost of care. Can the success of the statutorily implemented, public-sector Oregon Plan in meeting the public policy challenge be replicated in the private sector? Private plans have also struggled with the definition of medical necessity and medical appropriateness (Berghold 1995). How would Helga Wanglie's preferences be taken into consideration?

Constructing the Oregon Analog for the Private Sector

We have repeatedly pointed out that even where an objective determination of probabilities can be made, clinicians, patients, and families may disagree among themselves and with each other on the weight or value to be placed on those probabilities, thus leading to different treatment choices. Value judgments abound in the ICU. ICU care is capable of prolonging life, but it is also capable of prolonging the dying process. It is often a thin line that separates these poles, and where one draws that line is very much a value judgment. To some, staying in the ICU on a ventilator for a month or more hoping for a recovery in spite of a 2 percent or less chance of it may be entirely worth the effort. To others it may not be. In the Oregon Plan, community values substitute for individual values and preferences.

Practice Guidelines

Numerous studies show that physicians do a poor job in understanding patient values and acting upon patient preferences. One of the lessons of the SUPPORT study is that profound change in organizational structure and culture is necessary to change physician behavior and decision making at the end of life. Bernard Lo (1995), as we mentioned in Chapter 4, suggests that approaches to reduce ineffective, expensive interventions include (1) cutting the supply of intensive care specialists and intensive care beds thereby diminishing the technological imperative, and (2) placing intensive care specialists as well as hospitals at financial risk. We have noted that these are just the kinds of changes that are likely to be ushered in under managed care. This trend will be accelerated as the Medicare population moves toward capitation and risk HMOs. However, we have also warned that changing financial incentives and/or imposing constraints on supply may diminish rather than enhance patient involvement in decision making and replace the ethical dilemmas of overservicing the patient with that of underservicing the patient. Hence the greater the urgency to find mechanisms to counterbalance these tendencies.

Can practice guidelines play a constructive role in minimizing both overservicing and underservicing the patient? Based on professional norms and evidence from outcomes studies, they have been created to advise physicians, serve as payment screens, and inform utilization review and quality assurance. There is still a long way to go to achieve these expectations. Most practice guidelines, however, do not recognize a legitimate role for the patient in the decision-making process. It is extremely difficult to systematically structure a decision process that facilitates a discussion of the risk-benefit probabilities and an articulation of patient values and preferences. Nevertheless, some progress has been made. Barry et al. (1995) describe a method that incorporates, through interactive video, patient preferences in the area of benign prostatic hyperplasia, a high-variation condition with regard to treatment choice. David Eddy (1996), in a series of essays in the *Journal of the American Medical Association* in 1990–91, explains the formidable methodological challenges and suggests some approaches and solutions. Wennberg (1990) suggests that if patients' preferences were incorporated into decision making, the demand for invasive high-technology medicine would be reduced, especially with regard to care near the end of life, where patients might prefer less rather than more care.

The Insurance Policy Approach: Adding an Economic Dimension

To provide for consumer input and to create an economic dimension missing from the above discussion on guidelines and patients' preferences, Clark Havighurst (1995) argues that we could look to the insurance contract as the vehicle to legitimize a health plan's economizing actions in the eyes of the community and the law. Havighurst (1992) conceptualizes health insurance policies as agreements by which members of a covered group mutually elect:

> to be bound in order that the fund created by their contributions would be sufficient to cover their essential needs and would not be squandered on

nonessential, inefficacious, or overly costly services demanded by an individual. Under this view, an insurer rationing health care financing by invoking a coverage restriction can be seen as serving consumer interests as well as its own (p. 1771).

To be useful, the contract would have to offer the provider protection against law suits for personal injuries caused by the economizing choices of subscribers. On this issue, the Oregon Plan has laid the groundwork with its liability shield.

Along these same lines, Michael Rie proposes using the market to sort out tradeoffs among cost, quality, and access by bringing an economic dimension to the way patients exercise their preferences. Presumably, in a market system, there would not be universal entitlement to unlimited consumption of ICU services. As Rie (1989) argues, in a system designed to maximize consumer choice, a buyer should be able to purchase insurance coverage that is linked to a certain level of benefit (services), not unlike homeowners' insurance coverage. For example, some may not wish to purchase coverage guaranteeing access to marginally beneficial therapies and, therefore, would not be entitled to them. (Presumably the money they save from cheaper insurance premiums would be spent on endeavors more worthwhile to them). Others (e.g., Mrs. Wanglie) may wish to purchase extra coverage even for what many would consider marginally beneficial or futile services. Government (e.g., Oregon) may provide a basic level of coverage for the indigent and the uninsured, thus establishing a floor for the bottom tier of our multi-tier system.

How will insurance policies reflect individual consumer preferences? Rie (1995) offers a sample policy:

> This policy limits payments for futile and inappropriate critical care. For the purposes of this contract, futile care is defined by the signatories as a prognostic prediction of death of 95% probability after seven days of ICU care. It is recognized that patients may wish to have more or less degrees of probability attached to the determination of this finding. Accordingly, this contract offers a series of probability tolerances to the certitude of the ultimate diagnosis of futility. The basic package of ICU benefits in this health plan carries a probability variance of X percent. Should one decide, as a purchaser, that one wants a higher level of certainty attached to these outcomes, you may elect these degrees of probability as expressed in the premium surcharge table defined by this health insurance policy's actuaries. These option packages are available annually, at the renewal of the contract, and may not be changed during a covered benefit year (p. 159).

Rie's conceptual construct is inspired by the Oregon Plan; he refers to his proposal as the "Oregonian ICU." Like the Oregon Plan, it would require significant statutory change to implement. For example, a statute would be required for malpractice tort exemption to protect providers when not providing care that is not part of the insurance policy.

Thus far, Rie's "Oregonian ICU" policy proposal has not received substantial public attention. As we discussed in Chapter 5, serious question remains whether the task of enabling consumer choice can be effectively fulfilled by current prognostic tools and scoring systems. Beyond these technical issues, there is also considerable skepticism and resistance in the legal and political communities to allow the health insurance policy to play an economizing role. However, in spite of these obstacles, as cost-containment and the particular problems generated by managed care rise on the public agenda, it is inevitable that Rie's proposal, along with those by Havighurst (1995) and Morreim will receive increased public scrutiny. The interest in these proposals will be in part generated by the decreasing public confidence in managed care gatekeeping and physician gatekeepers who act in their own financial self-interest under risk-sharing or in the interest of the managed care plan. Physician gatekeepers are particularly sensitive to the dilemma of playing two contradictory roles. Robert Veatch (1986) warns of the consequences of asking the physician to be society's cost-containment agent, to replace the Hippocratic Oath with a warning: "I will generally work for your interests, but in the case of marginally beneficial care, I will abandon you in order to serve as their cost-containment agent" p. 84.

Zawacki (1985) attempted to address this dilemma. Drawing on the ideas of Mulley (1984), he proposed the institutionalization of the triage officer/gatekeeper role to represent society as microallocational decision maker and, in a larger sense, as conservator of societal resources. In this proposal, attending physicians would advocate for their patients as if in court. They would not bear the consequences, as do their British counterparts, of being their patient's physicians, the rationers of care, and society's cost-containment agents. In the British hospital there is no "official" analogous to the triage officer; physicians implicitly ration within the fixed budget and resources of the hospital (Aaron and Schwartz 1984). The consequences of the tradeoffs either remain invisible to individual patients or, as Zawacki says, physicians are engaged in "rationalization designed to make the denial of potentially beneficial care seem either routine or optimal for the patient." Of course, in the British hospital of the National Health Service there is limited fee-for-service, limited participation of primary physicians in hospital treatment, and limited malpractice claims. At least with regard to the first two characteristics, similarity exists to the closed ICU.

Under the Zawacki proposal, the opportunities for rationalization or implicit rationing are far fewer. The conceptualization of the gatekeeper function and the role of the triage officer/gatekeeper as part of the apparatus of the administrative state elevates the status of the individual patient to "citizen" with rights in relationship to the state.

The specter of patient-citizen battling the all-powerful and persuasive state has been challenging democratic theorists for years. Redford (1969) summarizes the traditional protections that should inform administrative decision making and embody democratic ideals:

1. Right to know—to be alerted to activity that affects interests, e.g., notice.
2. Right to be heard—to have access to and a hearing before the decisional authority that allocating benefits and disadvantages.
3. Right to a fair (unbiased) forum.
4. Right to appeal and independent review (e.g., the courts).

In the Zawacki model, the protection of the patient is to be assured by an adversarial relationship between the patient's physician (acting as fiduciary agent and "defense lawyer") and the clearly identified state agent/bureaucrat.

The consequence of the Zawacki model with the triage officer/gatekeeper as "agent of the state" is a heightened expectation of procedural due process guided by explicit standards for resource allocation in the face of scarcity. This expectation is not normally operating in the British National Health Service, which relies on implicit rationing within a context of fixed resources (Baker 1992). (Of course the centrally imposed resource constraints ration the supply of health services: with fewer resources, there is a lower expectation and less opportunity to recognize situations of denial or diminishment of benefit.) However, this expectation is operating in the United States. It takes on new urgency, not necessarily with regard to the citizen battling the all-powerful state, but with regard to the member (the covered life) vis-à-vis the managed care plan. How and where will the margins be drawn on the high-tech and expensive, marginally beneficial care that is rendered in the ICU? In particular, where will the margins be drawn in closed ICUs embedded in managed care systems, where capitation has transformed revenue generating activities into cost generating ones and where large integrated financial and clinical databases facilitate the incorporation of cost-effectiveness considerations into decision making? While health systems have done a better job of measuring costs of care, plan members will inevitably be concerned that important dimensions of benefit will not be captured by their measurements (Strosberg and Teres 1996).

Today, over a decade after Zawacki made his proposal, it is becoming more and more difficult to see how physicians practicing in a managed care environment can fulfill the patent advocacy role as he envisioned it. Nevertheless, the concerns remain. The AMA Council on Ethical and Judicial Affairs (1995), in its report, "Ethical Issues in Managed Care," recommends that physicians avoid making ad-hoc rationing decisions at the bedside. These types of decisions are better made according to guidelines established at a "higher policy making level" within managed care organizations. The policymaking process should include mechanisms for taking into account the preferences and values of plan members. Full disclosure of policies should be made. Physicians should make patients aware of alternative treatment options. Appeals mechanisms should be available. Furthermore, the AMA Council also recommends that physicians disclose financial incentives that might serve to limit care.

Sorum (1996) recommends that patient values and preferences be expressed through a policy committee structured to enable representatives of plan members as well as physicians to negotiate over the rules affecting the provision of services. The extent to which plan members become stakeholders could become an important selling point as plans compete for new members in the marketplace.

Rie and others suggest a much more formalized set of procedures which control "entitlement" to treatment. Rie's Oregonian ICU proposal calls for the establishment of a Humanism and Technology Usage Committee (HTUC). This legally constituted watch-dog committee would be composed of patient subscribers, hospital and medical staff representatives, intensivists, and payors. Rie describes it as "a conceptually new version of a medicolegally binding ethics committee organized to function within a hospital but under the purview of a health insurance plan." Attached to the HTUC would be salaried QCCPs, direct employees of the plan, who function as managers of critical care and gatekeepers. Primary physicians would directly participate in care, but the QCCP would have final authority for deciding whether the limitations of the policy as spelled out in the insurance contract had been reached. Rie describes how the arrangement might work:

> From time to time, a patient (identified through computerized entitlement limitation resource consumption screens) will have exceeded his/her limit. At such a point, automatic notice of this circumstance would be communicated formally to the primary physician advocate and to the patient or his/her legal surrogate. An appropriate period of time (within defined limits) for independent personal response from the patient and the physician advocate would then be permitted.
>
> In such cases, the critical care consultant gatekeeper has no discretion as to what the screens would be, as they would have already been decided in the health insurance policy. The authority of the gatekeeper is circumscribed in terms of notification of entitlement limitation excess by the rules of the health plan. As

the original model (given as an example only [see above]) already contains the health plan's definition of futile or inappropriate care, it will be difficult for individual patients of physicians to make appeals that would have standing in the health insurance plan.

The appellate process is designed to assure that all of the necessary information gathered by the critical care gatekeeper and the HTUC is factually correct. When that discovery process has been exhausted, a decision will be made (usually by the gatekeeper), and if contested, then by the HTUC. In this system, the committee's decision is final after the individual discovery appellate process has been concluded and all funding for curative critical care will be terminated (p. 162).

The proposals of Rie, Havighurst, and Morreim are aimed at the reformulation of the health insurance policy to provide an ethical and accountable way of expressing the values and preferences of the individual purchaser. Their proposals will be viewed as radical by many. Without a doubt, substantial legal and operational technicalities must be overcome. Also, critics claim that the proposals would create and legitimate a socially disruptive multi-tiered system with a divided standard of care. The Oregon Plan also was criticized on these grounds. Interestingly, in spite of this criticism, both sides of the political spectrum saw the plan as advancing their particular position. Liberals viewed the Oregon Plan not only as a way to expand access but also as a potential first step toward a universal, single-tiered system (Wyden 1992). On the other hand, conservatives (Englehardt 1992; Morreim 1992) viewed it as the public construction of the basic healthcare plan and the subsequent legitimization of multi-tiered healthcare.

The GUIDe approach, in contradistinction, by building a community consensus for the definitions of appropriate critical care, maintains a unitary standard of care. Consensus-building of this type is aimed at all four levels (a, b, c, and d) of the draft SCCM Futility Guidelines.

Both the insurance policy approach and the community consensus approach require support from the judiciary and the legislature. With regard to the latter approach, more court cases like the Catherine Gilgunn case will be needed to convince physicians, hospitals, and their attorneys that the community standard of care has provided them with legally defensible resource allocation policies. It is likely that there will be more court cases in this area.

What are the prospects for the insurance policy approach? Little can be said with certainty except to point out the obvious. Legal and operational obstacles remain. On the other hand, in the increasingly competitive market, healthcare is increasingly treated as a commodity like anything else exchanged in the marketplace. The writing of insurance contracts cannot help but reflect the commodification of healthcare, although it is difficult to predict the form the contracts will take.

What can be said with certainty is that more efforts will be undertaken to facilitate communication and understanding among physicians, nurses, patients, families/surrogates, especially in light of the disturbing findings of the SUPPORT study. In this context, the claims for the role of the QCCP are very compelling. As was discussed in Chapter 5, the SCCM considers the QCCP, by medical training and practice, to be in the best position to "help patients and their families measure the benefits of current and future therapies, make appropriate choices and preserve costly resources for those who can benefit."

Triage/Comparative Entitlement

Thus far we have been discussing ways to enhance the legal and ethical support for gatekeeping in the non-triage mode. It should be pointed out that the critical care gatekeeper, deciding on entitlement to treatment and operating within the framework of Rie's HTUC, had only limited discretion in carrying out his or her function. The gatekeeper is in effect a bureaucrat harnessed into office by the rules of the plan. What about triage-mode gatekeeping when comparative entitlement is at issue? At this level, where triage decisions have to be made in a timely fashion, there is need for an independently functioning triage officer to rapidly collect and interpret complicated information, apply rules, exercise discretion when necessary, and make authoritative bed allocation decisions based on physiological and organizational variables. Most triage policies recognize that triage officers must exercise a degree of discretion. But they recognize the potential conflict of interest when the physician acts as both healthcare provider and triage officer, and they urge the separation of these roles where possible. They also recommend the establishment of procedural protections for the patient and attending physician including appeals mechanisms, oversight, and the public announcement of policies. The implementation of this set of prescriptions is best exemplified by the polices covering the rationing of organs for transplantation.

Rules for ICU Triage: The Model of Organ Transplantation

Whether or not an individual is entitled to a particular organ transplant procedure is a matter of such considerations as the explicit contract language in the insurance policy, HCFA coverage determinations for Medicare patients, and, in the case the Oregon Medicaid population, the cut-point in a rank-ordered list of conditions/treatments. Entitlement to organ transplantation does not guarantee that an organ will be available.

Nationally recognized policies regulating the allocation of scarce organs for transplantation (United Network for Organ Sharing 1993) can provide lessons for the allocation of scarce ICU beds in that they limit discretion of individual physicians advocating for their patients while at the same time facilitating systemwide (nationwide) accountability (Benjamin, Cohen, and Grochowski 1994). In the United States, organs are allocated according to criteria that balance likely medical success, time on the waiting list, and urgency of need. These criteria explicitly recognize micro tradeoffs—saying no to one patient means saying yes to a more-deserving patient. The benefits of the tradeoff are realized on a national level as opposed to the level of a single ICU. Individual physicians generally accept the legitimacy of these criteria even though transplants may be denied or delayed to their patients. Complexity is greatly reduced while at the same time the discretion of central decision makers is limited.

The SCCM triage guidelines (1994) contains language that in many respects parallels national transplantation policy with regard to the admission of ICU patients.

> The demand for medical services such as critical care is likely to often exceed supply. In the setting of these constraining conditions, institutions and individual providers of critical care must use some moral framework for distributing the available resources efficiently and equitably. Guidelines are therefore provided for triage of critically ill patients. There are several general principles that should guide decision making: providers should advocate for patients; members of the provider team should collaborate; the restriction of care is necessary in an equitable system; decisions to give care should be based on expected benefit; mechanisms for alternative care should be planned; explicit policies should be written; prior public notification is necessary (p. 1200).

Major differences exist in the level of difficulty in designing allocation rules for scarce organs as opposed to scarce ICU beds. First of all, there is greater agreement on the definition of need for transplantation and on the criteria for rank ordering candidates. Secondly, scarce organs exist in the context of a naturally closed system; the supply of organs is truly limited and the shortage is persistent. In contrast, the supply of ICU beds or alternative beds is frequently stretchable and the shortage is intermittent. Furthermore, a large pool of patients awaits transplant and therefore a withholding decision is required. The choice in the ICU is often between a patient waiting for a bed and a person already in a bed and therefore a withdrawal decision must be considered (Truog 1992).

Significant obstacles remain, thus inhibiting adherence to the principles in the SCCM triage guidelines, in particular with regard to the establishment of explicit triage policies based on expected benefit and prior public notification. As was mentioned in Chapter 4, there is an unresolved controversy over the relative weights to be given to first-come, first-served (squatters' rights) versus other ethically relevant criteria such as urgency of need, likelihood of benefit, improvement in quality of life, and duration of benefit. Accordingly, the triage officer is unable to render a technical and impartial judgment on comparative entitlement because there is dispute concerning the criteria for such a judgment. Furthermore, while first-come, first-served is an easily understood, articulated, and applied criteria, hospitals have been unable to concretize urgency of need, quality of life, and ability to benefit into a set of easily understood and applied decision rules. The SCCM is reluctant to define benefit and futility "because they are subjective, value-laden terms for which there is no agreement" (1994). The more recent draft Consensus Statement on Futile and Other Possibly Inadvisable Treatments defines futility in such a narrow sense to be of little help in triage. The anxiety-provoking questions of legal liability inhibit full disclosure of gatekeeping policies to the public or to individual patients. With the exception of the von Stetina case (discussed in Chapter 4), the courts have provided little guidance or protection for the triage officer. It is much easier for a gatekeeper to follow the arrows on Dawson's flowchart (Exhibit 3.6). In summary, as opposed to the bureaucratically structured gatekeeping role of the HTUC, the triage officer finds himself or herself in a much different predicament. These gatekeepers have no choice but to exercise discretion in an environment where rules are often ambiguous or inconsistent. There are those who argue that decision makers facing comparative entitlement decisions should implicitly ration. Guido Calabresi and Philip Bobbitt (1978) make one such argument. They hold that so-called "tragic choices" should be hidden from public view to "preserve the moral foundations of social cooperation" (p. 18). However, most ethical and legal systems require public announcement and full disclosure. Both the SCCM and the AMA emphasize these requirements.

Gatekeeping and Hard Choices: The Emerging Crisis

In Exhibit 6.1, we conceptualize gatekeeping in terms of a four quadrant matrix. The upper two quadrants characterize decision making that is ad-hoc and political in nature, while the bottom quadrants characterize decision making that is bureaucratic (i.e., clear rules, stability, fairness, predictability) (Pfeffer 1981). Most of the decision making associated with the rounds and cases discussed throughout this book would fall in the upper two quadrants.

In this chapter we have discussed some of the approaches by which society might make the tradeoffs among risks, benefits, and costs of critical care while at the same time addressing the legal and ethical concerns of patients, surrogates, physicians, and other professionals. The approaches, listed in the bottom two quadrants, if carried through, would greatly enhance the effectiveness of ICU gatekeepers by helping to clarify and legitimize the three decision rationales for ICU gatekeeping: medical futility, non-triage mode/bed availability, and triage mode/comparative entitlement. But to provide the necessary legal framework through case law or statutory law that permits communities and institutions to set limits on treatments, allocate resources, and, when necessary, make comparative entitlement decisions will require hard choices on the part of governmental institutions. Thus far the hard choices, with a few exceptions, have not been made. The unresolved issues delineated earlier remain essentially unresolved.

Perhaps we can postpone making the hard choices. With managed care and competitive markets, many of the inefficiencies associated with the traditional practice of critical care medicine will be eliminated. Reengineered work processes with assembly-line production and fast-tracking will increase through-put and decrease length of stay. Advances in disease and severity modeling will increase the ability to exclude the too sick and the too well. Alternative settings (e.g., intermediate care units) will be available for these patients, including many of the high-risk monitor type. Patients, reflecting changing societal attitudes and encouraged to discuss what is meant by a "reasonable prospect for meaningful recovery," will desire less aggressive care. Demand for critical services will initially be reduced. Consolidation and downsizing will decrease the fixed costs of ICUs by eliminating excess beds and staff. What is the urgency in making hard choices?

First, as we have argued, it is likely that managed care will lead to the restructuring of ICUs from open and semi-closed units to closed units with the concomitant diminishment of the attending physician's role in gatekeeping. The combined role of the gatekeeper and attending physician will become more prevalent and raise ethical concerns. There is danger that the financial incentives of managed care will lead to an erosion of public trust in the attending physician and the gatekeeper. In gatekeeping, to whose benefit will the micro-tradeoffs accrue? This question is relevant even if the gatekeeper is the QCCP. And the QCCP-led ICU is by no means the norm in the United States.

Second, the rubber band of ICU resources has a limited amount of stretch and will be greatly reduced in the hospital of the future. Schwartz and Mendelson (1994) maintain that efficiency gains alone are

Exhibit 6.1 Gatekeeping: Current Practices (Upper Quadrants) and Potential Policy Improvements (Bottom Quadrants)

Decision-Making Style	NON-TRIAGE MODE	TRIAGE MODE
AD-HOC/POLITICAL Limited agreement on definition and application of decision criteria Locus of decision-making: at the bedside	• No agreed-upon legally sanctioned definition of benefit or futility and inconsistent application of criteria • Criteria may be constructed after-the-fact to rationalize action • Decision making using "Dawson Model" (see p. 82)	• Limited public announcement and understanding of triage policies • Limited legal guidance and protection for triage officer • Decision making using "Dawson Model" with street-level bureaucrats as decision makers in some instances • Covert rationing
BUREAUCRATIC Clear rules, stability, predictability Procedural rationality embedded in procedures Locus of decision making: at the level of public policy and at the bedside	• Community consensus on standards/Denver GUIDe approach • Community consensus on procedures/Houston City-Wide Taskforce approach • Massachusetts General Hospital Optimum Care Committee Approach (Gilgunn case) and/or • Insurance policy contract/"Oregonian ICU" approach (Rie)	• Case law giving clearer guidance in support of triage (von Stetina case, see page 135)

No Clear-Cut Delineation →

← *Clear-Cut Delineation*

not likely to solve the problem of rising health expenditure. After we squeeze out inefficiencies, the development of new technologies and the aging of the population will place pressure on hospital utilization and expenditure, including critical care (Aaron 1986). Advances in noncritical care medical and surgical techniques will expand the population of "potentially salvageable patients"—future candidates for the ICU (Kalb and Miller 1989).

What should be done in the meantime, as we wait for society to address the hard choices? We suggest that at least some of this trust and confidence can be maintained in a managed care-dominated health system by the institution of oversight mechanisms in conjunction with the QCCP-led ICU.

At the hospital level, we recommend the Rapid Ethics Evaluation Process, which has the advantage of community observers, independent from managed care organizations. At the level of the managed care plan, we see potential benefit in a policy committee designed to open channels for both patients and physician representatives to participate in negotiation over specific clinical guidelines that guide physicians in managing their patient's problems, compensation arrangements and financial incentives, and mechanisms for quality assurance (Sorum 1996). Physicians could also use these channels to express and address their ethical concerns. There is also a place for external monitoring (using prognostic models) by payors or independent oversight bodies. The JCAHO, the National Committee for Quality Assurance (NCQA), other accrediting bodies, and state departments of health can play a role. There is definitely a need for a public policy that encourages internal and external oversight.

One result of increased oversight activities of the hospital and managed care levels should be a greater recognition of the need to explore, assess, and document the lack of clarity and consistency in application of gatekeeping policies. We can confidently predict that overseers will find a discrepancy, particularly with regard to triage, between the requirements for full public announcement and disclosure of policies and the actual knowledge of individual patients.

Oversight will serve to bring the above concerns and quality deficiencies into legislative and judicial policy arenas, perhaps spurring a search for solutions lying along the paths we have discussed. But short of these measures, and in light of the reluctance to make hard choices, we would again raise the specter of the ICU gatekeeper as street-level bureaucrat functioning with much more limited resources than today, with ambiguous or contradictory performance criteria and expectations, and dispensing vital and even life-sustaining services.

References

Aaron, H. J. 1989. "Lessons from United Kingdom." In *Rationing of Medical Care for the Critically Ill*, edited by M. A. Strosberg, I. A. Fein, and J. D. Carroll, 24–31. Washington, D.C.: The Brookings Institution.

Aaron, H. J., and W. B. Schwartz. 1984. *The Painful Prescription: Rationing Hospital Care.* Washington, D.C.: The Brookings Institution.

American Medical Association Council on Ethical and Judicial Affairs. 1995. "Ethical Issues in Managed Care." *Journal of the American Medical Association* 273 (4): 330–35.

Asch, D. A., J. Hansen-Flaschen, and D. N. Lanken. 1995. "Decisions to Limit or Continue Life-Sustaining Treatment by Critical Care Physicians in the United States, Conflicts Between Physicians' Practices and Patients' Wishes." *American Journal of Critical Care Medicine* 151 (2.1) 288–92.

Baker, R., I. A. Fein, M. A. Strosberg, and M. H. Weil. 1988. "Caring for the Critically Ill: Proposals for Reform." In *Rationing of Medical Care for the Critically Ill*, edited by M. A. Strosberg, I. A. Fein, and J. D. Carroll, 87–91. Washington, D.C.: The Brookings Institution.

Baker, R. 1992. "The Inevitability of Health Care Rationing: A Case Study of Rationing in the British National Health Service." In *Rationing America's Medical Care: The Oregon Plan and Beyond*, edited by M. A. Strosberg, J. M. Weiner, and Robert Baker, 208–220. Washington, D.C.: The Brookings Institution.

Barry, M. J., F. J. Fowler, A. G. Mulley Jr., J. V. Henderson Jr., and J. E. Wennberg. 1995. "Patient Reactions to a Program Designed to Facilitate Patient Participation in Treatment Decisions for Benign Prostatic Hyperplasia." *Medical Care* 33 (8): 771–82.

Benjamin, M., C. Cohen, E. Grochowski. 1994. "What Transplantation Can Teach Us About Health Care Reform." *New England Journal of Medicine* 330 (12): 858–60.

Berghold, L. A. 1995. "Medical Necessity: Do We Need It?" *Health Affairs* 14 (4): 180–90.

Calabresi, G., and P. Bobbit. 1978. *Tragic Choices.* New York: W. W. Norton & Co.

Curtis, R., D. R. Park, M. R. Krone, and R. A. Pearlman. 1995. "Use of the Medical Futility Rationale in Do-Not-Attempt-Resuscitation Orders." *Journal of the American Medical Association* 273 (2): 124–28.

Eddy, D. M. 1996. *Clinical Decision Making: From Theory to Practice—A Series of Essays from the Journal of the American Medical Association.* Sudbury, MA: Jones and Bartlett.

Emanuel, E. J., and L. L. Emanuel. 1994. "The Economics of Dying: The Illusion of Cost Savings at the End of Life." *New England Journal of Medicine* 330 (8): 540–44.

Engelhardt, H. T. 1992. "Why a Two-Tier System of Health Care Delivery Is Morally Unavoidable." In *Rationing America's Medical Care: The Oregon Plan and Beyond*, edited by M. A. Strosberg, J. M. Weiner, and R. Baker, 196–207. Washington, D.C.: The Brookings Institution.

Engelhardt, H. T. and M. A. Rie. 1986. "Intensive Care Units, Scarce Resources and Conflicting Principles of Justice." *Journal of the American Medical Association* 255 (9): 1159–64.

Gradison, W. D. 1989. "Federal Policy and Intensive Care." In *Rationing of Medical Care for the Critically Ill,* edited by M. A. Strosberg, I. A. Fein, and J. D Carroll, 37–40. Washington, D.C.: The Brookings Institution.

Hadorn, D. C. 1994. "Who Really Needs to Be in the Intensive Care Unit: Using Clinical Guidelines to Define Healthcare Needs." *Critical Care Medicine* 22 (10): 1679–82.

Hadorn, D. C. 1991. "Setting Health Care Priorities in Oregon: Cost-effectiveness Meets the Rule of Rescue." *Journal of the American Medical Association* 265 (17): 2218–25.

Hall, M. A. 1989. "The Malpractice Standard Under Health Care Cost Containment." *Law, Medicine and Health Care* 17 (4): 347–55.

Havighurst, C. C. 1992. "Prospective Self-Denial: Can Consumers Contract Today to Accept Health Care Rationing Tomorrow?" *University of Pennsylvania Law Review.* 140 (5): 1755–1808.

Havighurst, C. C. 1995. *Health Care Choices: Private Contracts as Instruments of Health Reform.* Washington, D.C.: AEI Press.

Hirshfeld, J. D. 1990. "Economic Considerations in Treatment Decisions and the Standard of Care in Medical Malpractice Litigation." *Journal of the American Medical Association* 264 (15): 2004–12.

Houston City-Wide Task Force on Medical Futility. 1996. "A Multi-institution Collaborative Policy on Medical Futility." *Journal of the American Medical Association* 276 (7): 571–74.

Kalb, P. E., and D. H. Miller. 1989. "Utilization Strategies for Intensive Care Units." *Journal of the American Medical Association* 261 (16): 2389–95.

Kaplan, R. M. 1992. "A Quality-of-Life Approach to Health Resource Allocation." In *Rationing America's Medical Care: The Oregon Plan and Beyond,* edited by M. A. Strosberg, J. M. Weiner, and R. Baker. Washington, D.C.: The Brookings Institution.

Kitzhaber, J. 1991. "A Healthier Approach to Health Care." *Issues in Science and Technology* II (2): 59–65.

Kolata, G. 1995. "Withholding Care from Patients: Boston Case Asks Who Decides." *The New York Times,* April 3.

Lipsky, M. 1980. *Street-Level Bureaucracy: Dilemmas of the Individual in Public Services.* New York: Russell Sage Foundation.

Lo, B. 1995. "End-of-Life Care after Termination of SUPPORT." *Hastings Center Report.* November–December (Special Supplement): S6–S8.

Lubitz, J. D., and G. F. Riley. 1993. "Trends in Medicare Payments in the Last Year of Life." *New England Journal of Medicine* 328 (15): 1092–96.

Luce, J. M. 1995. "Physicians Do Not Have a Responsibility to Provide Futile or Unreasonable Care if a Patient or Family Insists." *Critical Care Medicine* 23 (4): 760–66.

Miles, S. H. 1991. "The Case of Helga Wanglie." *New England Journal of Medicine* 325 (7): 511–15.

Morreim, E. H. 1992. "Rationing and the Law." In *Rationing America's Medical Care: The Oregon Plan and Beyond,* edited by M. A. Strosberg, J. M. Weiner, and R. Baker, 159–184. Washington, D.C.: The Brookings Institution.

Morreim, E. H. 1989. "Stratified Scarcity: Redefining the Standard of Care." *Law, Medicine and Health Care* 17 (winter): 356–67.

Morreim, H. 1995. "Futilitarianism, Exoticare, and Coerced Altruism: The ADA Meets its Limits." *Seton Hall Law Review* 25 (883): 1–41.

Mulley, A. G., 1984. "The Triage Decision." In *The Machine at the Bedside,* edited by S. Reiser and M. Anbar, 221–26. Cambridge: Cambridge University Press.

Murphy, D. J., and Barbour. 1994. "GUIDe (Guidelines for the Use of Intensive Care in Denver): A Community Effort to Define Futile and Inappropriate Care." *New Horizons* 2 (3): 326–31.

New York Public Health Law. 1987. Article 29-B (L. 1987, Ch. 818).

Orentlicher, D. 1994. "Rationing and the Americans with Disabilities Act." *Journal of the American Medical Association* 271 (4): 308–14.

Peters, P. B. 1995. "Health Care Rationing and Disability Rights." *Indiana Law Journal* (Spring): 491–547.

Pfeffer, J. 1981. *Power in Organizations.* Boston: Pitman.

Redford, E. S. 1969. *Democracy in the Administrative State.* New York: Oxford University Press, 140.

Reinhardt, U. E. 1995. "Turning Our Gaze from Bread and Circus Games." *Health Affairs* 14 (1): 33–36.

Rie, M. A. 1995. "The Oregonian ICU: Multi-Tiered Monetarized Morality in Health Insurance Law." *Journal of Law, Medicine and Ethics* 23 (2): 149–66.

Rie, M. A. 1991. "The Limits of a Wish." *Hastings Center Report* 21 (4): 24–27.

Rie, M. A. 1989. "Professional Ethics and Political Power." In *Rationing of Medical Care for the Critically Ill,* edited by M. A. Strosberg, I. A. Fein, and J. D. Carroll, 82–86. Washington, D.C.: The Brookings Institution.

Schwartz, W. B., and D. N. Mendelson. 1994. "Eliminating Waste and Inefficiency Can Do Little to Contain Health Costs." *Health Affairs* 13 (1): 224–38.

Shoemaker, W., C. B. James, A. W. Fleming, E. Hardin, G. J. Ordog, R. Sterling-Scott, and J. Wasserberger. 1992. "DeFacto Rationing of Emergency Medical Services." In *Rationing America's Medical Care: The Oregon Plan and Beyond,* edited by M. A. Strosberg, J. M. Weiner, R. Baker, I. A. Fein, 151–56. Washington, D.C.: The Brookings Institution.

Society of Critical Care Medicine Ethics Committee. 1994. "Consensus Statement on the Triage of Critically Ill Patients." *Journal of the American Medical Association* 271 (15): 1200–03.

Society of Critical Care Medicine Ethics Committee. 1997. "Consensus Statement on Futile and Other Possibly Inadvisable Treatments." (Draft) Anaheim, CA: SCCM.

Society of Critical Care Medicine Task Force on Guidelines. 1988. "Recommendations for Intensive Care Unit Admission and Discharge Criteria." *Critical Care Medicine* 16 (8): 807–08.

Sorum, P. C. 1996. "Ethical Decision Making in Managed Care." *Archives of Internal Medicine* 156 (18): 2041–45.

Strosberg, M. A., and D. Teres. 1996. "Public Policymaking for Intensive Care Units." In *Intensive Care Medicine,* 3rd ed., edited by J. M. Rippe, R. S. Irwin, M. P. Fink, and F. B. Cerra, 2568–75. Boston: Little, Brown and Co.

Strosberg, M. A. 1995. "The New York State Do-Not-Resuscitate Law: A Study of Public Policy-Making." In *Legislating Medical Ethics: A Study of the New York State Do-Not-Resuscitate Law,* edited by R. Baker and M. A. Strosberg, 9–31. Dordrecht: Kluwer Academic Publishers.

Strosberg, M. A. 1992. "Introduction." In *Rationing America's Medical Care: The Oregon*

Plan and Beyond, edited by M. A. Strosberg, J. M. Weiner, R. Baker, I. A. Fein, 3–11. Washington, D.C.: The Brookings Institution.

Teno, J. M., D. Murphy, J. Lynn, A. Tosteson, N. Desbiens, A. F. Connors, M. B. Hamel, A. Wu, R. Phillips, N. Wenger, F. Harrell Jr., W. A. Knaus for the SUPPORT Investigators. 1994. "Prognosis-Based Futility Guidelines: Does Anyone Win?" *Journal of the American Geriatric Society* 42 (11): 1202–07.

Truog, R. D. 1992. "Triage in the ICU." *Hastings Center Report* (May–June): 13–17.

Truog, R. D., A. S. Brett, and J. Frader. 1992. "The Problem with Futility." *New England Journal of Medicine* 326 (23): 1560–63.

United Network for Organ Sharing. 1993. Bylaws and Policies. Policy 3.3.5.

Veatch, R. 1986. "The Ethics of Resource Allocation in Critical Care." *Critical Care Clinics* 2 (1): 73–89.

Wennberg, J. E. 1990. "Outcomes Research, Cost-Containment and the Fear of Health Care Rationing." *New England Journal of Medicine* 323 (17): 1202–04.

Wyden, R. L. 1992. "Why I Support the Oregon Plan." In *Rationing America's Medical Care: The Oregon Plan and Beyond,* edited by M. A. Strosberg, J. M. Weiner, R. Baker, I. A. Fein, 115–18. Washington, D.C.: The Brookings Institution.

Youngner, S. J. 1995. "Medical Futility and the Social Contract." *Seton Hall Law Review* 25: 1015.

Zawacki B. E. 1985. "ICU Physicians Ethical Role in Distributing Scarce Resources." *Critical Care Medicine* 13 (1): 57.

APPENDIX A

Guidelines on ICU Admission, Discharge, Triage, and Futility

1. Pages 205–208: Society of Critical Care Medicine. 1988. "Recommendations for Intensive Care Unit Admission and Discharge Criteria."
2. Pages 208–217: Society of Critical Care Medicine. 1994. "Consensus Statement on the Triage of Critically Ill Patients," *Journal of the American Medical Association* 271 (15): 1200–1203.
3. Pages 217–235: Council on Ethical and Judicial Affairs. "Ethical Consideration in the Allocation of Organs and Other Scarce Medical Resources Among Patients," *Code of Medical Ethics Reports* IV (2). © 1993 American Medical Association: Chicago.
4. Pages 236–244: Department of Medicine and the Center for Medical Ethics and Health Policy, Baylor College of Medicine. "A Multi-institution Collaborative Policy on Medical Futility," *Journal of the American Medical Association* 276 (7): 571–574. © 1996 American Medical Association.

1. Recommendations for ICU Admission and Discharge Criteria

Task Force Guidelines, Society of Critical Care Medicine

The Society of Critical Care Medicine, through its Task Force on Guidelines, has developed the following as a guide for hospitals in the formulation of admission/discharge policies for critical care units. Since each unit serves a different patient population, it will be necessary for each unit to develop an individualized policy using the model below only as a guide. In addition, each hospital should develop a policy for the accommodation of patients when the critical care unite is full.

Each critical care unit should develop admission and discharge policies and procedures. These policies and procedures should be developed by a multidisciplinary team representing medicine, nursing, and hospital administration. These policies and procedures should be reviewed and revised, as necessary, on a regular basis. compliance with these guidelines should be monitored by the multidisciplinary team.

Admission and Discharge Policy

An Intensive Care Unit provides services that include both intensive monitoring and intensive treatment. During times of high utilization and scarce beds, patients requiring intensive treatment (Priority 1) have priority over monitoring (Priority 2) and terminally or critically ill patients with a poor prognosis for recovery (Priority 3). Eligibility for ICU admission and discharge is also based upon reversibility of the clinical problem as well as the likely benefits of ICU treatment and expectation of recovery.

It is the responsibility of the patient's attending physician (or designee) to request ICU admission and to promptly transfer patients meeting discharge criteria.

It is the responsibility of the ICU director (or designee) to decide if the patient meets eligibility requirements for ICU. In case of conflict regarding admission or discharge criteria, the ICU director (designee) will decide which patient should be given priority. A procedure to implement this policy should be specified for each ICU. A mechanism should also exist to retrospectively review cases wherein the attending physician disagrees with the decision of the ICU director (designee).

Whenever possible, objective measures of illness and prognosis should be considered when reaching decisions to continue, limit, or terminate ICU support.

Admission Criteria

Priority 1 Patients: Critically ill, unstable patients in need of intensive treatment such as ventilator support, continuous vasoactive drug infusion, etc. Examples of such admissions may include, but are not limited to, post-open-heart cases, carotid endarterectomy patients receiving vasoactive drugs, or patients in septic shock. Priority 1 patients have no limits placed on therapy.

Appendix A

Priority 2 Patients: Patients who, at the time of admission, are not critically ill but whose condition requires the technologic monitoring services of the ICU. These patients would benefit from intensive monitoring (e.g., peripheral or pulmonary arterial lines) and are at risk for needing immediate intensive treatment. Examples of such admissions may include, but are not limited to, patients with underlying heart, lung, or renal disease who have a severe medical illness or have undergone major surgery. Priority 2 patients have no limits placed on therapy.

Priority 3 Patients: Critically ill, unstable patients whose previous state of health, underlying disease, or acute illness, either alone or in combination, severely reduces the likelihood of recovery and benefit from ICU treatment. Examples of such admissions may include, but are not limited to, patients with metastatic malignancy complicated by infection, pericardial tamponade, or airway obstruction, or patients with end-stage heart or lung disease complicated by a severe acute resuscitation.

Patients who do not meet routine admission criteria are:
1. Patients who have confirmed clinical and laboratory evidence of brain death (such patients can be admitted if they are potential organ donors but only for the purpose of life support prior to organ donation).
2. Competent patients who refuse life-supporting therapy.
3. Patients with nontraumatic coma causing a permanent vegetative state.

These patients would be admitted to the ICU only under unusual circumstances, at the discretion of the ICU director, and they should be discharged if necessary to make room for priority 1, 2, or 3 patients.

Discharge Criteria

Priority 1 patients are discharged when their need for intensive treatment is no longer present or when treatment has failed so that short-term prognosis is poor, and there is little likelihood of recovery or benefit from continued intensive treatment.

Priority 2 patients are discharged when intensive monitoring has not resulted in a need for intensive treatment and the need for intensive monitoring is no longer present.

Priority 3 patients are discharged when the need for intensive treatment is no longer present, but they may be discharged earlier if there is little likelihood of recovery or benefit from continued intensive treatment.

In consideration of the continuing and often specialized care needs of these patients, arrangements for appropriate non-ICU care will be made prior to ICU discharge.

Patients who are unlikely to benefit from continued ICU treatment include:
1. Patients of advanced age with three or more organ system failures who have not responded to 72 hours of intensive therapy.
2. Patients who are brain-dead or who have nontraumatic coma leading to a permanently vegetative state and a very low probability of meaningful recovery.
3. Patients who have had formal limits placed upon their care indicated by "comfort care only."
4. Patients with protracted respiratory failure who have not responded to initial aggressive efforts and who are also suffering from hematologic malignancy.
5. Patients with a variety of other diagnoses (advanced COPD, end-stage cardiac disease, or widespread carcinoma) who have failed to respond to ICU therapy whose short-term prognosis is also extremely poor and for whom no potential exists to alter that prognosis.
6. Physiologically stable patients who are at low risk of requiring unique ICU treatment. Examples of such low-risk monitor patients may include, but are not limited to, stable surgical patients recovering from carotid endarterectomy and aortofemoral bypass graft, and nonoperative patients with uncomplicated diabetic ketoacidosis, self-inflicted drug overdose, concussion, or mild CHF. These patients might be admitted to an intermediate care unit if such a unit exists.

Members of the Task Force on Guidelines include Carolyn E. Bekes, MD, Chairman; Robert W. Bayly, MD; Graziano C. Carlon, MD; R. Phillip Dellinger, MD; Burton A. Dole Jr.; I. Alan Fein, MD; David J. Fish, MD; Charles J. Fisher Jr., MD; Bernard H. Holzman, MD; H. Matilda Horst, MD; Michael S. Jastremski, MD; Albert S. Kyle; J. Michael Lonergan, MD; Philip D. Lumb, MB; John J. Mickell, MD; William New Jr., MD; Thomas G. Rainey, MD; Judith Snyderman; David B. Swedlow, MD; Robert W. Taylor Jr., MD; John D. Ward, MD; Jack Wolfsdorf, MD; and Jack E. Zimmerman, MD.

2. Consensus Statement on the Triage of Critically Ill Patients

Society of Critical Care Medicine Ethics Committee
It is likely that the demand for health care services will always exceed the supply. In this context of relative scarcity, it is appropriate to develop

Appendix A

explicit guidelines to help facilitate the fairest use of these services. This statement offers critical care providers principles and guidelines for the distribution of intensive care resources among individual patients.

Justification

The United States and other countries face difficult questions regarding access to, delivery of, and payment for health care services, as well as the proportion of health care expenditures that should be appropriated for critical care. These issues are not likely to be resolved easily or quickly, nor will these general issues be addressed herein. Regardless of when and how these broader issues are resolved, individual health care organizations and providers will continually face a disparity between demand for and availability of critical care facilities. Demand is created by the inclination of critically ill patients and their families to seek, and their physicians to provide, intensive care. The advancing age of the population is likely to increase the demand for services as more elderly individuals who are frail, chronically ill, and subject to life-threatening illness become potential candidates for critical care. The development of new pharmaceutical products and technological devices often makes the care provided more expensive. At the same time that demand for and expense of care are increasing, the capacity to meet demand is constrained by inadequate reimbursement, restricted growth or health care facilities, and personnel shortages.

In the setting of these constraining conditions, individual institutions and individual providers of critical care must use some moral framework for distributing the resources at hand. Sometimes resources are more obviously limited than at other times, as evidenced by the absence of an available bed in the intensive care unit (ICU). The guidelines provided herein are intended to be applicable whether or not an immediate shortage is apparent, because their continuous use will lead to more consistently equitable and efficient critical care. It is recognized that limiting care of critically ill patients during acute shortages is more likely to result in adverse consequences for individual patients than limiting care during times without shortages.

While various terms such as "triage," "rationing," or "allocation of resources" have been used to describe the distribution of limited goods and services, we will use the term "triage." This term has been chosen because it conveys a well-established process in medicine of finding the most appropriate disposition for a patient based on an assessment of the patient's illness and its urgency. "Triage" derives from the French verb *trier* meaning to pick, to sort, or to select. The first medical application of the word was in the French military, where *hospital de triage* meant a sorting station for injured soldiers. There are at least six major types of triage, depending on the location of the patient: (1) prehospital, (2) catastrophic, (3) emergency department, (4) intensive care, (5) battlefield, and (6) waiting list for lifesaving treatments in short supply such as dialysis or organ transplantation. We particularly endorse this process when it is based on a sound understanding of the probable outcome of the patient's illness, the availability of therapeutic modalities, the impact of therapy on outcome, and a judgment of the benefits and burdens or the therapy for the patient, the patient's family, and society.

Triage of critically ill patients that may limit individual patient and physician choices is justified when (1) the policy is aimed at achieving benefits for individual patients, the health care institution, and society and (2) the policy is announced in advance to notify the public.

Principles

General Principles

Guidelines should be formulated for expected categories of triage that may reasonably be anticipated. They should articulate the principles, justifications, and mechanisms pertaining to each situation as explicitly as possible.

Notwithstanding the pressures exerted on health care providers to limit resource consumption during real or perceived conditions of scarcity, physicians should remain staunch advocates of their patients' best interests. Conflicts of interest between the health care provider's role as gatekeeper and patient advocate may occur and should be anticipated. Because conflicts of interest cannot be altogether eliminated, institutions should attempt to separate the roles of gatekeeper and advocate when possible.

Physicians, nurses, and administrative staff should collaborate in framing guidelines and recommendations for the prudent use of scarce resources in their own institutions. The formulation and promulgation of explicit triage policies should help to minimize the necessity for ad hoc triage decisions in individual cases.

Health care providers, patients, policymakers, and the public at large must recognize that various treatments, including life-prolonging treatments, may be denied. Health care institutions may justifiably restrict the availability of certain services to use limited resources more effectively or to enhance equity in allocating them.

Priorities for patient selection for triage should be reflected in ICU policies. Priorities should weigh the scope of services available, patient inclusion and exclusion criteria, and institutional triage policies. Established standards of critical care should not be compromised.

Critical care units should, in general, be reserved for those patients who have a "reasonable prospect of substantial recovery." An exception may be patients being supported for organ donation. The scope of ICU services should be limited to diagnostic and therapeutic procedures from which a benefit is anticipated.

Each hospital should develop a policy for the accommodation of critically ill patients when all ICU beds capable of being staffed are full. This overflow policy should be prepared in advance so as to identify suitable areas for temporary overflow.

If sufficient ICU beds are not available and appropriate triage does not resolve the shortage, every effort should be made to provide the analogous levels of care in other settings. Hospitals should provided alternative solutions for patients in need of life support and/or monitoring who can be reasonably cared for outside the ICU setting.

Basic ICU services of known therapeutic benefit should receive priority over investigational ICU services that are not of proven value.

Specific Principles

The foremost consideration in triage decisions is the expected outcome of the patient in terms of survival and function, which turns on the medical status of the patient. In general, patients with good prognoses for recovery have priority over patients with poor prognoses. While uncertainty of prognosis is a crucial problem in critical care, providers should utilize predictive instruments with a full understanding of their strengths and limitations. Decisions to be made between patients with equivalent prognoses should be made on a first come, first served basis.

Priority for admission to an ICU should correlate with the likelihood that ICU care will benefit the patient substantially more than non-ICU care. Patients with very poor prognoses and little likelihood of benefit should not be admitted. Patients with very good prospects with or without ICU care also should not be admitted.

Benefit and futility have been variously defined by authors based on the goals of therapy and the likelihood of success. They are not specifically defined because they are subjective, value-laden terms for which there is no agreement. Factors that should be considered in determining benefit and utility for triage decisions include the following:

- likelihood of a successful outcome;
- patient's life expectancy due to disease(s);
- anticipated quality of life of the patient;
- wishes of the patient and/or surrogate;

- burdens for those affected, including financial and psychological costs and missed opportunities to treat other patients;
- health and other needs of the community; and
- individual and institutional moral and religious values.

All triage decisions made for individual patients on grounds of scarcity must be made explicitly, fairly, and justly. Triage decisions should not be made in an arbitrary or prejudiced fashion. Ethnic origin, race, sex, creed, social worth, sexual preference, and ability to pay should never be factors in determining triage decisions.

Triage policies should be disclosed in advance to the general public and, when feasible, to patients and surrogates on admission. Triage decisions may be made without patient or surrogate consent. Disclosure of triage decisions may help to facilitate communication, understanding, and cooperation among patients, surrogates, and physicians.

As a general rule, obligations to patients already hospitalized in an ICU who continue to warrant ICU care outweigh obligations to accept new patients. There may be circumstances, however, when it is justified to discharge a patient from the ICU to admit another patient (see next section). If admission of a new patient is likely to adversely affect the outcomes of patients already under care, then that admission is ordinarily justified only if the benefit to the new admission is significant and quite likely and the adverse effects on the present ICU patients are either conjectural or unlikely to be significant.

Criteria for ICU admission, discharge, and exclusion should be explicitly described. Patients who have do-not-resuscitate orders (no cardiopulmonary resuscitation, no chest compression) may still have compelling reasons for admission to an ICU and should not be automatically excluded. Patients with little or no anticipated benefit from further ICU treatment may be discharged or transferred from the ICU. Patients with terminal, irreversible illness who face imminent death should be excluded from the ICU. Very elderly individuals who are failing to thrive due to irreversible, chronic illness should not be encouraged to use intensive care. The decision to exclude or discharge a patient from the ICU may appropriately be made despite the anticipation of an untoward outcome.

Examples of terminally ill patients who *may* be excluded from the ICU, whether beds are available or not, include those with severe, irreversible brain damage or irreversible multiorgan failure and those with metastatic cancer unresponsive to chemotherapy and/or radiation therapy unless the patients are in specialized ICUs or on specific protocols.

Examples of patients who *should* be excluded from the ICU, whether beds are available or not, include those who competently decline intensive care or request that invasive therapy be withheld; those declared brain dead who are not organ donors, and those in a persistent vegetative or permanently unconscious state.

However, religious or moral convictions may legitimately be the basis for the provision of treatment to such patients if the costs are not borne by the general society and the provision of such services does not foreclose the treatment of other patients who would benefit from critical care.

Although triage decisions in military and disaster situations may mandate prioritizing care on the basis of potential contribution to military goals or the saving of other lives, such considerations are not ordinarily applicable to the civilian ICU setting. Hospitals should have a separate policy to handle civilian disasters.

A patient's personal behavior should not influence triage decisions if it does not affect the patient's outcome.

Patients, their surrogate, or others may not compel a physician to provide treatment that the physician believes is not medically indicated.

Mechanisms

Institutional Responsibilities

Hospitals are responsible, acting through ICU directors, for setting policy and implementing triage decisions in ICUs.

This responsibility will ordinarily be implemented by the critical care unit (ICU) committee. Depending on the administrative structure of the hospital, this responsibility may be overseen by other committees and/or individuals. The mechanism chosen will depend on each institution's view of the best method to discharge this responsibility.

Because of the complex medical, ethical, and legal issues involved in ICU triage, the ICU committee should include a broad range of health care professionals and other appropriate individuals. When appropriate, the ICU committee should seek the advice of members of the medical and nursing staffs, hospital administration, hospital ethics committee, patient advocacy representatives, and/or legal advisers.

The ICU committee should have medical oversight and responsibility for triage decisions. In addition, it should be vested with authority to implement these decisions.

The ICU committee should institute a mechanism for postponing elective operations and procedures requiring subsequent ICU care when ICU beds are not available.

The ICU committee should assess outcomes on a regular basis to ensure that policies do not lead to inappropriately restrictive ICU admission policies, premature discharge policies, misuse of ICU facilities, unwarranted morbidity and mortality, or inappropriate costs.

In its oversight role regarding triage, the ICU committee has the following responsibilities:

- evaluation of backup capacity, such as the capacity of the postanesthesia care unit or the emergency department to handle an overflow of critically ill patients;
- review of policies related to intermediate care or step-down units and their capacity and function;
- review of interactions among different ICUs and between these ICUs and other units;
- maintenance of a program for regional cooperation among hospitals during periods of overload;
- oversight of the functioning of the triage officer in relation to ICU admission and discharge policies and the triage of individual patients; and
- education of members of the institutional staff about triage issues and policies through appropriate mechanisms.

The Triage Officer

On a daily basis, a single individual should have the authority to implement hospital triage policy.

When all critical care units are filled to capacity, the hospital triage officer, with the cooperation of the ICU directors, should have access to all critical care units and have responsibility and authority to admit patients to and discharge patients from these units. The triage officer has the ultimate responsibility and discretion to implement hospital policy by arranging transfer of patients in and out of ICUs.

If there is an irreconcilable disagreement between the triage officer and other interested parties, the ICU committee should have a mechanism for reviewing appeals.

The triage officer should be a senior, experienced, and respected physician. The officer may delegate routine decisions to other physicians and nonphysicians as appropriate. The officer should make decisions in consultation with others who have appropriate expertise.

When a physician acts as both health care provider and triage officer, conflicts of interest are inevitable. Physicians serving in both roles must be aware of possible conflicts. Where adequate facilities exist to assign different personnel to each role, institutions should do so. When dual assignments are unavoidable, triage officers should balance both responsibilities impartially and should seek the advice of others. The triage officer's decisions may have to be monitored by the ICU committee.

Agreements between physicians and their patients regarding availability of ICU care are subject to the oversight and possible modification of the triage officer.

Hospital triage officers should have general knowledge of the various conditions treated in the hospital's ICUs, treatments commonly employed, and their associated range of outcomes. They should also be familiar with the various prognostic models and their uses and limitations.

Regardless of the patient's circumstances, the process of triage has the following common elements:

- patient assessment;
- urgency determination;
- priority of care based on urgency;
- resource analysis;
- documentation; and
- disposition.

Triage involves a common logic that includes probability estimates of outcomes; judgments of the benefit and burden to the patient and the system; and judgments of the value of the outcome to the patient and to the system.

Methods of Communication

The hospital should keep those who need to know informed about the status and availability of ICU beds. Physicians whose patients may require ICU services have a responsibility to know what is available and communicate their patients' needs to the appropriate individual.

Hospital triage officers should communicate effectively with those caregivers affected by triage decisions. The triage officer should engage in active and explicit negotiation and consultation with other caregivers when making decisions that may include postponing elective procedures for patients who normally require assignment of ICU beds.

Members of the Society of Critical Care Medicine Ethics Committee are as follows: Cochairman, Charles L. Sprung, MD, JD, FCCM, Hadassah-The Hebrew University of Jerusalem (Israel); cochairman, Marion Danis, MD, University of North Carolina at Chapel Hill; Associate Justice Christopher Armstrong, The Appeals Court, Commonwealth of Massachusetts, Boston; Mary Ann Baily, PhD, George Washington University, Washington, DC; Donald B. Chalfin, MD, Winthrop University Hospital, Mineola, NY; T. Forcht Dagi, MD, The Kennedy Institute of Georgetown University, Washington, DC; Fidel Davila, MD, Texas A & M University College of Medicine-Temple Campus; Michael DeVita, MD, University of Pittsburgh (Pa) School of Medicine; H. Tristram Engelhardt, Jr., PhD, MD, Baylor College of Medicine, Houston, Tex; Ake Grenvik, MD, University of Pittsburgh (Pa) School of Medicine; Paul B. Hofmann, MPH, Stanford (Calif) University Center for Biomedical Ethics; John W. Hoyt, MD, St. Francis Medical Center of Pittsburgh (Pa); Andrew Jameton, PhD, University of Nebraska Medical Center, Omaha; W. Andrew Kofke, MD, University of Pittsburgh (Pa); Joanne Lynn, MD, Dartmouth-Hitchcock Medical Center, Hanover, NH; Mary Faith Marshall, PhD, Medical University of South Carolina, Charleston; Rev. James J. McCartney, PhD, Villanova (Pa) University; Robert M. Nelson, MD, Medical College of Wisconsin, Milwaukee; Nicholas Ninos, MD, US Army Medical Corps (Ret). Palm Springs, Calif; Russell C. Raphaely, MD, Children's Hospital of Philadelphia (Pa); Frank Reardon, JD, Hassan and Reardon, Boston, Mass; Michael A. Rie, MD, University of Kentucky College of Medicine, Lexington; Stanley H. Rosenbaum, MD, Yale University School of Medicine, New Haven, Conn; Henry Silverman, MD, University of Maryland School of Medicine, Baltimore; Frank D. Sottile, MD, St. Vincent's Hospital, Worcester, Mass; Allen Spanier, MD, Jewish General Hospital of Montreal (Quebec); Avraham Steinberg, MD, The Hebrew University of Jerusalem (Israel); Rabbi Moses D. Tendler, PhD, Yeshiva University, New York, NY; Daniel Teres, MD, Baystate Medical Center, Springfield, Mass; Robert D. Truog, MD, Harvard Medical School, Boston, Mass; Thomas E. Wallace, MD, JD, University of Tennessee at Memphis; Ginger Wlody, RN, MS, University of California-Los Angeles School of Nursing; Timothy S. Yeh, MD, The Children's Hospital of Oakland (Calif).

References

Thurow LC. Learning to say no. *N Engl J Med.* 1981; 311:1569–1572.

Evans RW. Health care technology and the inevitability of resource allocation and rationing decisions. *JAMA.* 1983; 249:2047–2053, 2208–2219.

Aaron HJ, Schwartz WB. *The Painful Prescription: Rationing Hospital Care.* Washington, DC: The Brookings Institution; 1984.

Fuchs VR. The 'rationing' of medical care. *N Engl J Med.* 1984; 311:1572–1573.

Berenson RA. *Intensive Care Units (ICUs): Clinical Outcomes, Costs and Decisionmaking.* Washington, DC: Office of Technology Assessment; 1984. Health Technology Case Study 28, US Congress OTA-HCS-28.

Hiatt H. *America's Health in the Balance: Choice or Chance?* New York, NY: Harper & Row Publishers Inc; 1987.

Churchill LR. *Rationing Health Care in America: Perceptions and Principles of Justice.* Notre Dame, Ind: Notre Dame Press; 1987.

Schneider EL, Guralnik, JM. The aging of America: impact on health care costs. *JAMA.* 1990; 263: 2335–2340.

Strauss MJ, LoGerfo JP, Yeltatzie JA, Temkin N, Hudson LD. Rationing of intensive care unit services: an everyday occurrence. *JAMA.* 1986; 255:1143–1146.

Engelhardt HT, Rie MA. Intensive care units, scarce resources, and conflicting principles of justice. *JAMA.* 1986; 255:1159–1164.

Kalb PE, Miller DH. Utilization strategies for intensive care units. *JAMA.* 1989; 261:2389–2395.

Rund DA, Rausch TS. *Triage.* St. Louis, Mo: CV Mosby Co; 1981.

Winslow GR. *Triage and Justice.* Berkeley, University of California Press; 1982.

Reagan MD. Health care rationing: what does it mean? *N Engl J Med.* 1984; 311:1572–1573.

Baker R, Strosberg M. Triage and equality: an historical reassessment of utilitarian analyses of triage. *Kennedy Inst Ethics J.* 1992; 2:103–123.

Teres D. Civilian triage in the intensive care unit: the ritual of the last bed. *Crit Care Med.* 1993; 21: 598–606.

President's Commission for the Study of Ethical Problems in Medicine and Behavioral Research. *Deciding to Forego Life-Sustaining Treatment: A Report on the Thical, Medical and Legal Issues in Treatment Decisions.* Washington, DC: US Government Printing Office; 1983:3.

Danis M, Churchill LR. Autonomy and the common weal. *Hastings Cent Rep.* 1991; 21:25–31.

Task Force on Guidelines, Society of Critical Care Medicine. Recommendations for intensive care unit admission and discharge criteria. *Crit Care Med.* 1988; 16:807–808.

Critical care medicine. *JAMA.* 1983; 250:798–804. NIH Consensus Conference.

Lantos JD, Singer PA, Walker RM, et al. The illusion of futility in clinical practice. *Am J Med.* 1989; 87:81–84.

Schneiderman LJ, Jecker NS, Jonsen AR. Medical futility: its meaning and ethical implications. *Ann Intern Med.* 1990; 112:949–954.

Truog RD, Brett AS, Frader J. The problem with futility. *N Engl J Med.* 1992; 326:1560–1564.

Olick RS. Brain death, religious freedom, and public policy: New Jersey's landmark legislative initiative. *Kennedy Inst Ethics J.* 1991; 1:275–288.

3. Ethical Considerations in the Allocation of Organs and Other Scarce Medical Resources Among Patients

Council on Ethical and Judicial Affairs, American Medical Association

In the past, scarce resources (such as organs and intensive care unit [ICU] beds) (*Wall Street Journal.* May 23, 1992:1) have been allocated according to a wide range of criteria, some appropriate and some not.[2-6] Wide variation in allocation criteria and procedures still exists,[7,8] inhibiting ethical distribution of resources according to "fair, socially acceptable, and humane criteria."[1]

In this report, the Council on Ethical and Judicial Affairs considers the ethical issues relating to the equitable allocation of organs and other scarce resources among patients, including the criteria by which scarce medical resources should be distributed and a suggested procedure for applying these criteria. In addition, the Council considers the appropriate role of physicians in allocating scarce resources.

Some argue that, in addition to such existing scarce resources as organs and ICU beds, a broader range of medical resources may become scarce in the future[7,9,10] as society rethinks its health care goals in the face of rising costs and competing social demands.[10] The debate over rationing and the setting of societal priorities in health care is beyond the scope of this report. However, should there ever be societal agreement to limit or deny medically effective care to some patients on the basis of cost, the allocation criteria discussed in this report might then be applicable to those limited resources as well.

Acceptable Criteria for Resource Allocation Among Patients

Five factors relating to medical need may appropriately be taken into account when organs or other scarce medical resources, such as spaces in the ICU, are allocated. These include (1) the likelihood of benefit to the patient, (2) the impact of treatment in improving the quality of the patient's life, (3) the duration of benefit, (4) the urgency of the patient's condition (i.e., how close the patient is to death), and in some cases (5) the amount of resources required for successful treatment. Each of these criteria serves to maximize the following three primary goals of medical treatment: number of lives saved, number of years of life saved, and improvement in quality of life (i.e., the criteria maximize quantity of life, quality of life, or both).

Likelihood of Benefit

Giving priority to patients with a greater likelihood of benefiting from treatment is necessary for any efficient use of medical resources.[6-11] Likelihood of benefit helps decision makers maximize the number of lives saved as well as the length and quality of life.

The major concern with a likelihood of benefit criterion is the uncertainty involved in outcome predictions. Given current knowledge and information, predictions of outcomes are necessarily imprecise. Because of this uncertainty, only very substantial differences in likelihood of benefit among patients are relevant to allocation decisions. The larger those differences are, the more relevant a likelihood of benefit criterion becomes. For example, in allocating kidneys for transplant, it would be more justified to prefer a patient with an 80% chance of graft survival over a patient with a 10% chance than it would be to prefer a 60% chance to a 40% chance. Small differences in probabilities should not be used to fine-tune allocation decisions when dealing with patients with fairly comparable chances of benefiting from treatment.

In the application of a likelihood of benefit criterion, care that has a low likelihood of benefiting the patient must be distinguished from care that is truly futile (e.g., care that cannot be expected to have any physiologic benefit for the patient).[12] Patients who do have some chance of benefiting, in whatever degree, cannot be ruled out in advance as inappropriate candidates for treatment. In addition, allocation decisions that rely on nonmedical contributions to a patient's likelihood of benefit should be approached cautiously because of the risk of arbitrariness and overgeneralization. Communication or transportation problems, for instance, may be mere inconveniences rather than insurmountable obstacles. Reliance on these factors may systematically disadvantage the least well-off members of society, who, because of poverty or other reasons, may tend to experience these kinds of problems more often than others. Other criteria, such as strength of character or a supportive home environment, may contribute to likelihood of benefit[11,17] but are difficult to define or apply to individuals.

In general, if patient traits or behaviors that may adversely affect the patient's likelihood of benefit are taken into account, at least two conditions should be met. First, reasonable extra efforts on the part of physicians or others must fail to overcome the obstacles posed by the patient's traits or behaviors; and second, the traits or behaviors must directly and substantially detract from the patient's likelihood of responding to treatment. For instance, an intravenous drug user who is a candidate for liver transplantation should not be denied consideration until the possibility of rehabilitation for drug addiction has been fully explored.

Change in Quality of Life

Benefit to patients will be maximized if treatment is provided to those who will have the greatest improvement in quality of life. The biggest difficulty in applying this criterion is deciding on a standard definition of quality of life.[18]

Conceptually, defining the benefit gained from treatment and determining its importance in a patient's life depend greatly on patients' individual, subjective values.[18-22] Prioritizing candidates for treatment on the basis of their subjective preferences, however, would be impossible in practice. It would be extremely difficult to assess patients' individual preferences, and even more difficult to make useful comparisons among patients on that basis. Some allocation systems have proposed relying on patient or public surveys to determine average quality of life ratings for different outcomes.[23] However, because an individual's quality of life depends on subjective experience and values, an individual's preferences may depart significantly from the average and yet still not be unreasonable or unworthy of respect.

While no approach is perfect, perhaps the best approach is to define quality of life in terms of functional status.[24] Improvements in quality of life would be measured for each patient by comparing functional status with treatment and functional status without treatment. Making quality of life judgments in terms of changes in functional status facilitates comparisons between patients by allowing decision makers "to assess quality of life independent of the patient's feelings."[24] Although defining quality of life as functional status precludes consideration of the nuances of individual preferences, it does allow for objective comparisons between patients that may be relevant when differences between patients are very substantial. In the context of scarcity, some idiosyncratic high valuations of very poor functional status outcomes are simply too dubious to honor at the expense of other needy patients.

In considering quality of life (as defined by functional status), the first priority should be to prevent an extremely poor outcome, such as death or a life of permanent unconsciousness or extreme pain and suffering. When patients are admitted to a crowded ICU, for instance, a patient who can be saved by treatment from entering a permanent vegatative state (and given a reasonably good outcome) should be favored over another patient who, if denied treatment, would suffer only a mild disability. Preventing an extremely poor outcome, such as a permanent vegatative state, should be given priority over preventing milder disabilities.

If none of the patients competing for spaces in the ICU faces an extremely poor outcome, or if the extremely poor outcome cannot be avoided even with treatment, then patients should be prioritized to favor those who will receive the greatest improvement in functional status, measured by the difference between functional status with treatment and functional status without treatment. However, differences in the magnitude of change in functional status among patients are ethically relevant only when they are very substantial. Measurements of chance in functional status are inherently imprecise. In addition, because patients' attitudes toward a given change in functional status can differ, considering small differences in functional improvement would often fail to maximize overall benefit to patients and would be unfair to those whose preferences deviate from the norm. Consideration of only very substantial differences allows room, within reasonable limits, for expression of the range of patient valuations of a given change in functional status.

A major concern in making quality of life decisions is the possibility of discrimination against the disabled population.[23,25] The Council's approach to quality of life decisions allows resources to be directed according to where they will do the most good, without discriminating against those with preexisting disabilities. There may be occasions where disabled patients receive lower priority because their potential improvement in functional status is limited by preexisting disabilities. However, since only very substantial differences in the change in quality of life may be considered ethically relevant, a disabled patient will be given a lower priority only when doing so allows others to receive a much greater improvement in quality of life. In addition, the provision giving highest priority to those who need treatment to prevent an extremely poor outcome protects all patients, including the disabled, from receiving low priority when their need is greatest.

Duration of Benefit

The length of time a patient benefits from treatment can, in certain situations, be an appropriate consideration in maximizing overall benefit to patients.

The duration of benefit a patient receives from treatment will in many cases be limited by the patient's life expectancy. It is not always appropriate, however, to give organs or other scarce resources to the patient with the longest expected life span. There is often a lack of certainty in predicting life spans, especially at the individual level, as well as a risk of engaging in inappropriate age-based discrimination.[26] When a duration of benefit criterion is applied, patients should be assessed according to their own medical histories and prognoses, not aggregate statistics based on membership in a group.

In addition, giving priority to those who will benefit longer may not always maximize overall benefit to patients. The degree to which a longer duration of benefit actually benefits the patient depends on the patient's subjective experience and values. However, as with the quality of life criterion, some claims to treatment that will bring only a small benefit to the patient are simply too tenuous to sustain in the face of scarcity. Hence, duration of benefit can be a legitimate consideration when the differences among patients are very substantial. For example, the difference between an organ graft that lasts 8 years and one that lasts 10 years is not relevant, whereas the difference between 2 years and 10 years is relevant.

Urgency of Need

Prioritizing patients according to how long they can survive without treatment can help achieve the goal of maximizing the number of lives saved, depending on the kind of resource involved.[27] For instance, since spaces in an ICU are ordinarily scarce only intermittently, giving priority to urgent cases is generally justifiable because less urgent cases can still gain timely access to the ICU once the scarcity subsides.[11] With heart or liver transplants, however, the persistent scarcity of organs entails that some patients on the waiting list will die before an organ becomes available for them. With cases of persistent rather than temporary scarcity, then, urgency of need should be given less consideration because it would determine merely *who will survive, rather than maximizing the number of survivors*.[27] Furthermore, an urgency criterion can detract from length and quality of benefit. If patients with a less urgent need are set aside until their condition deteriorates to the point of dire emergency, treatment may not be as beneficial as it would have been had it been begun much earlier.

In sum, while urgency is an important criterion, it must be tempered with other considerations, including likelihood of benefit, the persistent or temporary scarcity of the resource involved, and the length of time other patients can survive without causing them irreparable harm. Preventing death (by treating urgent cases first) should generally be given priority in allocation decisions, but not if the life saved would be of extremely poor quality or extremely short duration. Also, an urgency criterion should not be used to deny resources to current patients in the expectation that others with more urgent need may soon present themselves.

Amount of Resources Required

Occasionally, assigning higher priority to patients who will need less of a scarce resource maximizes the number of lives saved. Each patient treated would require relatively little of it, making it more available for others.[28]

Conscious attempts to conserve resources in the allocation process will in general prove unnecessary. Patients who would be favored because they would require very little of a resource will often have a very high (or perhaps very low) likelihood of benefit as well, making likelihood of benefit the relevant criterion. When all else is equal, however, taking into account very substantial differences in the amount of resources required can be useful in ensuring efficient allocation. For instance, given two heart transplant candidates who are equal in all other respects, it is justified to give lower priority to the patient who would also require a liver transplant. By doing so, two lives can be saved rather than one.

This criterion should not be used to deny care to current patients in the expectation that others who will need fewer resources may soon present themselves. Rather, only when it is reasonably certain that conserving resources will have a good chance of saving more lives should this criterion be considered relevant.

Inappropriate Criteria for Resource Allocation Among Patients

The Council believes that the following criteria, although often used in allocating scarce resources, are ethically unacceptable: (1) ability to pay, (2) contribution of the patient to society, (3) perceived obstacles to treatment, (4) contribution of the patient to his or her own medical condition, and (5) past use of resources. Omission from this list does not necessarily mean that a criterion is justified; the Council considers only these five because of their prevalence in the literature and in allocation decisions today.

Ability to Pay

This is perhaps the most ubiquitous allocation criterion employed today, yet from an ethical standpoint there is little to recommend it.[29] In the medical realm, consideration of ability to pay is more often considered a regrettable necessity than a positive ethical principle of distribution. If a patient cannot pay the full fee for care, many physicians will waive the fee or accept lesser payment.[30] When ability to pay does play a role in allocating scarce resources, it is usually at the point of access to health care.

Consideration of a patient's ability to pay is problematic in many areas of health care, but especially when it comes to scarce, lifesaving resources. In other areas, market mechanisms may accurately reflect individuals' different valuations of various goods and services. At present, though, income disparity across society distorts the accuracy of the market model as a fair tool for distributing scarce medical resources, for the amount an individual can spend to gain access to a needed treatment will often fall short of his or her actual valuation of it.

Physicians and institutions should continue to accept patients with limited abilities to pay and should not systematically deny needed resources to patients simply because of their lower economic status.

Social Worth

A patient's contribution to society—or social worth—should not be a factor in allocation decisions. Such judgments are usually defended as attempts to maximize the return on society's investment in medical resources.[27,31] One common use is to justify the denial of care to the elderly, who some argue no longer make a positive contribution to the social good.[6,32] The problems of age-based rationing have been discussed by the Council at length elsewhere and cannot be repeated in full here. Although age-based rationing has it supporters,[33] the Council's view is that such an approach "fails to take into account the heterogeneity within older age groups" and the "increasing proportion of the elderly population . . . still in the work force and leading active, productive lives."[26]

A social worth criterion can also be used to justify discrimination against the young and virtually any other group not actively invovled in the economic productivity of society, on the grounds that those who have put the most into society are entitled to get the most back out of it.[34,35] Distinctions can be made among economic contributors as well; for instance, white collar workers with higher salaries may be favored over blue collar workers or the working poor. Social worth can also be measured by noneconomic criteria. Artists, writers, musicians, and other cultural elite may be favored over average citizens, and people with dependents may be preferred over those without families.[36]

Because of the pluralistic values of society, any single definition of social contribution or social worth is inherently suspect. Social worth judgments often reflect the preferences and values of individual decision makers rather than any objective criteria.[37] In addition, by assuming that members of a certain group make greater social contributions than others, a social worth criterion ignores diversity and the value of each individual.

Above all, a social worth criterion is a marked departure from the traditional patient-centered orientation of the medical profession. Social worth considerations would destroy public confidence in physicians' abilities to place patients' interests above broad social utility. Medicine should continue to concentrate on the best interests of patients and avoid evaluations of social worth.

Perceived Obstacles to Treatment

This criterion would give lower priority to patients whose circumstances pose special challenges to successful treatment, including patients with multiple diseases, alcohol and other drug abusers, the indigent, the uneducated, patients with transportation problems or language barriers, and patients with antisocial or aggressive personalities. Perceived obstacles to treatment may cause an unconscious prejudice in the minds of decision makers, who may think their considerations relate only to more objective medical criteria, such as likelihood of benefit.

The danger is that some patients will be given lower priority who, with a little extra effort and support, could benefit greatly from treatment. Thus, rather than downrate alcohol and other drug abusers as candidates for treatment, decision makers should consider whether rehabilitation could be successful in improving the patient's chances of benefit. Similarly, arrangements can be made to help patients with transportation problems or to provide interpreters for patients with language barriers.

Potential recipients of scarce medical resources should not be downrated prima facie because of surmountable difficulties attendant to their cases. Rather, whenever possible, physicians should encourage their patients to use additional resources, such as social workers, private charities, rehabilitation clincis, and other support networks, to facilitate their care.

Patient Contribution to Disease

This criterion assigns lower priority to patients whose past behaviors contributed significantly to their present need for scarce resources. Examples include heart transplant candidates whose high-fat diets may have contributed to their condition, or liver transplant candidates whose alcoholism led to cirrhosis of the liver.[38] The reasoning is that patients who failed to take action to prevent their illness are partially to blame for their conditions[38] and thus have forfeited the right to be given the same priority for treatment as others.

This argument is flawed in two ways. First, it is not always clear which factors actually contribute to a disease, or which are more or less to blame than other contributing factors.[38] Second, of all the possible contributors to disease, only certain behaviors are singled out as justifications for denying treatment. Few would suggest giving lower priority to wealthy heart transplant candidates whose high-stress occupations contributed to their heart disease, or denying intensive care to sky divers or football players injured in the course of their sports. Rather, only certain socially unacceptable or morally suspect behaviors, like immoderate eating or drinking, are considered appropriate criteria for denying treatment. However, the use of judgments about patients' morals to allocate health care seems grossly inappropriate and inconsistent; physicians do not refuse to treat patients who engage in other immoral behaviors, such as adultry or tax evasion.[39]

Another problem with this criterion is its assumption that patients' past contributions to their own illnesses were voluntary actions.[39] For instance, giving alcoholics lower priority for liver transplants seems to ignore some reasons for drinking that are beyond an individual's control, such as family history of alcohol abuse or possible genetic predilections for alcoholism.[40] Some argue that it is the failure to seek treatment, rather than having the problem itself, that is morally blameworthy.[38] However, it seems unjust to punish further those who already have suffered greatly from chemical dependency, especially when many may have simply been unaware of treatment options or unable to seek out treatment. It would be fruitless and potentially devastating to allocate Medicaid resources on the basis of the perceived moral culpability of patients.

Past Use of Resources

It may be argued that patients who have had considerable access to a scarce medical resource in the past should be given lower priority than equally needy patients who have received little or none of that resource. A consequence of this view would be that some currently using a resource may be displaced by others who have not yet had access. A patient could be displaced from an ICU by another patient with the same prognosis but less past access, or a retransplant patient could be denied any chance at all of receiving additional organs.

A criterion involving past use of resources is inappropriate because it rests on a fundamentally flawed conception of equality among potential recipients of treatment. Equality does not impose an ethical requirement that equally suitable patients receive the same amount of care; indeed, scarcity makes such an obligation impossible to fulfill. The only requirement is that patients be judged equally according to their current needs, on the basis of their diagnoses and prognoses. Unlike the five ethically acceptable criteria discussed in this report—likelihood of benefit, duration of benefit, change in quality of life, urgency, and amount of resources required—past use of resources does not contribute to maximizing the number, quality, or length of lives saved. It does not contribute to maximizing overall benefit to patients.[41] In addition, the seemingly commonsense view that everyone deserves a turn at receiving scarce medical resources ignores inequalities in access to other goods that affect health, such as income, education, and access to primary care.[41] Any serious attempt to base allocation decisions on past access to medical resources would have to evaluate candidates' past access to these other goods as well,[41] a task for which medicine is ill equipped.

There may be cases in which a patient's past use of resources contributes to the patient's current likelihood of benefit, duration of benefit, or expected improvement in quality of life. For instance, a retransplant candidate will often be a poorer candidate for transplantation because of the failure of a previous graft.[41,42] If so, then the relevant allocation criteria justifying lower priority for that patient would be likelihood of benefit or perhaps duration of benefit, but not the mere fact of past access to an organ. Because past use is irrelevant to present need, it should not factor into allocation decisions.

Applying Allocation Criteria

All patients who desire treatment must be assessed according to all five of the ethically appropriate criteria defined earlier: likelihood of benefit, urgency, change in quality of life, duration of benefit, and (when applicable) the amount of resources each candidate requires. All of these criteria are appropriate in certain circumstances, but only when disparities between patients are very substantial.

Once all the potential recipients have been studied, decision makers should allocate resources to maximize the number, length, and quality of lives saved. Because each of the five ethical criteria contribute to this goal in different ways, none is inherently more important than the others. However, because of the intrinsic worth of all persons, maximizing the number of lives saved should generally take priority over other goals, as long as the patients saved would not suffer an extremely poor quality of life or extremely short duration of benefit. For instance, it is better to save two patients who could each live 5 years than to save one patient who could live 10 years. In addition, preventing extremely poor outcomes should take precedence over other efforts to enhance quality of life or duration of benefit. A patient who can go from 0% (i.e., death) to 50% of full functioning, for example, should be preferred over a patient who can go from 25% to 75% of full functioning.

In some cases, the five ethical criteria will not clearly identify which patients should receive highest priority for treatment. While there may be some patients who clearly should be preferred over others, there might still be a number of patients for whom there were no very substantial differences according to these criteria. When these five ethical criteria do not clearly identify the most appropriate patients for treatment, some other method must be employed that provides each appropriate candidate with an equal opportunity to receive the needed resources.

Equal opportunity would not be provided if one criterion were arbitrarily given precedence over the others or if small differences between patients were given more weight than is appropriate. Rather, equal opportunity should be provided through the use of a first-come-first-served approach. The first-come-first-served method should not be used to abdicate responsibility for making decisions when appropriate criteria can give a sound basis for preferring some patients over others. If employed only when uncertainty is too great or the differences among candidates too close to call, the first-come-first-served approach respects the equality of individuals who have equally strong claims to a scarce resource and provides each with an equal opportunity to receive scarce resources.[43]

To ensure that a first-come-first-served approach is truly equitable, all potential candidates must be able to present themselves for treatment in a timely fashion. For instance, if patients with insurance are likely to be diagnosed as having endstage organ failure earlier that similar patients without insurance, then a first-come-first-served approach would inappropriately favor insured patients over uninsured. Appropriate safeguards are needed to ensure that differences in patient access to diagnostic services are taken into account.

There are a number of ways this general approach could be implemented. The five ethical criteria could be used to identify three groups of patients: those who are clearly good candidates for treatment, those who are clearly poor candidates, and those who do not fall into either group.[27] Within each group, patients could then be prioritized according to the first-come-first-served method or some other equal-opportunity mechanism. Alternatively, the five criteria could be used to define a minimum threshold for receiving treatment, and all potential recipients who exceed this threshold would be prioritized according to the first-come-first-served approach. Defining the boundaries of these different groups, however, is problematic. When there is a large pool of patients competing for organs, for instance, patients who fall just below the minimum threshold level or just miss entry into the group of clearly good candidates will probably not be substantially different from some patients who do make it into those groups.

To avoid drawing lines that may be arbitrary, an alternative approach would be to rank all potential organ recipients according to a weighted formula.[27] Each patient would receive a chance at treatment commensurate with his or her prognosis and need, according to the five ethical criteria discussed earlier, but no candidates would be excluded entirely. Thus, the patients who are the most deserving of treatment according to the ethical criteria would have the best chance of receiving treatment. This approach would not always generate the most efficient allocation decisions; there would inevitably be cases in which a poor candidate would beat the odds and receive the scarce resource before other patients. However, because each patient would have some chance of treatment, this approach would have the advantage of nonabandonment. All of these strategies for implementing the five ethical criteria would be ethically acceptable; no single approach is ethically mandated.

Appropriate Decision Makers

Physicians have an irreplaceable role in making diagnoses, determining prognoses, calculating probabilities, exploring patients' goals and values, and advocating on behalf of their patients. However, physicians of patients competing for resources are generally not in the best position to make impartial allocation decisions. Out of loyalty, physicians might feel pressured to choose their own patients over others, and any choice involving two or more of a physician's own patients would constitute a serious conflict of interest. The physician's role as patient advocate would be jeopardized, and trust between physicians and patients would be undercut.[44] Although individual physicians may have to decide which patients receive needed immediate care in some emergency triage situations, in general physicians should not be forced to make the decision to deny potentially beneficial care to their own patients.

Allocation mechanisms should be objective, flexible, and consistent. Objectivity refers to the need for decision makers not to be personally involved with patients competing for a scarce resource. Flexibility requires decision makers to weigh carefully all the relevant facts of a case, and not reflexively to apply a blanket rule, such as an age cap, to all cases. Consistency requires decision makers to consider the same (appropriate) criteria, interpreted in the same way, to ensure that all decisions are fair to the patients involved.

Centralized allocation mechanisms, such as the organ allocation formulas employed by the United Network for Organ Sharing (UNOS),[45] would probably generate the most consistent decisions. Centralized formulas, however, generally lack flexibility. The particulars of individual cases may sometimes "slip through the cracks" in the formula. In addition, formulas may gloss over uncertainty in the assignment of discrete numbers that appear objective but still only reflect our best guess as to which factors are more significant, and to what degree. These seemingly objective point values may also serve to disguise ethical decisions about the relative importance of various factors in allocation decisions. For instance, assigning points for medical urgency in organ allocation involves ethical judgments about the importance of saving those who are closest to death vs those with the best chances of long-term survival. Because of uncertainty and the need to make ethical decisions transparent, all allocation formulas should be periodically reassessed to enure that they reflect the most current scientific and ethical consensus on allocation issues.

A more decentralized decision making process would not overcome the inevitable uncertainties involved in allocation decisions and would probably be more difficult to apply consistently across institutional lines. However, a decentralized approach might be more flexible and would not necessarily result in unjust or arbitrary decisions. A more expansive understanding of the ethical issues involved in resource allocation decisions can go far in encouraging reasoned, fair, and consistent choices based on careful evaluation of appropriate criteria.

The Council at this time does not advocate either centralized or decentralized approaches; further discussion of these issues will be necessary in the future.

Patient Information in Allocation Decisions

Physicians should explain the allocation criteria and procedure to their patients or designated proxies so that they understand their chances of receiving treatment and the method by which the decision is made. This is in addition to all the customary information regarding the risks, benefits, and alternatives to any medical procedure. Furthermore, patients denied access to resources should be informed by their physicians of the rationale behind such decisions.

Future Directions

The current lack of consensus on allocation decisions reflects in part deep disagreement over appropriate allocation criteria and in part a general unwillingness to face the problem of scarcity directly. More informed, public discussion of scarcity and allocation decisions will help ensure that access to scarce resources is provided equitably. The reality of scarce resources must be confronted not only by those who must make allocation decisions, but by all of society, which must live with the consequences of those decisions. Justice in this area will never be achieved until limitations imposed by scarcity are accepted by all, without attempts to circumvent the allocation process. Physicians, hospitals, and other institutions that control scarce medical resources should encourage public discussion of allocation issues. Allocation procedures should also be subject to peer review and public auditing on a regular basis. Not only will such discussion direct public attention to the problem of scarce medical resources, but it may also encourage a broader consensus on how scarce resources should be distributed.

Guidelines

1. Decisions regarding the allocation of scarce medical resources among patients should consider only ethically appropriate criteria relating to medical need. (a) These criteria include likelihood of benefit, urgency

of need, change in quality of life, duration of benefit, and, in some cases, the amount of resources required for successful treatment. In general, only very substantial differences among patients are ethically relevant; the greater the disparities, the more justified the use of these criteria becomes. In quality of life judgments, patients should first be prioritized so that extremely poor outcomes are avoided; patients should then be prioritized according to change in quality of life, but only when there are very substantial differences among patients. (b) Research should be pursued to increase knowledge of outcomes and thereby improve the accuracy of these criteria. (c) Nonmedical criteria, such as ability to pay, social worth, perceived obstacles to treatment, patient contribution to illness, and past use of resources, should not be considered.

2. Allocation decisions should respect the individuality of patients and the particulars of individual cases as much as possible. (a) All candidates for treatment must be fully considered according to ethically appropriate criteria relating to medical need, as defined in guideline 1. (b) When very substantial differences do not exist among potential recipients of treatment on the basis of these criteria, a first-come-first-served approach or some other equal-opportunity mechanism should be employed to make final allocation decisions. (c) Although there are several ethically acceptable strategies for implementing these criteria, no single strategy is ethically mandated. Acceptable approaches include a three-tiered system, a minimal threshold approach, and a weighted formula.

3. Decision-making mechanisms should be objective, flexible, and consistent to ensure that all patients are treated equally. The nature of the physician-patient relationship entails that physicians of patients competing for a scarce resource must remain advocates for their patients and therefore should not make the actual allocation decisions.

4. Patients must be informed by their physicians of allocation criteria and procedures, as well as their chances of receiving access to scarce resources. This information should be in addition to all the customary information regarding the risks, benefits, and alternatives to any medical procedure. Patients denied access to resources have the right to be informed of the reasoning behind the decision.

5. The allocation procedures of institutions controlling scarce resources should be disclosed to the public as well as subjected to regular peer review from the medical profession.

6. Physicians should continue to look for innovative ways to increase the availability of and access to scarce medical resources so that, as much as possible, beneficial treatments can be provided to all who need them.

Ethical Issues in the Allocation of Intensive Care

In this section, the Council explores ethical dilemmas involved in the allocation of intensive care.

Admission to and Dismissal From the ICU in Periods of Scarcity

Physicians generally respond to a scarcity of ICU beds by restricting admission to patients with more severe illnesses or dismissing earlier those patients whose conditions are stable enough to warrant a move out of the ICU,[46-48] such as patients who require monitoring only. Neither stricter admission criteria nor more liberal dismissal practices have resulted in any measurable increase in mortality among patients admitted to the ICU[46-48] or among those denied admission.[46,48]

Severity of Illness and Likelihood of Benefit

Restrictive admission and earlier dismissal reflect considerations of both medical urgency and patients' likelihood of benefiting from treatment. However, in many cases the use of these two criteria alone may not result in the most effective use of resources; triage physicians should give each potential recipient of intensive care full consideration according to all ethically relevant criteria discussed earlier. Whereas patients who are closer to death should be given higher priority when other patients are "too well" to benefit from the ICU to a comparable degree,[11] distinctions based on medical urgency cannot be made among patients when all are likely to have extremely poor outcomes if denied immediate intensive care. Distinctions may be made among equally urgent cases on the basis of likelihood of benefit, improvement in quality of life, duration of benefit, or the amount of resources each patient requires for successful treatment, but only when very substantial differences among patients exist.

Responsiveness to Treatment

In many cases, a patient's prognosis will become more evident once treatment is initiated and the physician can evaluate the patient's response to therapy. In times of scarcity, however, it may be impossible to test the responsiveness of each patient to treatment. In such cases, the triage physician must make a choice as to which patients should be admitted while realizing that the crucial information necessary to make the very best choices—the responsiveness of the patients to treatment—is not yet available. In such circumstances, if the prognostic uncertainties are so great that ethically relevant distinctions cannot be made among patients, then patients should be admitted in the order in which they presented. When patients in need of intensive care exceed the spaces available, patients who do not respond to treatment, or who respond only poorly, should not remain in the ICU. Allocation of intensive care must be an ongoing process; patients' responsiveness to treatment should be regularly reevaluated so that the most appropriate candidates can be ensured access according to the five criteria discussed in this report.

Conclusions—Allocation of Intensive Care

The council encourages triage physicians to consider the following in allocating intensive care.

1. During times of scarcity, triage physicians should give each potential recipient of intensive care full consideration according to all ethically relevant criteria, including urgency of need, likelihood of benefit, change in quality of life, duration of benefit, and in some cases the amount of resources required for successful treatment. All of these criteria can be relevant in different cases, but only when the differences among patients are very substantial. When quality of life judgments must be made, patients should first be prioritized so that extremely poor outcomes are avoided; patients should then be prioritized according to change in quality of life, but only when there are very substantial differences among patients.

2. When no relevant ethical distinctions can be made among patients, priority should be given according to the order in which patients present to the ICU.

3. In many cases, testing a patient's responsiveness to treatment can be useful in allocating intensive care, for it enables the physician to confirm or refine a patient's prognosis.

4. Allocation of intensive care during times of scarcity must be an ongoing process; patients' responsiveness to treatment should be regularly reevaluated so that the most appropriate patients can be ensured access.

Members of the Council on Ethical and Judicial Affairs at the time of this report included the following: Oscar W. Clarke, MD, Gallipolis, Ohio, Chair: John Glasson, MD, Durhan, NC, Vice Chair: Charles H. Epps, Jr. MD, Washington, DC; Charles W. Plows, MD, Anaheim, Calif; Victoria Ruff, MD, Columbus Ohio; Allison August, Chicago, Ill; Craig M. Kliger, MD, Huntington Beach, Calif; George T. Wilkins, Jr, MD, Edwardsville, Ill; James H. Cosgriff, Jr, MD, Buffalo, NY; David Orentlicher, MD, Jd, Chicago, Secretary and Staff Author: Karey Harwood, Chicago, Staff Associate; Jeff Leslie, Chicago, Staff Associate and Staff Author.

References

1. Opinion 2.03: allocation of health resources. In: *Current Opinions of the Council on Ethical and Judicial Affairs.* Chicago, Ill: American Medical Association; 1992.
2. Kilner JF. Limited resources. In: *Who Lives? Who Dies? Ethical Criteria in Patient*

Selection. New Haven, Conn: Yeale University Press; 1990: chap 1.

3. Dossetor JB. Principles used in organ allocation. In: Land W, Dossetor JB, eds. *Organ Replacement Therapy: Ethics, Justice, and Commerce.* Berlin, Germany: Springer-Verlag; 1991:393–398.
4. Evans RW. Health care technology and the inevitability of resource allocation and rationing decisions: part 2. *JAMA.* 1983; 249:2208–2219.
5. Perkins HS, Jonsen AR, Epstein WV. Providers as predictors: using outcome predictions in intensive care. *Crit Care Med.* 1986; 14:105–110.
6. Kalb PE, Miller DH. Utilization strategies for intensive care units. *JAMA.* 1989; 261:2389–2395.
7. United Network for Organ Sharing. *Bylaws and Policies.* March 4, 1993. Policy 3.3.5.
8. US General Accounting Office. *Organ Transplants: Increased Effort Needed to Boost Supply and Ensure Equitable Distribution of Organs.* Washington, DC: US General Accounting Office; April 1993. Publication GAO/HRD-93-56.
9. McGregor M. Technology and the allocation of resources. *N Engl J Med.* 1989; 320:118–120.
10. Callahan D. Rationing medical progress: the way to affordable health care. *N Engl J Med.* 1990; 322:1810–1813.
11. Truog RD. Triage in the ICU. *Hastings Cent Rep.* May/June 1992; 22:13–17.
12. Council on Ethical and Judicial Affairs. Guidelines for the appropriate use of do-not-resuscitate orders. *JAMA.* 1991; 265:1868–1871.
13. Kilner JF. Psychological ability. In: *Who Lives? Who Dies? Ethical Criteria in Patient Selection.* New Haven, Conn: Yale University Press; 1990: chap 8.
14. Thompson ME. Selection of candidates for cardiac transplantation. *Heart Transplant.* 1983; 3:65–69.
15. Leenen HJ. Selection of patients. *J Med Ethics.* 1982; 8:33–36.
16. Jonsen AR. Selection of recipients for cardiac transplantation. In: Evans R, ed. *National Heart Transplantation Study.* Washington, DC: Health Care Financing Administration, US Dept of Health and Human Services: 1984; 4:36-1–36-8.
17. McKevitt PM, et al. The elderly on dialysis: physical and psychosocial functioning. *Dialysis Transplant.* 1986; 15:130–137.
18. Edlund M, Tancredi LR. Quality of life: an ideological critique. *Perspect Biol Med.* 1985; 28:591–607.
19. Kilner JF. Quality of benefit. In: *Who Lives? Who Dies? Ethical Criteria in Patient Selection.* New Haven, Conn: Yale University Press; 1990: chap 14.
20. Lo B. Quality of life judgments in the care of the elderly. In: Monagle D, Thomasma JF, eds. *Medical Ethics: A Guide for Health Professionals.* Rockville, Md: Aspen Publishers; 1988:140–147.
21. Smith A. Qualms and OALYs. *Lancet.* 1987; 1:1134–1136.
22. Ferrans CE. Quality of life as a criterion for allocation of life-sustaining treatment: the case of hemodialysis. In: Anderson G, Glesnes-Anderson V, eds. *Health Care Ethics: A Guide for Decision Makers.* Rockville, Md: Aspen Publishers; 1987:109–124.
23. Menzel PT. Oregon's denial: disabilities and quality of life. *Hastings Cent Rep.* November/December 1992; 22:21–25.

24. Dracup K, Raffin T. Withholding and withdrawing mechanical ventilation: assessing quality of life. *Am Rev Respir Dis.* 1989; 140:S44–S46.
25. Orentlicher D. Rationing and the Americans With Disabilities Act. *JAMA.* 1994; 271:308–314.
26. Council on Ethical and Judicial Affairs. Ethical implications of age-based rationing of health care. In: *Code of Medical Ethics: Reports.* Chicago, Ill: American Medical Association; 1992; 1:53–56.
27. Brock, DW. Ethical issues in recipient selection for organ transplantation. In: Mathieu D, ed. *Organ Substitution Technology: Ethical, Legal, and Public Policy Issues.* Boulder, Colo: Westview Press; 1988:86–99.
28. King TC. Ethical dilemmas of restricted resources. In: Herter F, Forde K, Mark L, De Bellis R, Kutscher A, Selder F, eds. *Human and Ethical Issues in the Surgical Care of Patients With Life-Threatening Disease.* Springfield, Ill: Charles C Thomas Publisher, 1986:169–175.
29. Callahan D. Symbols, rationality, and justice: rationing health care. *Am J Law Med.* 1992; 18:1–13.
30. Council on Ethical and Judicial Affairs. Caring for the poor. *JAMA.* 1993; 269:2533–2537.
31. McIntyre KM, Benfari RC, Battin MP. Two cardiac arrests, one medical team. *Hastings Cent Rep.* 1982; 12:24–25.
32. Kilner JF. Age. In: *Who Lives? Who Dies? Ethical Criteria in Patient Selection.* New Haven, Conn: Yale University Press; 1990:chap 7.
33. Callahan D. *Setting Limits: Medical Goals in an Aging Society.* New York, NY: Simon & Schuster, 1987.
34. Brody B. *Ethics and Its Applications.* New York, NY: Harcourt Brace Jovanovich; 1983.
35. Kilner JF. Social value. In: *Who Lives? Who Dies? Ethical Criteria in Patient Selection.* New Haven, Conn: Yale University Press; 1990:chap 3.
36. Winstow GR. *Triage and Justice.* Berkeley, Calif: University of California Press; 1982.
37. Evans RW, Blagg CR, Bryan FA Jr. Implications for health care policy: a social and demographic profile of hemodialysis patients in the United States. *JAMA.* 1981; 245:487–491.
38. Moss AH, Siegler M. Should alcoholics compete equality for liver transplantation? *JAMA.* 1991; 265:1295–1298.
39. Cohen C, Benjamin M. Ethics and Social Impact Committee of the Transplant and Health Policy Center. Alcoholics and liver transplantation. *JAMA.* 1991; 265:1299–1301.
40. Starzl TE, Van Thiel D, Tzakis AG, et al. Orthotopic liver transplantation for alcoholic cirrhosis. *JAMA.* 1988; 260:2542–2544.
41. Ubel PA, Arnold RM, Caplan AL. Rationing failure: the ethical lessons of the retransplantation of scarce vital organs. *JAMA.* 1993; 270:2469–2474.
42. Evans RW, Manninen DL, Dong FB, McLynne DA. Is retransplantation cost effective? *Transplant Proc.* 1993; 25:1694–1696.
43. Beauchamp TL, Childress JF. *Principles of Biomedical Ethics.* 3rd ed. New York, NY: Oxford University Press; 1989:290–302.
44. Levinsky NG. The doctor's master. *N Engl J Med.* 1984; 311:1573–1575.

45. United Network for Organ Sharing. *Bylaws and Policies.* March 4, 1993. Policy 3.0–3.11.3.
46. Singer DE, Carr PL, Mulley AG, Thibault GE. Rationing Intensive care: physician responses to a resource shortage. *N Engl J Med.* 1983; 309:1155–1160.
47. Strauss MJ, LoGerfo JP, Yeltatzie JA, Temkin N, Hudson LD. Rationing of intensive care unit services. *JAMA.* 1986; 255:1143–1146.
48. Selker HP, Griffith JL, Dorey FJ, D'Agnostino RB. How do physicians adapt when the coronary care unit is full? *JAMA.* 1987; 257:1181–1185.

4. A Multi-institution Collaborative Policy on Medical Futility

An infant born with multiple congenital abnormalities that rendered survival unprecedented required high-dose vasopressors to maintain blood pressure. After several days, gangrene developed in the extremities, and the parents sequentially demanded amputations of several limbs in an attempt to "do everything." The surrogate decision maker for a comatose woman dying of multisystem organ failure in an intensive care unit (ICU) was her estranged husband; they separated because of repeated spousal abuse. Despite many conferences with the husband recommending comfort measures and a do-not-resuscitate order, the husband demanded that the medical staff "do everything to my wife." A public hospital serving an indigent community of several hundred thousand had a full ICU, and 3 patients were being kept in the emergency department on ventilators. One of the patients in the ICU was a gentleman who had been ventilator dependent and unresponsive for 4 1/2 months after a cardiac arrest; his daughter insisted on full support because she was hoping for a miracle.

Common to all 3 cases was a health care team that believed that continued aggressive support was inappropriate or futile and a surrogate decision maker who insisted on "everything" being done for the patient. These cases clearly differ from the traditional right-to-die cases in which treatment is refused by the patient or surrogate decision maker and are not easily handled by existing hospital policies. As opposed to cases such as *Quinlan* and *Cruzan*, which had surrogate decision makers trying to limit physician-driven overtreatment, these 3 cases involve physicians trying to limit surrogate-driven overtreatment. These cases, drawn from the experiences of ethics committees at 3 Houston, Tex, hospitals and others from around the country, have caused medical futility to become 1 of the dominant topics in medical ethics in recent years.

By the early 1990s, most of the major hospitals in Houston had experienced difficult cases such as the 3 described above, but none had formally adopted a policy on medical futility or had created a mechanism to override what were perceived to be inappropriate patient or surrogate requests. Discussions at the monthly meetings of the Houston Bioethics Network, a consortium of representatives of ethics committees in the greater Houston area, revealed that many institutions were interested in pursuing such policies. However, the legal and ethical uncertainties and the confusing array of proposed futility definitions discouraged institutions from proceeding alone. In August 1993, we convened an ad hoc group with representatives from most of the major Houston hospitals. This article reports on the creation of a multi-institution futility policy in the greater Houston area that is based on a new approach to dealing with these problematic cases.

Old Approaches and Common Problems

Many different bodies of organized medicine,[1-4] ethicists,[5-6] and legal commentators[7-8] have offered various definitions of futility that range from lack of intended physiologic effect to low likelihood of survival to discharge, to low likelihood of surviving for more than a few months, to poor quality of life or permanent dependence on intensive care. In addition, various permutations of these definitions serve as the basis for many individual hospital policies.[9-11] However, careful review of either the supporting futility definitions or the details of the policies reveals 3 common problems: (1) the futility definitions are flawed, (2) the processes of determining futility are flawed because they are insufficiently open and raise concerns of fairness, and (3) there is no ethical framework to ground the physician-institution opposition to the requested intervention.

Flawed Definitions

We have previously categorized 4 conceptual types of futility definitions found in the literature: physiologic futility (the intervention does not have its intended physiologic effect), imminent demise futility (the patient will die before discharge regardless of the intervention), lethal condition futility (the patient has an underlying disease that is not compatible with long-term survival, regardless of the intervention, even if the patient could survive to discharge from this hospitalization), and qualitative futility (the resultant quality of life is too poor).[12] We also offered a set of criteria to determine if an effective operational futility policy could be derived from and supported by a particular definition. The 4 criteria are (1) the futility determination must be made prospectively,

(2) the determination must be precise enough to apply to individual cases, (3) the determination must be socially acceptable, and (4) the determination must be applicable in a sufficient number of cases to warrant the attention and efforts required to create such policies. We concluded, with supporting evidence on the incidence of futility reported elsewhere,[13,14] that none of the definitions satisfied all of the criteria and that any futility policy based on any substantive definition was unworkable.

That is not to argue that the concept is unworkable. The basic problem is that the clinical reality of the uniqueness of patients and diseases results in judgments of futility that are not easily formulated into a general substantive definition. We concluded that we need to treat futility as the courts treat pornography, acknowledging that while it cannot be defined, we certainly know it when we see it. This approach to value-laden, context-dependent judgment has recently been eloquently defended.[15] In this conclusion, we concur with the recent American Medical Association Council on Ethical and Judicial Affairs opinion that futility "cannot be meaningfully defined" but that "denial of treatment should be justified by openly stated ethical principles and acceptable standards of care."[16]

Flawed Process

The second major problem with many of the proposed futility policies is that both the process of creating the initial policy and the process of determining futility in an individual case are flawed because of limited viewpoints in policy creation or limited patient involvement in policy implementation.

With few exceptions, notably the Denver, Colo-based GUIDe program,[17] most of the futility definitions or processes that have been proposed reflect a fairly narrow spectrum of opinions, usually coming from an individual hospital. A community-wide effort involving many different types of institutions representing a full spectrum of societal health care choices, by its very nature, would have an enormous advantage over efforts by a single institution in that it would allow consideration of and reflection on a diverse and more representative set of values in the policy creation stage.

More important, limited viewpoints often result in implementation of processes of determining futility that are insufficiently open or raise questions of fairness. Some policies allow for individual physician determination of futility without adequate instructional review. Others do not allow patient participation or input in the decision-making process. Still others make no provision for the right of patient transfer. Finally, many policies do not address the continuing need for a comprehensive care plan despite nonprovision of the futile intervention and thus potentially result in patient abandonment.

Ethical Framework

The third major problem with most published futility policies is that they are not grounded in ethical concerns that are adequate to justify overruling patient autonomy. A defensible ethical basis for a futility policy is essential to respond to the many critics of the entire concept of futility who argue that futility is indefensible because of imposed values.[18] We agree that no futility policy is, or can be, value free. We also agree with Tomlinson and Brody that it should not be.[19] However, it is also a value judgment, itself unfounded, that patient autonomy is always inviolate and must always be valued over other legitimate competing values. Our policy proposes a fair process that balances the competing values of respect for patient autonomy with respect for professional and institutional integrity. Our concept of integrity is discussed more fully below.

The Houston Policy

Emerging from the above criticisms of the various proposed futility policies were 3 points that guided the Houston task force. The first is that rather than relying on a substantive definition of futility, the policy should rely on a procedural approach that recognizes the importance of thorough institutional review of each case. The second is that the policy should be based on open and fair processes involving patients, physicians, and institutions. The third is that the policy should be clearly grounded on professional integrity and institutional integrity as a balance to patient autonomy.

These 3 points emerged at the initial meetings of the task force. It then formed a drafting subcommittee that created a first draft that was circulated to participating institutions for comment in January 1994. After comments were collected from all of the participating institutions, the task force met to synthesize the various comments into a second working draft. This process was repeated several times until a final working draft, "Guidelines on Institutional Policies on the Determination of Medically Inappropriate Interventions," was presented for institutional approval in early 1995.

The first major advantage of the Houston policy is that it is a procedural policy. By creating a process that gives voices to all the parties involved in the dispute, rather than by attempting to define futility, the task force was able to create a document that satisfied the above-mentioned American Medical Association Council on Ethical and

Judicial Affairs guidelines.[16] More important, by emphasizing process, it also called for a review of each case that allows for consideration of the subtleties and nuances that are the hallmarks of caring for actual patients.

The second advantage of the Houston approach is that it grew out of a diverse group of institutions. Participating institutions included teaching and nonteaching hospitals, not-for-profit hospitals, and for-profit hospitals, public hospitals and private hospitals, and religious order hospitals and secular hospitals. In all, institutions accounting for a majority of the greater Houston hospital bed capacity participated. Participating institutions were represented by a diverse group of individuals including physicians, nurses, social workers, attorneys, chaplains, administrators, and ethicists.

While no document or process can satisfy every need or desire of every individual, by including many voices, the Houston task force was able to create a fair and open process that minimizes 4 problems encountered by some policies: nonparticipation by the patient or surrogate, unilateral physician action, ignoring patient transfer options, and the potential for patient abandonment. While minimizing these problems by fair process requires additional time and effort, the task force concluded that fairness outweighted rapidity.

1. The Houston policy requires that patients or their surrogates are included from the beginning. Steps 1 through 3 of the process require the responsible physician to involve them in the decision-making process and to explain to them the various options. In addition, steps 5 and 6 encourage the patient or surrogate to be present at the institutional review mechanism to express their views and also provide them with adequate preparation time.

2. The Houston policy insists that physicians may not act unilaterally. Any conflict between the responsible physician and the patient that cannot be resolved by informal discussions including the use of institutional resources such as social workers or chaplains must, according to step 4, be referred to an interdisciplinary review mechanism within the isntitution. In addition, the responsible physician is charged with the duties of obtaining a second opinion and providing the review body with pertinent clinical and scientific information. No final determination of medical inappropriateness can be made without concurrence of the institutional review body.

3. The Houston policy also clearly preserves the patient's right to be transferred. The second step of the process requires the responsible physician to discuss the option of patient transfer to another physician within the institution or to another institution. Even after an institutional determination of futility has been reached, step 8 bans only intrainstitu-

tional transfers to another physician to obtain the futile intervention. We recognize that the possibility of transfer may be limited by reimbursement limitations or by the unwillingness of other providers to accept difficult, very sick patients. Still, the option deserves to be explored and may be possible in some cases. However, we firmly believe that professionals and institutions should not be required to provide treatments that violate their integrity if patients cannot or will not arrange transfer. We are not alone in making this judgment.[20]

4. Finally, the Houston policy avoids patient abandonment by either the physician or the institution. An institutional determination that a particular intervention is inappropriate results in only the discontinuation or withholding of that intervention; all other interventions that are medically appropriate for the care of the patient are continued. The task force felt that stressing the ongoing necessity of appropriate care was important enough to warrant specifically requiring in step 7 that a plan of care that emphasized comfort measures and preservation of patient dignity must be established if a particular intervention were found to be inappropriate.

The third advantage of the Houston approach is that it is firmly grounded on ethical principles such as professional and institutional integrity that serve to balance patient autonomy. These values are introduced in the preamble to the policy. The value of patient autonomy is widely recognized as grounding a prohibition on clinicians and institutions forcing unwanted treatments on patients. The values of professional and institutional integrity should be recognized as grounding a prohibition on patients and families forcing clinicians and institutions to provide treatments they judge to be inappropriate.

Our conception of integrity involves 3 new aspects: (1) institutional as well as individual professional integrity, (2) an account of some of the reasons why an intervention may violate integrity, and (3) an explanation of how resource allocation may be relevant to judgments of futility based on the value of integrity. As each of these aspects are new, further explanation is necessary.

Both the physician who brings the case for review and the institutional review mechanism must consider whether providing the intervention in question is compatible with the maintenance of integrity. Providing these interventions requires the joint efforts of many professionals and the support of extensive institutional resources. The individual physician who brings the case for review must consider whether providing the intervention is compatible with his or her professional integrity. Equally, the institutional review mechanism, representing the full set of professionals who efforts would be involved and the institution whose resources must be employed, must consider whether providing the intervention is compatible with the values of these individuals and of the institution. If it is not, then it will not be provided in the institution in question, even if some physician is willing to write the orders to provide it. This is why our policy bans intrainstitutional transfers after an institutional determination of futility.

Many factors must be considered in making these judgments; our policy mentions 3 we find particulary relevant. The physician and the review mechanism must consider the traditional medical question of whether in their judgment the intervention harms patients without compensating benefits (e.g., the case of the abusive husband). This type of consideration is stressed by Tomlinson and Czlonka.[20] They must also consider the question of whether in their judgment it constitutes the provision of unseemly care. As the multiple amputations case illustrates, such judgments are not irrelevant. Finally, they must consider the question of whether in their judgment it represents an inappropriate stewardship of resources (e.g., the vegetative patient in the ICU). In our approach, this is a way that allocation of resources can sometimes be the basis for a futility determination.

The principle of justice or appropriate allocation of scarce resources has been championed by some as the basis for futility policies, and has been rejected by others such as Jecker and Schneiderman[21] as confusing futility with rationing. We concur that futility policies cannot be based solely on resource considerations since issues of resource allocation have nothing to do with many futility cases. Our policy maintains, however, that appropriate stewardship of institutional resources may be the basis in some cases for the judgment that provision of the disputed intervention is inappropriate. Because we recognize that this is an extension of the notion of futility, we use the language of medical inappropriateness throughout the policy. Whatever the language used, the crucial point is that the intervention is not provided because provision would conflict with professional and institutional integrity.

The ultimate question is not whether our futility policy is value free, but whether it is based on defensible values. We believe that it is because it provides the appropriate balance between patient autonomy and professional and institutional integrity.

Conclusion

Currently, most of the major hospitals in the greater Houston area (including several not involved in the drafting effort) have supported these guidelines in principle as has the Harris County (Texas) Medical

Society. Three institutions have approved them for use and a fourth hospital has nearly completed the process of doing so. However, none has yet had a case that went beyond step 3. At least in this regard, the process has been a success as it has created a de facto community standard, grounded in professional and institutional integrity, to deal with individual cases of demands for futile interventions.

We recognize that our policy was primarily developed by institutional representatives without extensive explicit community-wide involvement. We would argue, however, that there was substantial community input into the process because the ethics committees of the various institutions and their boards of directors, which had to approve the policy, contain extensive community representation from the diverse constituencies that these institutions serve. Further community input was obtained at a public symposium conducted in early 1994 by the Houston Bioethics Network, which was attended by more than 150 individuals. These inputs helped produce the many procedural safeguards described above.

There is still residual uncertainty about the legal standing of such a policy in light of the *Baby K* decision,[22] which mandated life support for an anencephalic infant at parental request despite physician and institution insistence that such interventions were futile. Moreover, several of the participating institutions desire an amendment to the Texas Natural Death Act codifying such a futility mechanism with others would like to see similar process-based policies developed in other cities and states. So there is more work to be done. Part of that work is tracking the use of this policy in Houston so that others can learn from our experience.

We believe that the Houston approach of an open and fair process of determining futility, which balances patient autonomy with professional and institutional integrity, can be a useful tool to resolve the type of disagreements raised by our 3 cases and countless others around the country.

Amir Halevy, MD
Baruch A. Brody, PhD
for the Houston City-Wide
Task Force on Medical Futility

References

1. Council on Ethical and Judicial Affairs, American Medical Association. Guidelines for the appropriate use of do-not-resuscitate orders. *JAMA*. 1991; 265:1868–1871.
2. Ethics Committee. American College of Physicians Ethics Manual. *Ann Intern Med.* 1992; 117:947–960.
3. American Thoracic Society. Withholding and withdrawing life-sustaining therapy. *Am*

Rev Respir Dis. 1991; 144:726–731.
4. Society of Critical Care Medicine, Task Force on Ethics. Consensus report on the ethics of foregoing life-sustaining treatments in the critically ill. *Crit Care Med.* 1990; 18:1435–1439.
5. Schneiderman LJ, Jecker NS, Jonsen AR. Medical futility: its meaning and ethical implications. *Ann Intern Med.* 1990; 112:949–954.
6. The Hastings Center. *Guidelines on the Termination of Life-sustaining Treatment and the Care of the Dying.* Bloomington: Indiana University Press; 1987.
7. Grant ER. Medical futility: legal and ethical aspects. *Law Med Health Care.* 1992; 20:330–335.
8. Daar JF. Medical futility and implications for physician autonomy. *Am J Law Med.* 1995; 21:221–240.
9. Sadler JZ, Mayo TW. The Parkland approach to demands for 'futile' treatment. *HEC Forum.* 1993; 5:35–58.
10. Santa Monica Hospital Medical Center. Futile care guidelines. *Med Ethics Advisor.* 1993; (October suppl):9.
11. Waisel DB, Truog RD. The cardiopulmonary resuscitation-not-indicated order: futility revisited. *Ann Intern Med.* 1995; 122:304–308.
12. Brody BA, Halevy A. Is futility a futile concept? *J Med Philos.* 1995; 20:123–144.
13. Halevy A, Neal RC, Brody BA. The low frequency of futility in an adult intensive care unit setting. *Arch Intern Med.* 1996; 156:100–104.
14. Sachdeva R, Jefferson L, Coss-Bu J, Brody B. Resource consumption and the extent of futile care among patients in a pediatric intensive care unit setting. *J Pediatr.* 1996; 128:742–747.
15. Gewirtz P. On 'I know it when I see it.' *Yale Law J.* 1996; 105:1023–1047.
16. Council on Ethical and Judicial Affairs, American Medical Association. *Code of Medical Ethics.* Chicago, Ill: American Medical Association; 1994.
17. Murphy DJ, Barbour E. GUIDe (Guidelines for the Use of Intensive Care in Denver): a community effort to define futile and inappropriate care. *New Horizons.* 1994; 2:326–331.
18. Truog RD, Brett AS, Frader J. The problem with futility. *N Engl J Med.* 1992; 326:1560–1564.
19. Tomlinson T, Brody H. Futility and the ethics of resuscitation. *JAMA.* 1990; 264:1276–1280.
20. Tomlinson T, Czlonka D. Futility and hospital policy. *Hastings Cent Rep.* 1995; 25:28–35.
21. Jecker NS, Schneiderman LJ. Futility and rationing. *Am J Med.* 1992; 92:189–196.
22. *In the matter of Baby K,* 16 F3d 590 (4th Cir, 1994).

APPENDIX B

BAYSTATE MEDICAL CENTER
Intensive Care Unit Structure Standards

Admission Criteria

Addendum C

I. *Sources of Admissions to ICU*
   A. Emergency Department - The Emergency Room physician will admit patients directly to the ICU in accordance with the established guidelines.
   B. In-house Transfers - Requests for transfer of in-house patients to the ICU will be made by the attending physician/resident to the ICU resident assigned to such duty.
   C. Direct Admissions - These patients will come from physician's offices, clinics, other medical facilities. These patients will require approval of the attending triage officer prior to acceptance.
   D. Inter-hospital Transfers - These patients will require the approval for admission by the attending triage officer.

II. *Admission Criteria to ICU*
   A. Level I - Critically ill patients with unstable vital signs requiring high intensity nursing services and special diagnostic, therapeutic, and pharmacological interventions such as:
      1. Titratable vasoactive infusions (pharmacological manipulation of cardiac output).
      2. Hemodynamic evaluation requiring the use of specialized ICU monitoring and frequent nursing interventions:

a) frequent vital signs q30 minutes or more often
b) pulmonary artery wedge pressure readings q1/2 hours
c) cardiac output determinations q1–2 hours
3. Significant hypotension accompanied by impending secondary organ failure as defined:
   a) hypoxic encephalopathy with altered levels of consciousness
   b) myocardial depression and/or life threatening arrhythmias
   c) impairment of renal function progressing to acute renal failure requiring intervention.
   d) persistent hemorrhage requiring frequent blood products or Blakemore tube for variceal bleed
   e) respiratory failure or early ARDS
4. Mechanical ventilatory support with high levels of PEEP and presence of hypoxemia.
5. Induced paralysis for ventilatory control.
6. Impending respiratory failure
   a) compromised airway
   b) status asthmaticus with potential for further consideration
   c) respiratory insufficiency requiring continuing presence and observation
   d) aggressive treatment to avoid need for instrumentation and further respiratory support
7. Post extubation for a subset of patients (COPD) for a period of two hours (observation)
8. Patients requiring aggressive pulmonary hygiene associated with critical hypoxemia and/or the need for frequent suctioning q15minutes - 60 minutes; frequent CPT q1H.
9. Recurrent life-threatening arrhythmias requiring bolus IV infusion, cardioversion/defibrillation, pacemaker insertion, CPR, vasopressor support.
10. Intracranial hypertension or deteriorating level of consciousness requiring aggressive brain therapy for the control of intracranial pressure. Such therapy may include but not limited to:
    a) inducing barbiturate coma
    b) frequent administration of diuretics
    c) paralysis
    d) ICP monitoring
11. Status epilepticus requiring:
    a) intubation, mechanical ventilation

       b) sedation
       c) paralysis or induced coma
       d) induce paralysis for ventilatory control
    12. Brain death with preparation for organ donation.
    13. Unstable burn patients requiring aggressive fluid resuscitation.
B. Level II - Patients acutely ill with stable vital signs requiring minimal pharmacologic support or being weaned from pharmacologic support; may or may not require mechanical ventilatory support.
    1. Comatose, intubated patients or stable vital signs with improving or stabilizing neurostatus and/or minimal treatment to control ICP.
    2. Patients not requiring mechanical ventilation with stable vital signs with:
       a) altered level of consciousness
       b) questionable volume status (renal failure, pulmonary edema requiring vital signs q1–2hours).
       c) pulmonary edema
       d) patients with potential development of ARDS requiring monitoring and measurement of respiratory parameters
       e) immediate post-op craniotomy, altered level of consciousness
    3. Metabolic abnormalities:
       a) Diabetic ketoacidosis
       b) Hyperosmolar coma
       c) Hepatic coma
       d) Any life-threatening electrolyte disturbance with or without arrhythmias (i.e., hypocalcemia, hypercalcemia, hypokalemia, hyperkalemia).
    4. Medical conditions:
       a) acute, complicated pancreatitis
       b) meningoencephalitis with stable vital signs
       c) thyroid storm, adrenal insufficiency, myxedema coma
       d) severe pneumonia with hypoxemia not requiring mechanical ventilatory support
       e) brain death determination
       f) progressive neurodysfunction, i.e., Guillian Barre, myasthenia gravis.
       g) Head trauma, stable vital signs without invasive monitoring.
C. Level III - Stable, high risk patients requiring care/observation beyond the limitations of general floor nursing.

1. Patients with reversible airway disease requiring bronchodilators and/or steroids to maintain respiratory status.
2. Pulmonary embolus
3. Stable, controlled hypoxemia
4. Stable postoperative patients requiring close observation without need for mechanical ventilation or invasive monitoring (complicated/frequent dressing changes, multi-drain monitoring).
5. Chronic, stable long-term ventilatory patients.
6. Routine abdominal surgery, uncomplicated or complicated with need for observation only.
7. Metabolic dysfunction not effecting organs.
8. Stable spinal fracture requiring a Stryker. These patients will be transferred to the floor when condition is manageable by general nursing.
9. Stable patient requiring respiratory therapy or frequent turning of Rotorest trauma bed to maintain pulmonary hygiene.

Triage

Resident physicians receive requests from either inside or outside the institution. All potential ICU admissions will be discussed with the designated medical staff triage officer who is a member of the Division of Critical Care Medicine. Transfers from outlying hospitals will be directly referred to this triage officer.

Multiple requests for admission require triage coordination between the Charge RN and the triage officer. The attending triage officer will have final authority in all disputed cases. Patients will be assigned priority levels I, II and III by the attending triage officer upon presentation to the unit for admission. Priority for admission will be I greater than II, and II greater than III.

Upon admission approval, the responsibility of coordinating all transfers of patients to the ICU rests with the ICU charge nurse.

III. *Fast Track Admissions*
  A. The following patients will be accepted to the ICU after telephone contact with the ICU Resident by the Emergency Department attending physician. If a patient has a private physician, the Emergency Department attending will also contact the private physician (should be done in any case). The patient will be transported as soon as possible to the ICU once the nursing report is given. All critically ill patients that are transported to the ICU will be transported with a nurse,

physician (when needed), respiratory therapist (when needed), and full resuscitative equipment.
1. Intubated overdoses
2. Overdoses that have significant risk for rapid deterioration, i.e., MAO overdose, tricyclic antidepressants, etc.
3. Respiratory failure requiring intubation (asthma, COPD, pneumonia, etc.) or impending respiratory failure.
4. Diabetic ketoacidosis with an initial pH less than 7.1 or an initial bicarbonate level less than 11.
5. Septic shock (after an appropriate fluid challenge, usually 2 liters in urosepsis.
6. Acute ongoing GI bleeds or an acute GI bleed that is hemodynamically unstable or has the potential for rapid deterioration.
7. CCU overflow - MI's thrombolysis patients, intubated CHF.
8. Hypertensive crisis with end-organ damage on a vasoactive drip.
9. Chronic renal patients who require urgent dialysis.

IV. *Certain patients who fall into one of the above categories will need to be discussed with the ICU attending. Examples are severe dementia, hopelessly ill, or DNR. These of themselves are not exclusions to ICU admittance, but must be discussed with the ICU attending.*

V. *Exclusion Criteria* - Patients that would not ordinarily be considered for admission to the ICU
   A. Irreversible primary pathology, such as terminal cancer, end-stage HIV infection, multiple organ failure without expectation of recovery, and CNS pathology which will cause the patient's demise during the current hospitalization.
   B. Patient under the age of 15.
   C. Patients not requiring critical care nursing, i.e., expectation of less than 1:3 nursing care as contrasted with the criteria for 1:1, 1:2, or 1:3 nursing.
   D. Diagnostic and therapeutic procedures including but not limited to bronchoscopy and endoscopy in patients with no other risk factors.

BAYSTATE MEDICAL CENTER
Intensive Care Unit Structure Standards

Discharge/Transfer Criteria

Addendum D

I. *Discharge Criteria from ICU*
   A. Patients no longer require high-intensity nursing services and special diagnostic, therapeutic, monitoring and/or pharmacologic interventions.
   B. Patient is breathing spontaneously:
      1. without mechanical ventilation for at least 4–6 hours
      2. with a stable airway
      3. with an intact cough
      4. respirations are without signs of muscle fatigue, i.e., accessory muscle use, paradoxical breathing
      5. care on general nursing floor requires:
         a) suctioning every 4 hours or less
         b) vital signs every 4 hours or less
         c) neurological signs every 4 hours or less
   C. Mechanically ventilated patient who has previously been assigned a DNR status when continuation of other ICU support/services is no longer needed.
   D. Patient who is mechanically ventilated with a high probability for rehabilitation and has been accepted by RICP (refer to C.O. #1.620).
   E. Patient who is mechanically ventilated with a low probability for rehabilitation (refer to C.O. #1.620).
   F. Patient is no longer receiving titration of either parenteral vasoactive drugs or antihypertensive agents for a minimum of 3 hours.
      1. inotropes
      2. alpha agents
      3. antihypertensives
   G. Patient who is hemodynamically stable and being maintained on IV fluids less than 250cc/hr and
      1. mean BP greater than 65 and/or
      2. mean BP within 10mmHg of the patient's normal and/or
      3. urine output greater than 0.55 cc/kg/hr except for those patients in acute or chronic renal failure.
   H. Patient who does not require hemodynamic evaluation, i.e.,
      1. Swan-Ganz and/or

Appendix B

2. CAVH and/or
3. ETCO2 measurements and/or
4. rapid electrolyte replacement

II. *Triage from The Adult Intensive Care Unit*
   A. Triage situation exists when accelerated discharge has reached the maximum by the previously stated discharge criteria. (*For time of high hospital census and high level triage, refer to C.O. #1.350 for administrative responsibilities*).
      1. Critical Care service is at operating capacity and a bed is needed for another patient who requires urgent or emergency care.
      2. All efforts will be made to provide additional support as appropriate for the triage patients on the general patient care units.
      3. Patients who meet Baystate Medical Center's criteria for brain death (refer to C.O. #9.300) will ordinarily remain in the Intensive Care Unit.
         a) Full criteria for brain death met:
            (1) Continuation of the organ procurement process OR
            (2) Discontinuation of mechanical ventilation.
         b) Full criteria for brain death not met:
            (1) Patient may be triaged out of the Intensive Care Unit and placed on a general patient care unit where mechanical ventilation may or may not be continued.
      4. Patients who fail to respond to intensive care therapy and are considered unsalvageable will not be kept in the Intensive Care Unit.
         a) Clinical determination made by triage officer.
         b) Triage officer will coordinate discharge planning with attending physician and family.
            (1) Documentation of discussion by triage officer with the family must be included in the medical record.
      5. Determination of patient triage status will be made by the triage officer.
         a) Decision to triage a patient out of the Intensive Care Unit shall rest exclusively with the triage officer or his/her designate.
         b) Requests for admission to the Intensive Care Unit must be made directly to the triage officer.
         c) Elective admissions will be suspended.
         d) All surgical cases previously booked and in progress will be evaluated by the triage officer for the Intensive

Care Unit, the surgical Intermediate Care Unit, or a general patient care unit.
(1) Those booked and not yet anesthetized shall be held.
e) Triage officer will inform the Medical Director or the Operating Room to determine care order and/or cancellations.
(1) Cases which proceed without receiving bed confirmation from the triage officer cannot be accommodated in the Intensive Care Unit.
f) Patients remaining in Post-Anesthesia Care Unit for an extended period of time refer to C.O.#1.350.
(1) Coordination for this extended period will occur among the triage officer, medical director of the Post-Anesthesia Care Unit, attending anesthesiologist and the nursing staff of the Intensive Care Unit and Post-Anesthesia Care Unit.
g) Intensive Care Unit triage officer shall contact the cardiovascular triage officer to coordinate use of available critical care beds.
h) Intensive Care Unit triage officer shall also contact the medical director of the Post-Anesthesia Care Unit and the Nursing Director of Critical Care if a patient is to utilize a Post-Anesthesia Care Unit bed.

III. *Transfer to Other Hospitals*
A. Need for special services not available in Baystate Medical Center Intensive Care Unit.
1. Patients will be evaluated for specialized referrals on a case-by-case basis.
2. Liver, heart or lung transplantation.
a) Appropriate Baystate Medical Center Consultants will discuss possible options with patient and family (or health care surrogate).
b) Transplant service will be contacted by telephone to describe the patient's clinical status.
c) Intensive Care Unit at Baystate will be responsible for transporting the patient to the appropriate referral center with documentation from the medical record. Burn capacity exceeded
d) Brigham & Women's Hospital or the Shriners' Burn Hospital will accommodate our overflow of patients.
3. Selected spinal injury patients may be referred and transferred to a spinal injury center as coordinated by

Trauma Service in conjunction with Neurosurgery and Orthopedics.
4. Social Services will actively participate in coordination of high level transfers.
5. Patients requesting transfer to a hospital providing a comparable level of care closer to their home.
   a) Arrangements will be made on a case by case basis.
   b) Transfers will be made when there is an identified physician who will accept the transfer.
   c) Patient must be stable.
   d) Accepting physician must have sub-specialty training appropriate to the patient's major problems.
   e) Possible risks will be explained to the patient and surrogate decision-maker.
   f) Controlled transfer will be put into effect by the Baystate Intensive Care Unit.
      (1) Needs assessment for accompanying personnel, i.e., paramedic, intensive care nurse, respiratory therapist or physician (PGY 2 or higher) will be made by Baystate Medical Center Intensive Care Unit.

APPENDIX C

Admission and Discharge Criteria Assessment Scale

Institute For Healthcare Improvement*

Score 1: Non-discriminating
       – very general admission guidelines
       – no priority categories
       – no criteria for discharge
       – no screening of admissions
       – no exclusions
       – no triage statement

Score 2: General with Some Discriminating Guidelines
       – general admission guidelines
       – some prioritization
       – no limited criteria for discharge
       – no clear screening
       – some exclusion criteria
       – no triage statement

Score 3: Good
       – objective admission criteria with some quantification
       – detailed prioritization
       – some criteria for discharge
       – daytime screening

- exclusions stated
- triage described

Score 4: Strong
- objective admission criteria fully quantified
- medical and nursing discharge criteria defined
- detailed prioritization
- 24 hour physician screening
- special care unit committee provides regular oversight function
- conflict resolution available
- detailed triage plan described

Score 5: Outstanding
- admission and discharge criteria fully quantified
- patients evaluated by ICU physician prior to ICU admission, 24 hours per day
- detailed prioritization, including exclusions
- qualified critical care physician coordinates care
- special care unit committee provides close oversight
- detailed triage plan, including canceling elective OR cases and diverting ambulances, if necessary
- clear policy to share resources among all ICUs.

---

* Presented by Daniel Teres at "Breakthrough Series on Reducing Costs and Improving Outcomes in Adult Intensive Care," Institute for Healthcare Improvement, July 30, 1996, Boston, Mass.

APPENDIX D

Components of Rapid Ethics Evaluation Process for ICU Patients with High Probability of Mortality

I. **Assess the patient** (It is understood that most patients in the ICU setting have diminished mental capacity due to primary disease process and sedative or pain medication used in the ICU.)
   ⇒ Evaluate patient's capacity to:
   - Understand information
   - Reason and deliberate
   - Apply a set of values
   - Communicate decisions and choices

   ⇒ Are there any advance directives?
   - Health proxy
   - Living will
   - Durable power of attorney
   - Statements

II. **Assess the patient and family together**
   ⇒ Identify support systems
   ⇒ Examine family unit's decision-making capacity:
   - What is role of family relative to the patient?
   - Who will make decisions for the patient?
   - Who will receive information?
   - How will information be disseminated through the family?

   ⇒ Assess the family unit's value system and culture regarding:

- Life and death
- Religion
- Disability
- Pain and Suffering
- Etc.

⇒ What is the relationship with the medical attending physician, house staff, and nursing team?
- Trusting?
- Good relationship?
- Long-standing?
- Skeptical?
- Mixed messages?

III. Assess the medical team
⇒ Diagnosis, prognosis, treatment plan
- Clear understanding by attending physician
- Clear understanding by medical team and consultants
- Clear understanding by nursing, respiratory therapy, social service

⇒ Pain and anxiety management
⇒ Contingency, if patient's status deteriorates
⇒ Have any limitations on case been discussed with ———?
- CPR, DNR (no CPR)
- Intubate, re-intubate
- Surgery

⇒ Has there been a family conference?
- Early on?
- Recently?
- Any conflicts?

IV. Review information with the patient and family
⇒ Diagnosis and prognosis
⇒ Treatment and non-treatment options:
- Likelihood of success
- Degree of invasiveness
- Side effects and complications versus potential benefits
- Potential morbidity, including pain, emotional suffering, and possible disabilities
- Potential mortality
- Alternatives
- Non-financial costs

⇒ Pain management
⇒ Quality of life

⇒ Ascertain what other factors may influence decisions

V. **Assess the interaction between patient, family, and medical team**
  ⇒ Determine if there is agreement regarding:
  - Diagnosis
  - Prognosis
  - Treatment plan
  - Pain management
  - Expectations of outcome
  ⇒ Determine if there are any differences in value judgment and, if so, where they occur
  - Explore possible explanations for aspects of disagreement, including medical and non-medical reasons
  ⇒ Determine if there are any conflicts regarding quality of care

VI. **Write concise note in the medical record in a timely fashion**
  ⇒ Complete recommendations checklist
  - Send to Ethics Committee
  - Send to medical and nursing directors of ICU, chair of Special Care Unit Committee

Appendix D

Recommendations Checklist

What are recommendations of the Rapid Ethics Evaluation Process?

	Yes	No
There is a good working relationship between family/patient and medical/nursing team	☐	☐
Family needs more information	☐	☐
Physician-family conference should be scheduled	☐	☐
Need to involve:		
Hospital Chaplain	☐	☐
Social Worker	☐	☐
Family minister/priest/rabbi (clergy person)	☐	☐
Formal ethics case review	☐	☐
Risk manager	☐	☐
Acute paliation referral (hospice)	☐	☐
There is a need for a formal second medical opinion	☐	☐
Physician counseling or guidance suggested	☐	☐
Nurse counseling or guidance suggested	☐	☐

Patient ID #: _____

Team Members: _____

_____

_____

_____

_____

Daniel Teres, M.D., FCCM
Director
Center for Health Services Research
Baystate Medical Center
Associate Professor of Medicine and Surgery
Tufts University School of Medicine

APPENDIX E

Role Playing the Simulation and Suggestions for New Rounds

Instead of reading the cases presented in Chapter 4 of this book, why not role play them? The decision rounds are designed to encourage this type of activity. Here's how it might work:

A role player considers requests to admit patients to a hypothetical 12-bed medical-surgical ICU on the basis of physiological and organizational information that is given by the "simulation" (i.e., the book). Provided is information on the number of staffed beds available, characteristics of patients in those beds, a set of admission-discharge policies and other guidelines, and information on organizational characteristics of the hospital and the ICU. The introductory case as presented in Chapter 1 provides the context for the simulation as it begins in "Round 1."

In each round a decision must be made. Readers may place themselves in the role of triage officer who, after taking into consideration the perspectives of other decision makers including the attending physician, nurse manager, and the administrator, makes the decision.

Or individuals in groups may play the roles of the four decision makers (triage officer, attending physician, nurse manager, administrator). Collectively, through discussion and negotiation, they will try to reach a consensus. If a consensus cannot be reached, the triage officer will make the decision.

After the role players make their decision for the round, the simulation will reveal its decision based on the particular dynamics of Anywhere Hospital. The organizational rationale behind the decision will then be given, followed by a discussion of the important issues raised by the decision.

Role players may wish to obtain the services of a facilitator to extract and present appropriate materials from the book and to manage the simulation exercise. The facilitator can also act as discussion leader at end-of-round intervals. Also needed is a technical consultant with ICU experience who can clarify assumptions and answer questions in an authoritative manner.

The facilitator should divide participants into groups of up to four and assign the different roles. Role descriptions (pages 61–64) should be distributed and read carefully. The facilitator may wish to reinforce role behaviors by distributing badges with role labels.

The cases themselves may be distributed for the participants to read or the facts can be verbally presented by the facilitator. The disposition of beds at the beginning of rounds should be presented as an overhead projection. Erasable marking pens can be used to change disposition of beds from round to round.

After the group(s) has presented its decision and rationale, the facilitator should present the simulations's decision and the organizational rationale behind that decision. Drawing upon materials in the book, the facilitator may wish to lead a discussion highlighting key issues.

With regard to ethical dilemmas that arise from the cases, the participants may wish to discuss the degree of conflict among four widely-recognized ethical principles (Beauchamp and Childress 1994): beneficence (helping people in need), nonmaleficence (doing no harm), autonomy (respecting patients' rights to make choices regarding their health care), and justice (treating everyone in a fair manner).

Although the rounds of the simulation can be played by role players, they will more likely be read as a series of case studies. Whatever the approach, clinicians, healthcare managers, and students are encouraged to raise what if questions by changing the decision variables. Or better yet, they can design their own simulation to model actual decisions and constraints faced by a particular ICU and hospital.

Suggestions for new rounds

Add new role players, change the characteristics of the current ones, or change the mix of decision makers. For example, the triage officer could become a full-time, salaried intensivist totally based in the ICU, with no other patient care responsibilities. The attending physician could be the primary care physician gatekeeper of an HMO. Instead of role playing the hospital administrator, the player could represent the CEO of an integrated delivery network servicing a variety of capitated managed care contracts.

Another way of approaching the modification of the decision rounds is to use the six improvement levers presented by Shortell et al. (1992) and discussed in Chapter 5, as guideposts for constructing new scenarios:

1. Patient Characteristics: prognostic probabilities, type of illness (e.g., AIDS, cancer, cardio-vascular disease), age, advance directives, decision-making capacity, socio-economic status, type of insurance coverage, presence of family member or surrogate, level of agreement among family members, religious background.

2. Provider Characteristics: availability of qualified ICU-based intensivists, availability of qualified nurses and allied health personnel, reimbursement arrangements, level of agreement among physicians and nurses.

3. Unit Characteristics: type and size of unit, staffing patterns, technology, availability of alternative care sites, policy on allowing mechanical ventilators on the floors. Availability of a working medical director and triage officer, organizational structure of unit (open vs. closed), employment arrangements for ICU-based physicians (salary, fee-for-service, hybrid), if available.

4. Hospital Characteristics: size, teaching status, population served, relative power of medical staff, hospital market share, importance of elective surgery, financial health, role of ethics committees (proactive providing timely consults or reactive), role of risk management.

5. Inter-organizational Characteristics: presence of contracts to treat certain groups of patients (e.g., cardiac surgery) and other managed care arrangements, utilization controls for managed care patients (e.g., primary care physician as gatekeeper).

6. Environmental Characteristics: degree of regulatory constraints and competitive pressures, malpractice experience, and ethical norms (patient autonomy vs. physician paternalism).

References

Beauchamp, T. L., and J. F. Childress. 1994. *Principles of Biomedical Ethics.* Oxford: Oxford University Press.

ABOUT THE AUTHORS

Martin A. Strosberg, Ph.D., is currently Professor of Management and director of the Graduate Program in Health Administration at Union College in Schenectady, NY. He is the author of numerous articles on the management of intensive care units and on public policy for the allocation of scarce resources. For many years, he codirected Managing Critical Care Units, a national management seminar for physicians, nurses, and administrators.

Daniel Teres, M.D., FCCM, is currently medical director of Health Services Research at Baystate Medical Center in Springfield, Mass. The hospital is the western campus of Tufts University School of Medicine where he is Associate Professor of Medicine and Surgery. Dr. Teres was director of Adult Critical Care for many years and has been actively involved in the development and applications of ICU severity models, including the Mortality Probability Model and Logistic Organ Failure Model.